METABOLIC BONE DISEASE IN CHILDREN

Clinical Pediatrics

Series Editor: Fima Lifshitz
Cornell University Medical College, New York, New York
North Shore University Hospital, Manhasset, New York

Volume 1 Common Pediatric Disorders: Metabolism, Heart Disease, Allergies, Substance Abuse, and Trauma, *edited by Fima Lifshitz*

Volume 2 Congenital Metabolic Diseases: Diagnosis and Treatment, *edited by Raul A. Wapnir*

Volume 3 Pediatric Endocrinology: A Clinical Guide, *edited by Fima Lifshitz*

Volume 4 Antimicrobial Therapy in Infants and Children, *edited by Gideon Koren, Charles G. Prober, and Ronald Gold*

Volume 5 Food Allergy: A Practical Approach to Diagnosis and Management, *edited by Lawrence T. Chiaramonte, Arlene T. Schneider, and Fima Lifshitz*

Volume 6 Metabolic Bone Disease in Children, *edited by Salvador Castells and Laurence Finberg*

Volume 7 Pediatric Endocrinology: A Clinical Guide, Second Edition, Revised and Expanded, *edited by Fima Lifshitz*

Other volumes in preparation

METABOLIC BONE DISEASE IN CHILDREN

EDITED BY

Salvador Castells

Laurence Finberg

Department of Pediatrics
SUNY Health Science Center at Brooklyn
Brooklyn, New York

MARCEL DEKKER, INC. New York and Basel

Library of Congress Cataloging-in-Publication Data

Metabolic bone disease in children / edited by Salvador Castells
Laurence Finberg
p. cm.-- (Clinical pediatrics ; v. 6)
Includes bibliographical references.
ISBN 0-8247-8153-8
1. Bones--Diseases. 2. Metabolic disorders in children.
I. Castells, Salvador. II. Finberg, Laurence. III. Series:
Clinical pediatrics (Marcel Dekker, Inc.) ; 6.
[DNLM: 1. Bone Diseases, Metabolic--in infancy & childhood. W1
CL761Y v. 6 / WS 270 M587]
RJ482.B65M48 1989
618.92'716--dc20
DNLM/DLC
for Library of Congress 89-23517
CIP

MARCEL DEKKER, INC.
270 Madison Avenue, New York, New York 10016

Current printing (last digit):
10 9 8 7 6 5 4 3 2 1

PRINTED IN THE UNITED STATES OF AMERICA

About the Series

Clinical Pediatrics is a series of books designed to continuously update the knowledge of the practicing pediatrician in diverse areas of the specialty. Each volume in the series addresses rapidly developing topics which are changing the attitudes and treatment approaches of the clinician. The chapters comprising the volumes represent the state of the art on the various subjects from the vantage point of recognized experts in the field.

The first book in the series, *Common Pediatric Disorders*, deals with diseases of metabolism, cardiology, allergies, substance abuse, and trauma. The second volume, *Congenital Metabolic Diseases*, reviews a field which recently celebrated the 75th anniversary of the first treatise on this theme written by Sir Archibald Garrod. The third book, *Pediatric Endocrinology*, is devoted in its entirety to endocrine disorders in children. The fourth book, *Antimicrobial Therapy in Infants and Children*, delineates the principles of antibiotic therapy in the pediatric population and includes the most recent developments in this field. The fifth title, *Food Allergy*, represents one of the most important areas of clinical allergy and it covers the clinical picture, immunologic mechanisms, and treatments. The present volume, *Metabolic Bone Disease in Children,* reviews the current understanding of this complicated problem afflicting children with diverse diseases. An additional book, the seventh of this series, *Pediatric Endocrinology*, Second Edition (in press), is an updated, improved, and greatly expanded version of the third volume of the same title which was published in 1985. These seven books serve as the foundation for the volumes that will follow, each complementing the other, and together, constituting a comprehensive review of the most recent developments in the area of pediatrics.

Fima Lifshitz

Preface

Metabolic bone disease includes all disorders of the mineral skeleton in which there is a generalized disorder of the processes of bone formation and dissolution. In children these conditions differ from those of adults in that growth is in progress and, of course, the skeleton is the major determinant of linear growth. Recent discoveries make this topic a dynamic one; its evolution brings new implications for clinical action.

We have assembled here a series of reviews of recent advances that will bring the reader up to date, allowing for some lag time from submission to publication. We begin with a general review of the biochemical transformations and the physiological roles of vitamin D by Hector DeLuca, who, more than anyone else, has helped to formulate this exciting story.

The application of new knowledge to the role of the kidney in regulating calcium and phosphorus excretion is admirably described by Russell Chesney from his perspective as a pediatrician, nephrologist, and cell transport physiologist. The rhythmic hormonal control of calcium and phosphorus in the plasma is elaborated next by the elegant studies of Morri Markowitz and John Rosen.

The following three chapters review the current epidemiology, chemical problems, and their management. One of these is from Reginald Tsang and his colleagues at Cincinnati, whence many studies have emanated and enriched our understanding of problems in the low-birthweight infant and in the newborn period generally. The other two are from our own clinical experiences with the modern incidence and management of rickets in a pediatric department.

Stephen Marx then develops further the contributions of his laboratory to the newly understood role of receptors in varieties of clinical rickets. At last there really is a "vitamin-D-resistant" rickets in a fundamental sense. Harold Harrison adds another contribution to his long list of publications by looking at unusual responsiveness to vitamin D metabolites.

Among the most important problems in metabolic bone disease confronting clinicians today are those arising as a consequence of the prolongation of life in chronic renal disease by dialysis and transplantation programs, the latter attended by the side effects of immunosuppressive therapy. Richard Fine reviews these problems from his vantage point of vast experience. A special problem, that of aluminum toxicity induced by dialysis and antacid therapy, has been elucidated by Sharon P. Andreoli of the University of Indiana.

The next two chapters deal with specialized skeletal disorders of over- or undermineralization. The state of knowledge here remains more descriptive than in other disorders because our understanding of the mechanisms involved lag behind. The problems, which are well-presented here, provide a challenge for the near (we hope!) future.

Osteogenesis imperfecta and the skeletal deformations found in genetic disturbances of tissue structure represent another set of challenges currently being met by imaginative hypotheses of the dynamic events and by innovative surgical techniques. These events are covered from our own institutions by Drs. Castells and Spero, and by Cervantes and Lifshitz at neighboring North Shore University Hospital.

The field of mineral metabolism and metabolic bone disease now nears its adolescent growth spurt. The last two decades have shown an increasingly rapid advance. The next two should raise us to new levels of understanding, with clear clinical applications.

Salvador Castells
Laurence Finberg

Contents

Contributors

Sharon P. Andreoli, M.D. Assistant Professor of Pediatrics, Department of Pediatric Nephrology, James Whitcomb Riley Hospital for Children, Indiana University Medical Center, Indianapolis, Indiana

Carl Barbera, M.D. Assistant Professor of Surgery, SUNY Health Science Center at Brooklyn, Brooklyn, New York

Julia Barsony National Institute of Diabetes, Digestive, and Kidney Diseases, Bethesda, Maryland

William Bastian, M.D. Clinical Assistant Instructor, Department of Pediatrics, SUNY Health Science Center at Brooklyn, Brooklyn, New York

M. Michael Bliziotes National Institute of Diabetes, Digestive, and Kidney Diseases, Bethesda, Maryland

Maria Luisa Brandi National Institute of Diabetes, Digestive, and Kidney Diseases, Bethesda, Maryland

Salvador Castells, M.D. Professor of Pediatrics, Director, Unit of Growth and Metabolism, SUNY Health Science Center at Brooklyn, Brooklyn, New York

Cecilia D. Cervantes, M.D. Department of Pediatrics, North Shore University Hospital, Manhasset; Department of Pediatrics, Cornell University Medical College, New York, New York

Russell W. Chesney, M.D. Professor of Pediatrics, Department of Pediatrics, College of Medicine, University of Tennessee, Memphis, Memphis, Tennessee,

Hector F. DeLuca, Ph.D. Harry Steenbock Research Professor and Chairman, Department of Biochemistry, College of Agricultural and Life Sciences, University of Wisconsin-Madison, Madison, Wisconsin

Chas Eil Naval Hospital and Uniformed Services, University of the Health Sciences, Bethesda, Maryland

Laurence Finberg, M.D. Professor and Chairman, Department of Pediatrics, SUNY Health Science Center at Brooklyn, Brooklyn, New York

Richard N. Fine, M.D. Professor of Pediatrics, Department of Pediatrics, UCLA Medical Center, Los Angeles, California

Irma Fiordalisi, M.D. Clinical Associate Professor, Department of Pediatrics, SUNY Health Science Center at Brooklyn, Brooklyn, New York

Kevin E. Halbert, M.D. Fellow in Neonatology, University of Cincinnati College of Medicine, Cincinnati, Ohio

Harold E. Harrison, M.D. Professor of Pediatrics, Department of Pediatrics, The Johns Hopkins University School of Medicine, Baltimore, Maryland

Daniel Kaplan, M.D. Division of Orthopedics, Department of Surgery, UCLA Medical Center, Los Angeles, California

Brenda Kohn, M.D. Assistant Professor, Department of Pediatrics, Long Island College Hospital, and SUNY Health Science Center at Brooklyn, Brooklyn, New York

Uri A. Liberman National Institute of Diabetes, Digestive, and Kidney Diseases, Bethesda, Maryland and Beilson Medical Center, Petah-Tikua, Isreal

Fima Lifshitz, M.D. Associate Director of Pediatrics; Chief, Pediatric Endocrinology, Metabolism, and Nutrition; Chief, Pediatric Research, Department of Pediatrics, North Shore University Hospital, Manhasset; Professor, Department of Pediatrics, Cornell University Medical College, New York, New York

Morri E. Markowitz, M.D. Associate Professor of Pediatrics, Department of Pediatrics, Montefiore Medical Center and Albert Einstein College of Medicine, New York, New York

Stephen J. Marx, M.D. Chief, Mineral Metabolism Section, Metabolic Disease Branch, National Institute of Diabetes, Digestive, and Kidney Diseases, Bethesda, Maryland

Mark S. Nanes National Institute of Diabetes, Digestive, and Kidney Diseases, Bethesda, Maryland

William L. Oppenheim, M.D. Division of Orthopedics, Department of Surgery, UCLA Medical Center, Los Angeles, California

John F. Rosen, M.D. Professor and Head, Division of Pediatric Metabolism, Montefiore Medical Center and Albert Einstein College of Medicine, New York, New York

Isidro B. Salusky, M.D. Department of Pediatrics, UCLA Medical Center, Los Angeles, California

Binita R. Shah, M. D. Clinical Associate Professor, Department of Pediatrics, SUNY Health Science Center at Brooklyn, Brooklyn, New York

Charles R. Spero, M.D. Assistant Professor of Surgery, Kings County Hospital Center, Brooklyn, New York

Reginald C. Tsang, M.D. Professor of Pediatrics, Obstetrics, and Gynecology; Director, Division of Neonatology, University of Cincinnati College of Medicine, Cincinnati, Ohio

Israel Zelikovic, M.D. Department of Pediatrics, College of Medicine, University of Tennessee, Memphis, Memphis, Tennessee

METABOLIC BONE DISEASE IN CHILDREN

1

The Vitamin D Story

A Success of Basic Science in the Treatment of Disease

Hector F. DeLuca
University of Wisconsin-Madison, Madison, Wisconsin

I. INTRODUCTION

It is indeed rare and perhaps unexpected when an investigation of basic science provides so rapidly a practical application to medicine. Throughout the entire history of vitamin D, basic investigations have repeatedly yielded findings of great medical importance. Furthermore, the vitamin D investigations currently underway promise to yield still additional important medical benefits.

II. DISCOVERY OF VITAMIN D AND THE ELIMINATION OF RICKETS AS A MAJOR MEDICAL PROBLEM

Early in this century, rickets appeared in epidemic proportions in northern Europe, the northern United States, and northern Asia (1). We now know rickets to be a disease of vitamin D deficiency that affects rapidly growing, young animals, including humans. Although rickets was described in antiquity and clearly described in 1645 (2), its appearance in epidemic proportions correlated with the Industrial Revolution (1). Very likely, two factors contributed to this occurrence. The urbanization of a previously agrarian society very likely resulted in less exposure to sunlight, and second, industrialization brought about atmospheric pollution that was likely to limit the arrival of ultraviolet light on human skin, where we now know that vitamin D is produced. These factors, especially in low-sunlight areas, probably precipitated the high incidence of rickets.

In the field of nutritional biochemistry, attention was being focused on accessory food factors that were not described by carbohydrate, protein, fat, and minerals (3,4). These accessory food factors were obviously needed for growth and reproduction. Thus, the work of Hopkins, Funk, Holst, and Frolik and Eichman strongly suggested the existence of such factors (3,4). In the agricultural field, the single-grain experiment at the University of Wisconsin also demonstrated that analysis of feeds for carbohydrate, protein, fat, and minerals was insufficient to describe their nutritive value (5). This led McCollum in 1913 to demonstrate the existence of a lipid-soluble factor responsible for growth and reproduction, which he later called vitamin A (6,7). Both McCollum and Osborne and Mendel then demonstrated the existence of a water-soluble substance later called vitamin B that prevented neurological symptoms (7,8). Thus, many of the widespread diseases appeared to be of nutritional origin.

This led Sir Edward Mellanby to examine the question of whether rickets might be of nutritional origin. He, therefore, fed dogs a diet reminiscent of that consumed by Scottish residents. Unknown to him was the fact that he kept these dogs indoors and thus shielded from ultraviolet light (9,10). The dogs developed rickets and Mellanby cured the rickets by administration of cod liver oil. Since cod liver oil was the source of vitamin A used by McCollum, Mellanby concluded that this was another property of the fat-soluble nutrient, vitamin A. In later work, McCollum demonstrated that one could destroy vitamin A activity by oxidation and heating cod liver oil but retain the ability to heal rickets. Thus, a new vitamin was discovered called vitamin D (11).

Another important discovery was made by Huldshinsky, who demonstrated that children with rickets could be healed by exposing them to sunlight or artificially induced ultraviolet light (12). Thus, both ultraviolet light and cod liver oil could cure the same disease. Steenbock and associates demonstrated that ultraviolet light converts a precursor present in skin and food to vitamin D (13, 14). Food could be irradiated and vitamin D activity imparted to it. This important discovery not only led to the identification of vitamin D but also provided the means to eliminate rickets as a major medical problem. Thus we have the first application of basic investigations of vitamin D to the solution of major medical problems (15).

With the identification of vitamin D_2 by two groups in 1931 (16,17) and the chemical synthesis of vitamin D_3 (18), the form resulting from ultraviolet irradiation of skin (19,20), there became available substances that could be used to treat metabolic bone diseases. Thus, large doses of vitamin D came into common use for the treatment of a number of diseases presenting with rickets, osteomalacia, or hypocalcemic tetany (21).

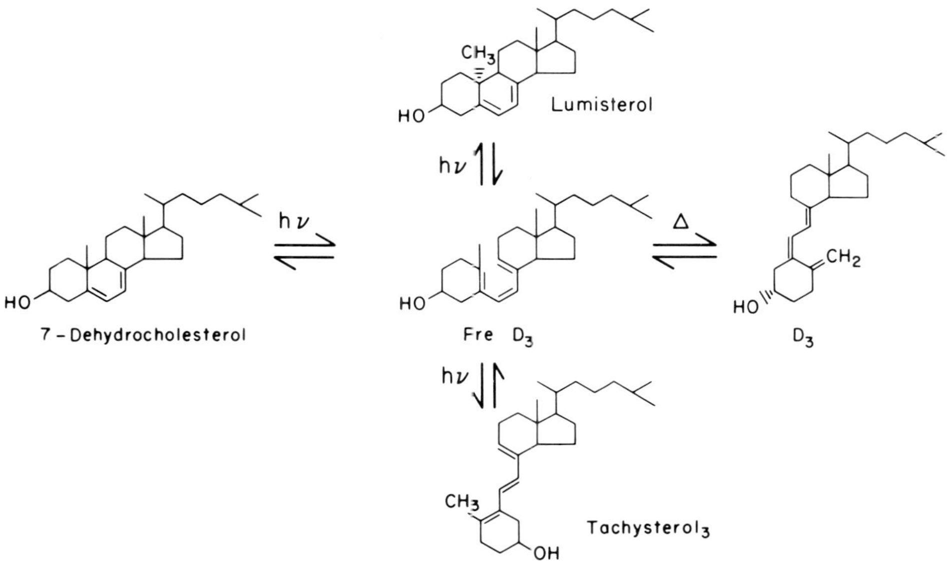

Figure 1 Production of vitamin D_3 by ultraviolet irradiation. Note that the intermediate is previtamin D, which can be isomerized further to lumisterol or to tachysterol as side reaction products. It is in thermal equilibrium with vitamin D_3.

The chemistry of the conversion of the precursor to vitamin D_3 remained uninvestigated until the work of Velluz and of Havinga (22,23), in which the chemical steps involved in the irradiation process were determined. More recent work has demonstrated that the biologically active material produced in skin by ultraviolet irradiation is indeed vitamin D_3 (19,20) and that an intermediate, previtamin D_3, is the actual irradiation product, as illustrated in Figure 1 (24). It slowly equilibrates at body temperature to the vitamin D_3 structure, which is recognized by the vitamin D transport protein and transported to the liver where it begins the sequence of metabolic activation. Previtamin D_3 is not recognized by the vitamin D transport protein and is essentially biologically inert until converted to vitamin D_3 (24). The irradiation process in which 7-dehydrocholesterol absorbs, through its chromophore, ultraviolet light of 282–290 nm does not involve proteins or enzymes since the same reaction occurs in organic solvents (24). The 7-dehydrocholesterol undergoes a rupture of the 9,10-bond and a 5,7-sigmatropic shift to produce the previtamin D. The equilibration to the vitamin D structure also does not involve proteins or enzymes and is a strictly chemical process. Thus, these steps are not regulated. However, it is clear that heavily pigmented skin or heavily tanned skin is less efficient at producing vitamin D (25), as is the skin of older people (26), and thus the incidence of ultraviolet light reaching the precursor can be limited by these factors. The photolysis reaction in skin is actually quite efficient; as little as 10–15 min of summer sun on hands and face is sufficient to produce the daily requirement of vitamin D, which is considered to be approximately 10 μg (27). The irradiation process in skin is often ignored but one that physicians should remember, since it is an excellent way to introduce vitamin D in subjects with intestinal malabsorption syndrome such as steatorrhea, Crohn's disease, and celiac disease. Introduction of vitamin D by this route eliminates the danger of intoxication brought about by large doses of vitamin D.

Vitamin D is, of course, toxic at higher doses (28). Some individuals show toxicity with as little as 5,000 units/day, whereas others do not show toxicity until doses of the order of 20,000 units/day are given (15,28,29).

III. THE CLASSIC FUNCTIONS OF VITAMIN D

Figure 2 illustrates in a diagrammatic fashion the known functions of vitamin D in the regulation of bone mineralization. Rickets and osteomalacia, the vitamin-D-deficiency diseases, are characterized by a failure of the organic matrix to acquire the hydroxyapatite mineral (1,15,16,30). The absence of mineral leaves the collagen fibrils in a soft and pliable state that gives rise to overt symptoms of rickets. Although it had been believed that some form of vitamin D worked

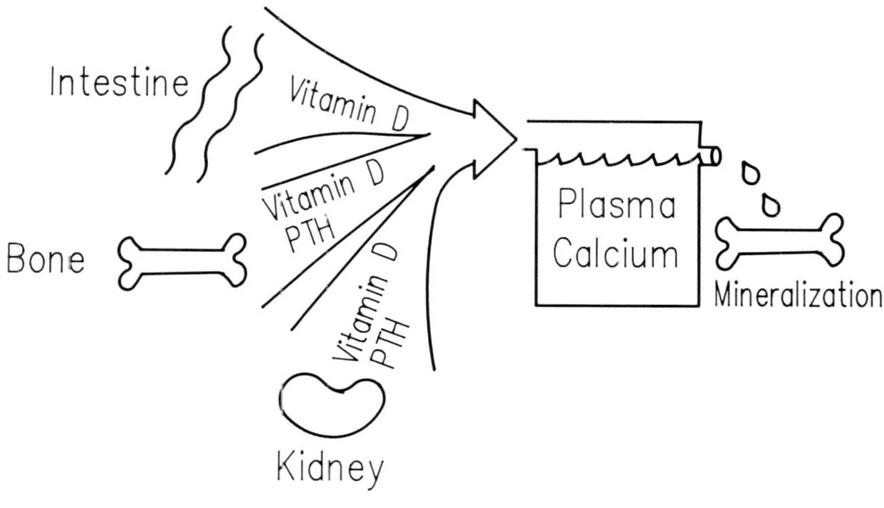

Figure 2 Diagrammatic representation of the classic functions of vitamin D.

directly on the bone-forming cells to play a role in the synthesis of the organic matrix of bone (31-33), and played a role in the mineralization process (34-36), recent work from two laboratories has clearly disproved this idea (37-39). Thus, the presence in the plasma of adequate amounts of calcium and phosphorus bring about normal bone growth and mineralization. This important fact is one in which basic science now instructs physicians as to how to manage a very difficult form of vitamin-D-resistant rickets, vitamin-D-resistant rickets type II, which is discussed later.

Vitamin D brings about mineralization of bone primarily by the elevation of plasma calcium and phosphorus to levels that are supersaturating and required not only for the mineralization of skeleton but also the prevention of hypocalcemic tetany, the most serious disorder brought about by deficiency of vitamin D (1,15,40). Low blood calcium levels result in the convulsive state called hypocalcemic tetany. This is life-threatening and thus calcium physiology is constructed to guard against this possibility. In the absence of vitamin D, however, the body cannot mobilize calcium and thus hypocalcemic tetany is a major deficiency disease (1).

Vitamin D brings about the elevation of plasma calcium and phosphorus levels by three basic mechanisms:

1. It is the only substance known to stimulate the enterocytes of the small intestine to transport calcium from the lumen to the plasma compartment (41). In the same cells, it brings about the transport of phosphorus into the plasma compartment (41).
2. Because the presence of calcium in the diet and hence intestine is not predictable, the body utilizes the skeleton as a ready source of calcium. To mobilize calcium from the skeleton, two hormones are involved: the vitamin D hormone and the parathyroid hormone working in concert (41,42). The mechanism by which they mobilize calcium from the skeleton is unknown. It is a very rapid process and probably does not involve osteoclastic-mediated bone resorption (43).
3. In the distal renal tubule, calcium is reabsorbed under the influence of parathyroid hormone and vitamin D (44,45). Again, both hormones function at this site, in contrast to the small intestine (46).

Plasma calcium and phosphorus levels are elevated because of these three actions and thus new bone is mineralized and hypocalcemic tetany is averted. In addition to these classic actions of the vitamin D system, new and unexpected sites of action of vitamin D are now being found as a result of basic science investigations. These will be described in a subsequent section.

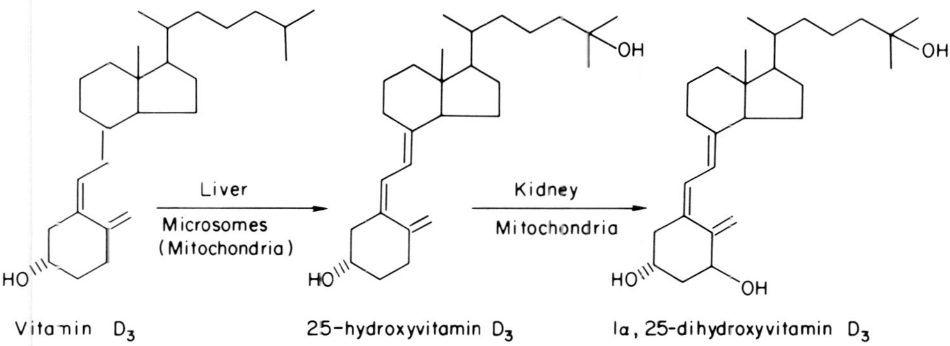

Figure 3 Metabolism of vitamin D_3 required for function.

IV. METABOLISM OF VITAMIN D REQUIRED FOR FUNCTION

Figure 3 illustrates a well-known series of reactions required for vitamin D to function. An important breakthrough in our understanding of the vitamin D system occurred in the mid-1960s, when it was learned that vitamin D must be processed metabolically before it can function (47), despite conclusions to the contrary in two different laboratories (48,49). Thus, vitamin D is first hydroxylated on carbon 25, primarily in the liver by a microsomal cytochrome P-450 system (50,51), and subsequently this product, 25-hydroxyvitamin D_3 (25-OH-D_3) is transported to the kidney where it undergoes 1α-hydroxylation to form the final active form of vitamin D, 1,25-dihydroxyvitamin D_3 (1,25-$(OH)_2D_3$) (52–54). The 25-OH-D_3 is the major circulating form of vitamin D_3, being present at a level of 25–30 ng/ml in normal human blood (55,56). Under conditions of low vitamin D intake, as for example in northern Europe, the levels may be less (15–20 ng/ml) (55). Deficiency of vitamin D becomes apparent when the level of this substance falls to a value of $<$10 ng/ml (57,58). Thus, measurement of this important metabolite has great medical importance and is another provision of basic science to the diagnosis of metabolic bone disease.

For all practical purposes in normal animals and humans, the kidney is the exclusive site of synthesis of 1,25-$(OH)_2D_3$ (59,60). There is no doubt that tissue culture preparations from a number of tissues can be induced to produce 1,25-$(OH)_2D_3$. For example, bone cells (61) and macrophages (62,63) can produce 1,25-$(OH)_2D_3$ in culture. In normal animals or in normal humans from which kidneys have only recently been removed, 1,25-(OH)-$_2D_3$ is not found in the circulation (64,65). On the other hand, sarcoid patients have high levels of 1,25-$(OH)_2D_3$ even in the absence of kidneys (66,67). Thus, the hypercalcemia of sarcoidosis is very likely the result of ectopic production of

$1,25\text{-}(OH)_2D_3$, probably in the granulomatous tissue (68). Thus a new understanding of disease results from this basic science investigation. Treatment involves vitamin D deprivation and control of dietary calcium levels until the ectopic production of $1,25\text{-}(OH)_2D_3$ can be controlled. The administration of glucocorticoids is often helpful in this disorder as well.

The placenta is also a site of production of $1,25\text{-}(OH)_2D_3$ and thus anephric pregnant animals will produce this important hormone (69,70). Why it is produced in the placenta is unknown at the present time, especially since it is known that rats can survive and reproduce under conditions of severe vitamin D deficiency (71). It is not clear what the need is for vitamin D during embryonic and neonatal development, and thus the question of why placenta produces the vitamin D hormone remains unanswered.

The discovery by Kodicek and his colleagues (72) that the compound later identified in our group as $1,25\text{-}(OH)_2D_3$ (52) is produced in the kidney was the basis for elucidation of the vitamin D endocrine system (73). It also provides an important new application of the vitamin D system in the case of the bone disease brought about by loss of renal function (74,75). This disease is known as renal osteodystrophy and is a complex mixture of disorders (76). Basically, two diseases are found, osteomalacia and osteitis fibrosa cystica, which is essentially a secondary hyperparathyroidism. One of the contributing features to this disease is the patient's inability to produce the vitamin D hormone. The administration of chemically synthesized $1,25\text{-}(OH)_2D_3$ is an obvious way to help in the treatment of the metabolic bone disease found in such subjects (75). A great deal of information is available on the treatment of renal osteodystrophy. The sequence of treatment seems to be as follows: (1) management of the plasma phosphorus levels by phosphate deprivation and administration of phosphate binders; (2) administration of $1,25\text{-}(OH)_2D_3$ or an analog that increases calcium absorption and utilization, and (3) it has recently been found that intravenous administration of $1,25\text{-}(OH)_2D_3$ is superior to an oral form in the treatment of this bone disease (77). The oral form is partly destroyed as it is absorbed across the small intestine and also tends to exert a preferential action on the small intestine. We now know that an important target site of $1,25\text{-}(OH)_2D_3$ is the parathyroid gland (78,79), in which the synthesis of parathyroid hormone appears to be suppressed (80). Thus, the discovery of the activation of vitamin D to its hormonal form has provided another important new medical application, namely the treatment of renal osteodystrophy. This treatment is especially important for children who present with severe renal rickets (81). These patients benefit very greatly by the administration of the vitamin D hormone. No child with renal osteodystrophy should be without this treatment, whether orally or intravenously administered.

A disease of considerable importance to the vitamin D endocrine system in terms of basic science is vitamin-D-dependent rickets type I. This disease called either pseudovitamin-D-deficiency disease or vitamin-D-dependency rickets, was discovered by Prader in Zurich in the early 1950s (82). Children with this condition present with severe rickets in the presence of normal vitamin D intakes. They can also be treated with large doses of vitamin D or 25-OH-D, and they then show approximately normal mineralization. With the chemical synthesis of 1,25-$(OH)_2D_3$, it was possible to test the nature of the defect in this disease. Thus, physiological amounts of 1,25-$(OH)_2D_3$ could completely heal this disease, as large doses of vitamin D or 25-OH-D (83). Measurement of blood levels in these patients illustrates that 1,25-$(OH)_2D_3$ is very low compared to normal (84). Thus, this disease is an autosomal recessive defect in 1α-hyroxylase, resulting in failure to synthesize the vitamin D hormone when normal amounts of vitamin D are present.

Why do large doses of vitamin D heal this disorder? The 25-hydroxylase is regulated only slightly, if at all, and thus large doses of vitamin D can be hydroxylated to form high blood levels of 25-OH-D (85,86). The intestinal receptor for 1,25-$(OH)_2D_3$ accepts 25-OH-D_3 as an analog (87,88). An approximately 20-fold excess of 25-OH-D_3 is required to compete for the binding site on the receptor. Thus, high blood levels of 25-OH-D_3 can serve to bypass 1α-hydroxylation in terms of intestinal calcium transport and absorption. The mineral can then come into blood and, because the mineralization process does not require any form of vitamin D, mineralization can proceed approximately normally. This disorder thus confirms in humans the basic science investigation of the vitamin D endocrine system. 1,25-$(OH)_2D_3$ is therefore the physiological approach to treatment of this rare disorder (83,89).

An important series of investigations provided definite proof that 1-25-$(OH)_2D_3$ or one of its metabolites is the metabolically active form. These experiments were carried out with anephric rats, who could be demonstrated as not responding to physiological amounts of 25-OH-D_3 in terms of intestinal calcium transport or bone calcium mobilization. The same animals respond normally to 1,25-$(OH)_2D_3$ whether or not they have kidneys (90,91). Ureteric ligated animals, although they have a high degree of uremia, will respond to physiological amounts of 25-OH-D_3 (90). These experiments permitted the conclusion that 1,25-$(OH)_2D_3$ or a further metabolite is the metabolically active form of vitamin D in its classic actions, and provided the basis for the conclusion that there is a vitamin D endocrine system in which the kidney serves as an endocrine organ that synthesizes the vitamin D hormone from the circulating form of vitamin D, 25-OH-D.

V. OTHER METABOLISM OF VITAMIN D

Some 33 metabolites of vitamin D have now been isolated and identified (92). Many of these had been isolated from in vitro incubation systems and from

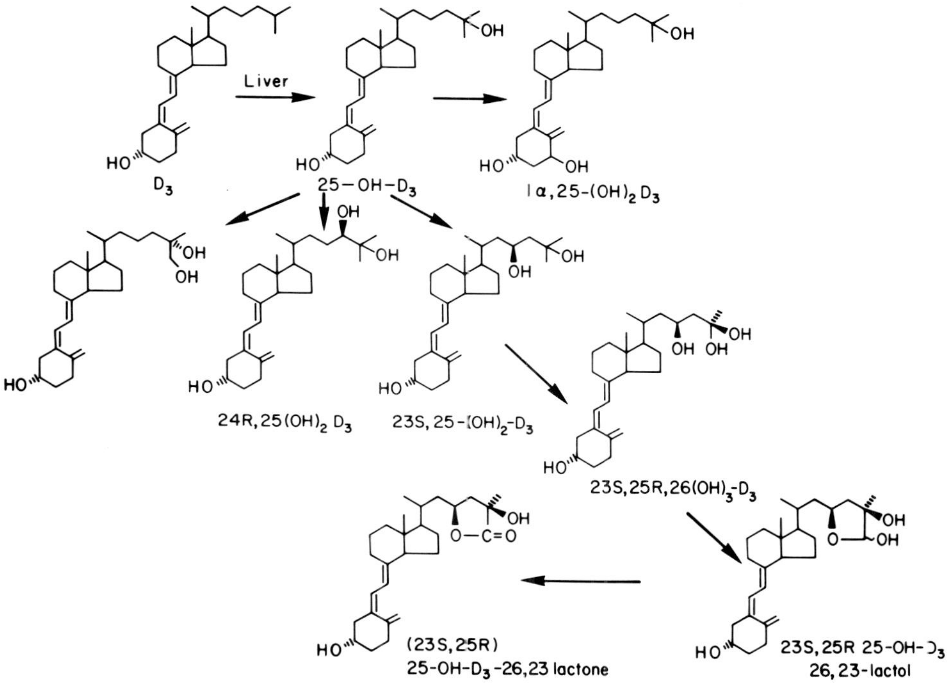

Figure 4 Physiological metabolism of vitamin D to the major circulating metabolites.

kidney perfusions or cell cultures. Often they are metabolites produced from very high concentrations of vitamin D and their physiological relevance remains largely unknown. However, some very clear pathways of vitamin D metabolism occur under normal circumstances in vivo. These are illustrated in Figure 4.

Two major pathways are of special importance. 23S-Hydroxylation of 25-OH-D produces essentially a biologically inactive form of vitamin D. This compound subsequently undergoes 26-oxidation to form a 26-aldehyde that cyclizes and becomes oxidized to a lactone. These compounds are all biologically inert, but they may provide some not yet discovered special function of vitamin D. Perhaps the most important pathway of metabolism other than 1α-hydroxylation is the 24R-hydroxylation to produce 24,25-$(OH)_2D_3$ (93). The 24-hydroxylase is induced under circumstances when 1α-hydroxylation is suppressed (94,95). Thus, 1,25-$(OH)_2D_3$ induces the 24-hydroxylase; the absence of parathyroid hormone causes the 24-hydroxylase to appear; conditions of high blood phosphorus will also bring about increased 24-hydroxylation at the same time that may suppress 1α-hydroxylation (95,96). It is unknown whether 24-hydroxyla-

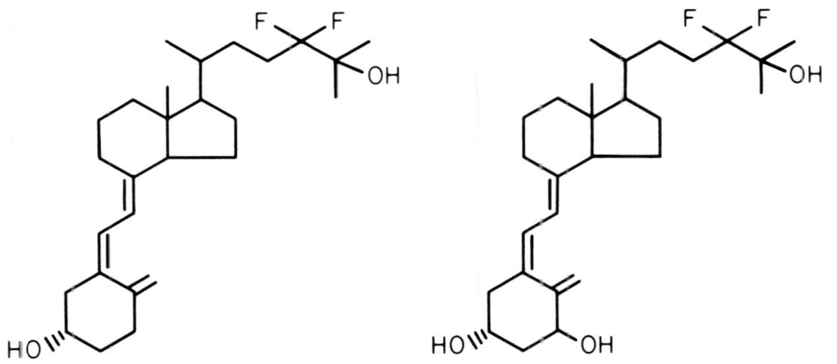

24,24-F_2-25-OH-D_3 24,24-F_2-1α,25$(OH)_2D_3$

Figure 5 Structure of the difluoro derivatives used to demonstrate the nonessentiality of 24-hydroxylation of vitamin D compounds to function.

tion, which is believed to be the initial event in inactivation of the vitamin D hormone (97,98). Much work remains to be done on the 24-hydroxylases to determine what their roles might be in degradation of the vitamin D hormone or, alternatively, why it 24-hydroxylases 25-OH-D_3.

Nevertheless, 24,25-$(OH)_2D_3$ has been examined as a possible alternative hormonal form of vitamin D. One investigator has concluded that this is a hatching hormone for birds (98,99). The same group has claimed that this substance is required for the regulation of plasma calcium (100,101). However, it is clear that 24,24-F_2-25-OH-D_3, illustrated in Figure 5, is fully able to satisfy all of the functions of vitamin D (102). In fact, two generations of animals have been grown with this compound as their sole source of vitamin D. These animals were completely normal in every respect (103–105). Furthermore, these compounds do not become 24-hydroxylated and the CF-bond is quite stable in this position (106). It has also been demonstrated that the binding proteins, namely the 1,25-$(OH)_2D_3$ receptor and the plasma transport protein, react to the 24,24-F_2 analogs as if the fluoro groups are hydrogen and not hydroxyl. The argument that the fluoro compounds mimic 24,25-$(OH)_2D_3$ is without chemical or physiological basis. Thus, 24,25-$(OH)_2D_3$ is not required for life and reproduction, refuting the claim that it is needed for bone or calcium regulation. It has also been demonstrated that 24,25-$(OH)_2D_3$ is not a hatching hormone (107–109). Thus, 24-hydroxylation likely plays a role in the elimination of vitamin D compounds. 23,23-F_2-25-OH-D_3 and 26,27-F_6-25-OH-

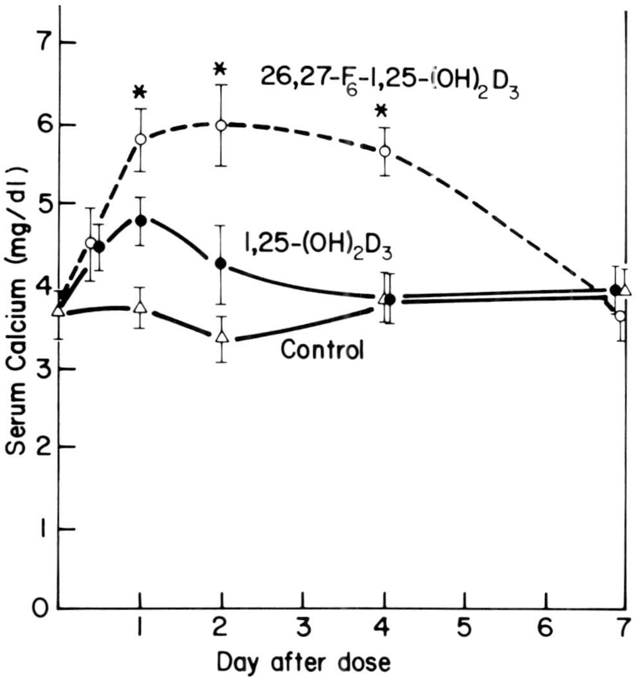

Figure 6 Time course of response of bone calcium mobilization to the 26,27-hexafluoro 1,25-$(OH)_2D_3$ compared to the native hormone, 1,25-$(OH)_2D_3$. Rats were fed a vitamin-D-deficient, low-calcium diet and then given a single injection of 650 pmol of either compound dissolved in propylene glycol. The control received the propylene glycol carrier. Serum calcium levels were measured at the times indicated. Vertical bars represent SEM for at least six animals. Asterisks indicate significantly different value from those engendered by 1,25-$(OH)_3D_3$ at $p < 0.001$.

D_3 have been prepared and used to demonstrate that hydroxylation of these carbons is not required for the normal functions of vitamin D (110,11).

Of considerable importance is that the fluoro derivatives are rapidly 1α-hydroxylated in vivo and the 1,25-$(OH)_2D_3$ fluoro derivatives represent interesting potential therapeutic agents (112,113). As illutrated in Figure 6, hexafluoro 1,25-$(OH)_2D_3$ is not only more biologically active but also has a longer-lasting activity than the native vitamin D hormone (117). The vitamin D hormone has a lifetime of 2–4 hr in human plasma (114) and thus its therapeutic effectiveness is limited by its lifetime. It is often necessary to give 1,25-$(OH)_2D_3$ at least twice daily for maximum therapeutic effectiveness. The fluoro derivatives are not only more active but also can be given once a day or less frequently and retain their therapeutic effectiveness. Thus, the side-chain fluoro compounds such as 24,24-F_2-1,25-$(OH)_2 D_3$ or the hexafluoro 1,25-$(OH)_2 D_3$ represents compounds potentially of considerable therapeutic importance.

VI. REGULATION OF THE VITAMIN D ENDOCRINE SYSTEM

Figure 7 provides a diagrammatic representation of regulation of plasma calcium concentration involving the vitamin D endocrine system. Regulation of the vitamin D endocrine system was elucidated in 1971 by Boyle et al. (94). Low plasma calcium levels stimulate the parathyroid glands to secrete parathyroid hormone (95). Parathyroid hormone binds to kidney and bone; it does not bind to the small intestine (116). In the proximal convoluted tubule cells of the kidney, this peptide hormone stimulates 1α-hydroxylation of 25-OH-D to produce the vitamin D hormone (117). In fact, stimulation of the vitamin D endocrine system by low calcium levels occurs largely through the parathyroid gland, although some evidence that there may be direct regulation by calcium has been produced but is still not convincing (118). The increased levels of 1,25-$(OH)_2 D_3$ stimulate the intestine to transport calcium and phosphorus (119). These levels stimulate the bone to mobilize calcium and phosphorus, and the distal renal tubule to reabsorb calcium (see above). This raises the blood calcium level, which then shuts down the parathyroid gland's actions which in

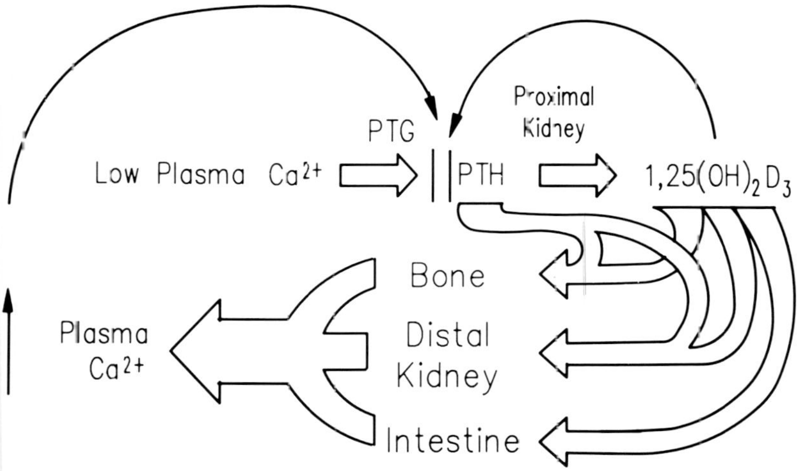

Figure 7 Diagrammatic representation of regulation of plasma calcium concentration involving parathyroid hormone and the vitamin D hormone.

turn shuts down production of the vitamin D hormone. Thus, the vitamin D endocrine system is intimately involved in the regulation of plasma calcium concentration. This regulation, however, cannot take place without the parathyroid system. The parathyroid system therefore represents a very quickly reacting messenger system (120,121). Furthermore, the parathyroid is required to mobilize calcium from bone (42). Certainly the vitamin D endocrine system cannot function or operate in the absence of parathyroid tissue. Loss of the parathyroid glands by surgery, autoimmune disease, or because of a genetic defect results in hypoparathyroidism: The body loses its ability to sense the drop in plasma calcium concentration and cannot react to produce either calcium-mobilizing hormone, parathyroid hormone or 1,25-$(OH)_2D_3$. Since parathyroid hormone is a peptide hormone, it cannot be administered orally. Furthermore, its lifetime can be measured in minutes. However, 1,25-$(OH)_2D_3$ can be given orally and will stimulate the intestine in the absence of parathyroid hormone (42). Thus, one can use dietary calcium to support plasma calcium concentration even in the absence of parathyroid hormone. A supply of chemically synthesized 1-25-$(OH)_2D_3$ plus large amounts of dietary calcium can result in management of hypocalcemia, hypoparathyroidism, and pseudohypoparathyroidism (122,123). Both dietary calcium and 1,25-$(OH)_2D_3$ are essential for this treatment.

In the past, large doses of vitamin D have been used for treatment of this disorder often with success but with the complications of vitamin D intoxication. Vitamin D in large doses is effective for the very same reason that it is effective in the treatment of vitamin-D-dependent rickets type I as described above: high circulating levels of 25-OH-D can serve as an analog of 1,25-$(OH)_2D_3$ in promoting intestinal calcium transport. It is, therefore, apparent that 1,25-$(OH)_2D_3$ or its analogs can be very useful in the management of a variety of hypocalcemic disorders.

VII. REGULATION OF INTESTINAL CALCIUM ABSORPTION AND ITS IMPORTANCE IN REGULATING BONE MASS

In the early 1930s, Steenbock and associates learned that calcium-deprived animals are much better able to utilize dietary calcium than are anomals with adequate amounts of calcium (124). This basic observation was largely expanded by Nicolaysen and his colleagues, who demonstrated that the intestine seemed to be informed of the skeletal needs for calcium (124,125). The ability to utilize or absorb calcium avidly from the small intestine remained active until their skeletons were completely mineralized. Thus, Nicolaysen postulated the existence of an "endogenous factor" that notified the intestine of the body's need for calcium (125). With the discovery of 1,25-$(OH)_2D_3$, we became aware that this factor might be 1,25-$(OH)_2D_3$ and the parathyroid system that signals production of the vitamin D hormone (119). It now is apparent that regulation of intestinal calcium absorption is a major function of $1,25\text{-}(OH)_2D_3$ and the parathyroid system. Thus, in animals requiring calcium or in which calcium is being utilized to mineralize the skeleton, plasma calcium levels will tend to fall slightly. The parathyroids react by increasing secretion of parathyroid hormone, which in turn stimulates production of the vitamin D hormone. This hormone in turn increases the efficiency of the intestinal absorption of calcium, thus providing calcium from the environment (126). This environmental source of calcium is then required to prevent continued use of bone calcium to support soft tissue needs. In animals deprived of calcium, although their intestines are stimulated to transport calcium by the vitamin D endocrine system, there is no calcium to be absorbed. Thus, calcium does not come in from the small intestine. The parathyroids will continue to be activated and thus high blood levels of $1,25\text{-}(OH)_2D_3$ and parathyroid hormone will result. This brings about a mobilization of skeletal calcium to provide calcium to prevent hypocalcemic tetany. Thus in the absence of dietary calcium, a normal animal will utilize its skeletal calcium to statisfy its soft tissue needs. If adequate dietary calcium is provided but the animal is unable to absorb calcium because some factor inhibits this, the parathyroids will likewise continue to agitate for bone calcium, bringing in skeletal calcium to meet soft tissue needs. An example is glucocorticoid treatment that inhibits intestinal calcium absorption (127). It is well known that glucocorticoid treatment brings about a loss of skeletal mass or osteoporosis (128). This is in part the result of its inhibition of intestinal calcium absorption, although it may also have other effects such as causing calcium excretion in the urine and may have direct actions on bone as well as suppression of hydroxylation of $1,25\text{-}(OH)_2D_3$ (129).

If inadequate calcium absorption could alone account for osteoporosis under a variety of circumstances, one could reason that merely increasing the intake of calcium might be sufficient to provide calcium to prevent osteoporosis. However, it is important to realize that the vitamin D hormone has important actions on the skeleton and elsewhere in the body. We have already discussed that an important site of action of the vitamin D hormone is the parathyroid gland, where it suppresses synthesis of parathyroid hormone (80). Of great importance is its role in the skeleton. It localizes in the osteoblasts and bone lining cells (130) where it is believed to play an important role in transporting calcium back into the plasma when stimulated by the parathyroid hormone. However, an important observation was made in basic science when $1,25\text{-}(OH)_2D_3$ was first isolated, identified, and synthesized. This was supplied to Drs. Raisz and Trummel, who demonstrated that $1,25\text{-}(OH)_2D_3$ at very low concentrations will cause embryonic bone to resorb in culture by an osteoclastic-mediated mechanism (131). This was also found by an in vivo/in vitro technique by Dr. John Reynolds in collaboration with our group (132,133). Thus, it might appear that

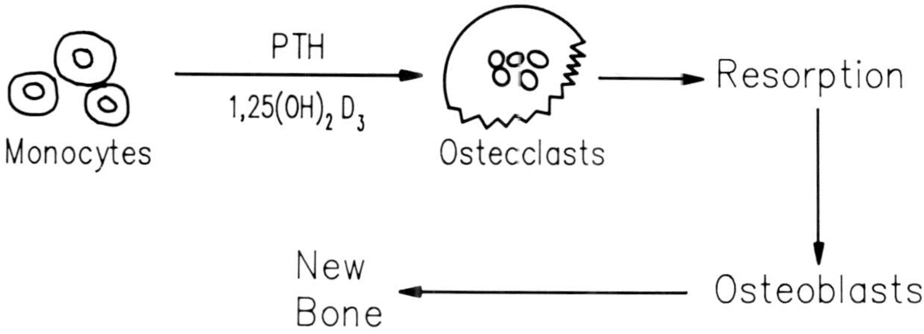

Figure 8 Diagrammatic representation of the process of bone remodeling.

vitamin D rather than increasing bone mass might well cause bone resorption. However, in vivo 1,25-$(OH)_2 D_3$ does not cause bone loss, but causes an increase in bone (134).

What is the meaning of the osteoclastic-mediated bone resorption response that has been studied so thoroughly? Very likely this represents an initial event in the bone remodeling system, which is illustrated in Figure 8. A major contribution was made by Frost and his colleagues, who demonstrated that bone is constantly turned over and remodeled by a remodeling system (135). Precursor cells, probably monocytes, are recruited to form osteoclasts and the hormones involved in this recruitment are parathyroid hormone and 1,25-$(OH)_2 D_3$ (136). It is not clear whether these two hormones further stimulate the osteoclasts after they are formed. These osteoclasts then resorb the bone surface; this resorption is required for new bone formation to occur. Formation of bone is tightly coupled to bone resorption in normal adult human beings (135). The remodeling process is needed to repair damage to the skeleton brought about by use and may well play an important role in maintaining skeletal mass. Thus, it is clear that vitamin D and parathyroid hormone may play an important role in the synthesis of new bone, which results from the remodeling process by activating the resorption process, which is a precursor for bone formation. Thus, if one were to give calcium to an osteoporotic subject and the calcium were absorbed, it would suppress parathyroid secretion and in turn suppress 1,25-$(OH)_2 D_3$ production. The absence of these two hormones would shut down the resorption process and thereby retard bone remodeling. Without the resorption surface being present, new bone could not be formed in adults. The administration of calcium to osteoporotic subjects therefore might not be beneficial. In fact, it has been shown that calcium in the diet alone cannot prevent the bone loss characteristic of the postmenopausal state (137,138).

Since 1,25-$(OH)_2 D_3$ can promote calcium absorption and increase bone remodeling, it might be useful in the treatment of osteoporosis. Administration of the vitamin D hormone could increase calcium absorption and increase the

Table 1 Postmenopausal Osteoporosis: Treatment with 1,25-$(OH)_2D_3$

	Baseline	6–8 Months	2 Years
Ca absorption (%)	7	27[a]	27[a]
Ca balance (mg/day)	-59	2[b]	-27
Trabecular bone volume (%)	11.3	13.4	16.2[b]
Urinary hydroxyproline (mg/day)	26.3	21.1[b]	22.0[b]

[a]$p < 0.001$
[b]$p < 0.01$
Study included 30 patients, approximately age 55, with at least one crush fracture and other evidence of osteoporosis. Fifteen were treated with 0.5 μg of 1,25-$(OH)_2D_3$ for the 2 year period as indicated (139).

resorption surfaces upon which new bone can be formed. It is thus possible that bone mass can be rebuilt by administration of 1,25-$(OH)_2D_3$ from exogenous sources. Preliminary results by double-blind trials at the Mayo Clinic under the direction of Drs. Riggs and Gallagher (139) and at Creighton University under the direction of Drs. Gallagher and Recker (unpublished results), have provided such information. Bone mass is increased when 0.5 μg or more are given per day to patients who have normal calcium intake. Furthermore, the fracture rate in postmenopausal women with osteoporosis has been reported to be reduced. Table 1 illustrates the data obtained in the Mayo Clinic study.

Very low doses of 1,25-$(OH)_2D_3$ are not helpful in the treatment of osteoporosis (140). A dosage of 0.25 μg/day is far below the amount normally made in humans (1.7 μg/day) and thus represents a homeopathic dosage). More recently, in the laboratory of Aloia, additional confirmatory results have been obtained in which 0.5–0.75 μg of 1,25-$(OH)_2D_3$ per day markedly improved calcium retention and bone mass in postmenopausal women with osteoporosis (141). Thus, the use of this compound in the treatment of osteoporosis is very promising but will not likely be approved by the Food and Drug Administration for use in the United States since patent protection is too short to permit the investment of funds required for its approval. On the other hand, 1α-OH-D_3 has been in use in Japan for several years for the treatment of osteoporosis with an apparent high degree of success.

Older animals and humans have a reduced ability to absorb calcium (142, 143). This can be exactly correlated with plasma levels of 1,25-$(OH)_2D_3$ (143, 144). Furthermore, administration of parathyroid hormone to elderly subjects is unable to stimulate production of the vitamin D hormone, whereas when 1,25-$(OH)_2D_3$ is given to elderly subjects, increased calcium absorption has been found (145). Thus, the intestine retains its responsiveness to the hormone but there is an age-related defect in production of the vitamin D hormone (143,144). Age-related osteoporosis may well be the result of the defective production of $1,25\text{-}(OH)_2D_3$ and $1,25\text{-}(OH)_2D_3$ may be an important agent for use in prevention of hip fractures in the elderly (146).

VIII. MOLECULAR MECHANISM OF ACTION OF $1,25\text{-}(OH)_2D_3$

A great deal of work has been carried out to understand how $1,25\text{-}(OH)_2D_3$ functions in its target organs. Perhaps the largest amount of work has been centered on the small intestine. When radiolabeled $1,25\text{-}(OH)_2D_3$ is administered to vitamin-D-deficient animals, within one-half hour the radiolabel is localized in the nuclei of the enterocytes of the small intestine but not in the nuclei of goblet cells, submucosa, or smooth muscle of the small intestine (78). Similar nuclear localization is found in osteoblasts and bone lining cells but not osteclasts (130). It also occurs in distal renal tubule cells, in parathyroid tissue, and in a variety of other tissues discussed in a subsequent section. This steroid hormone is localized in the nucleus and one might expect it to function by a mechanism similar to that of other steroid hormones. A nuclear receptor for $1,25\text{-}(OH)_2D_3$ has been described by Brumbaugh and Haussler (147) and by Kream et al. (148). Since these earlier discoveries, a large number of papers have appeared on the receptor (149). The receptor for $1,25\text{-}(OH)_2D_3$ in the small intestine can be demonstrated by sucrose density gradient sedimentation, as illustrated in Figure 9, and by Scatchard analysis. This receptor has a high-affinity, low-capacity binding site with a K_D of 5×10^{-11} and, furthermore, it is highly selective for $1,25\text{-}(OH)_2D_3$ compared to other steroids and vitamin D metabolites (149). Among the metabolites, the closest competitor for $1,25\text{-}(OH)_2D_3$ is $1,24,25\text{-}(OH)_3D_3$, which is one-tenth as active than the native hormone (150). The $26,27,F_6\text{-}1,25\text{-}(OH)_2D_3$ and the $24,24\text{-}F_2\text{-}1\alpha,25\text{-}OH\text{-}D_3$ have approximately equal activity to $1,25\text{-}(OH)_2D_3$ in binding to the receptor (112,113,151). The precursor, $25\text{-}OH\text{-}D_3$, is one-twentieth as active, $24,25\text{-}(OH)_2D_3$ is one-thousandth as active, and so on (Link and DeLuca, unpublished results). Thus, the receptor is quite selective for the hormonal form of vitamin D.

The question is: How important is this nuclear receptor for $1,25\text{-}(OH)_2D_3$ to its function? It appears that it is essential. Vitamin-D-dependent rickets type II, which is discussed subsequently, involves target-organ resistance to $1,25\text{-}(OH)_2D_3$. One subgroup of these patients has a clear defect in the receptor, illustrating that the receptor is required for $1,25\text{-}(OH)_2D_3$ to function (152). Furthermore, neonatal rats fail to respond to $1,25\text{-}(OH)_2D_3$ until approximately 16–18 days postpartum, precisely when this receptor makes is appearance in the small intestine (153). Glucocorticoids cause a precocious appearance

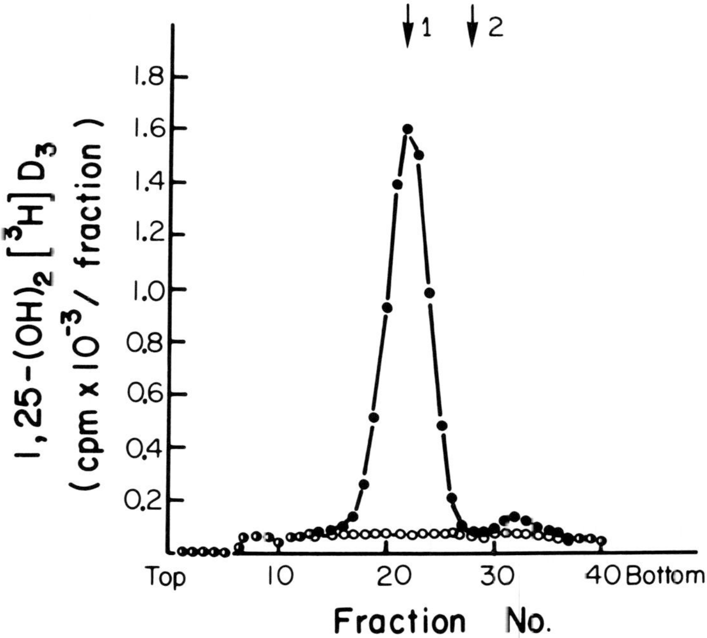

Figure 9 Sucrose density gradient sedimentation demonstration of the rat intestinal receptor for 1,25-$(OH)_2D_3$. Whole cell extract prepared in high-salt buffer was labeled with radiolabeled 1,25-$(OH)_2D_3$, treated with dextran-coated charcoal to remove unbound labeled sterol, then layered over a 10–20% Sucrose gradient and spun for 18 hr at 80,000 g. Fractions were collected from the bottom of the tube and counted. Clear circles represent cytosol incubated together with radiolabeled 1,25-$(OH)_2D_3$ and a 10-fold excess of 1,25-$(OH)_2D_3$. Arrow 1 represents the sedimentation of bovine seurm albumin; arrow 2 is ovalbumin.

Table 2 Purification of the Porcine 1,25-$(OH)_2D_3$ Receptor Protein

	Specific Activity (pmol/mg)	Purification (X)	Yield (%)	Purity (%)
Nuclear extract (10)[a]	0.635	1	100	0.0035
DNA cellulose (10)	47.2	74	51	0.26
$(NH_4)_2SO_4$ ppt (10) and size exclusion HPLC (25)	629	990	37	3.8
DEAE Sepharose (6)	4170	6600	23	24

[a]( ) = number of batches or columns (157,158).

of the receptor in neonatal rats, whereas adrenalectomy delays the receptor's appearance (154). These maneuvers also affect the intestinal calcium transport in the same way. Thus, there is an exact correlation between receptor and calcium transport response of the small intestine in the neonatal rat to 1,25-$(OH)_2D_3$. It is, therefore, unlikely that the so-called rapid and non-nuclear reactions of 1,25-$(OH)_2D_3$ are important to the basic function of 1,25-$(OH)_2D_3$.

A great deal of effort has been expended to purify the receptor. Simpson et al. (155) and Pike et al. (156) have purified the receptor from chick small intestine, although the amounts produced are rather small. Furthermore, it is not clear exactly how pure these preparations might be, although the intestinal preparation from the chick was shown by Coomassie staining to be homogeneous by Simpson et al. (155). Because the quantities produced were small, our group turned to a better source, the young pig, which has very large amounts of the receptor in its small intestine, providing approximately 2,000 fmol/mg protein of binding activity as compared to 500 fmol/mg found in the chicken (157, 158). The receptor was highly purified, as illustrated in Table 2 (158). However, it was not homogeneous and, in fact, silver-nitrate-stained gels of the peak tubes showed that several protein bands were still present (157). When the preparation was renatured, a protein band of 55,000 molecular weight was the only one that renatured into hormonal binding activity (157). This band also reacted to monoclonal antibodies we produced to the receptor. Thus, the molecular weight of the mammalian receptor is 55,000. We used this preparation to generate monoclonal antibodies and develop screening for such antibodies (158). We obtained 24 monoclonal antibodies, of which 17 were well characterized; the characteristics are shown in Table 3. With the use of competition studies, we could show that these are found in four epitope groups, with two of the epitope groups overlapping.

What can be learned with these monoclonal antibodies? First, by immobilizing an antibody on Sepharose CL6B, an immunoaffinity resin can be prepared that can be used to purify the receptor to homogeneity. We can now obtain quantities of the receptor that are a single band on sodium docedyl sulfate (SDS) gels and are being used for protein sequencing work (Brown and DeLuca, unpublished results). Furthermore, the receptor antibodies have been used in a lambda GT11 expression library system to clone a cDNA to the receptor. Cloning of the chicken receptor has been reported by Pike et al. (159) using a monoclonal antibody directed to the chick receptor. Our group has also been able to obtain a cDNA clone for the rat receptor. Through this route the detailed chemical structures of the receptor will be obtained, including the topology: where the receptor binds to DNA and where on the receptor the hormone binds. The antibodies can be used in immunoblots or Western blotting to detect the forms of the receptor (160). With the use of one-dimensional gel electrophoresis, we can demonstrate that fresh tissue provides only 55,000 Da species as the highest

Table 3 Monoclonal Antibodies to the Porcine Intestinal Receptor

	Clone Designation	Clone Reactivity—Intestinal Receptor					Immunoblot
		Pig	Monkey	Human	Rat	Chicken	
Mouse: NS-1	IVA7E7	+	+	+	+	+	+
	IVB12G12[a]	+	+	+	+	+	+
	IVG8C11	+	+	+	+	+	+
	VA3C12	+	+	+	+	+	−
	VB3F12	+	+	+	+	+	−
	VD2F12	+	+	+	+	+	+
	VIIA1E9A7	+	+	+	+	+	−
	VIIIB8B2A9	+	+	+	+	+	−
	VIIID8C12	+	+	+	+	+	+
	VIIIF7E12	+	+	+	+	+	−
	IXD5F10	−	−	−	+	+	−
	XA9E8	+	+	+	+	+	−
	XH12G11	+	+	+	+	+	+
	XIID9G5D6	+	+	+	+	+	−
	XVA9A7B6	+	+	+	+	+	−
	XVIE6E6G10[b]	+	−	−	−	−	+
	XVIE10B6A5	+	−	−	−	−	+
Rat: NS-1	IXC1H5	+	+	nd	−	+	+

[a]$IgA_{,k}$; all other mouse hybridomas $IgG_{1,k}$.
[b]Protein-A-binding antibody (158).

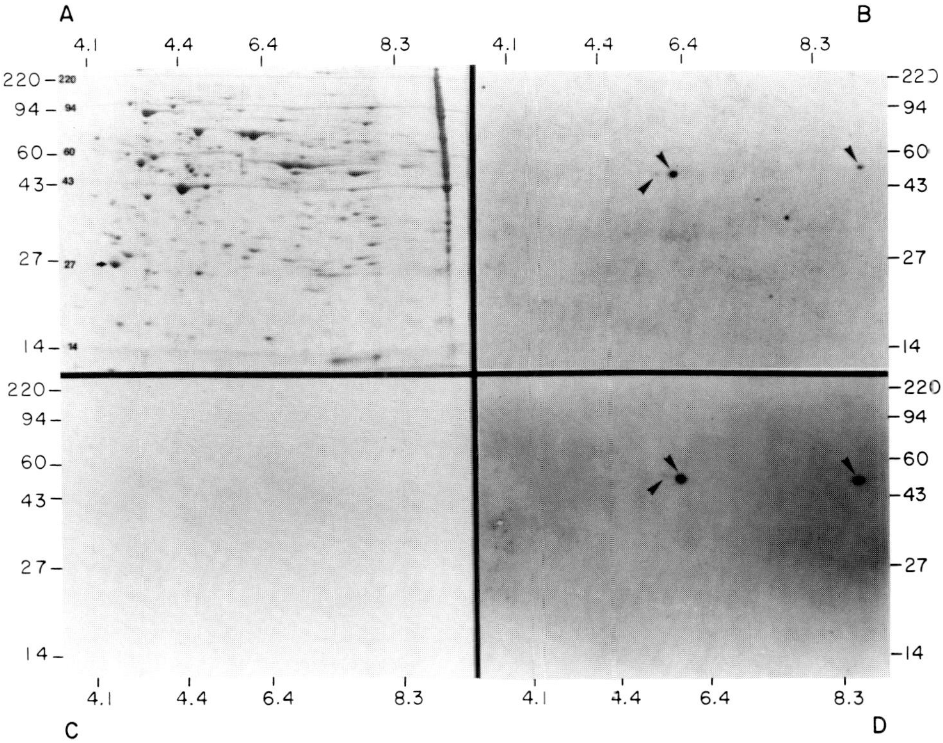

Figure 10 Two-dimensional immunoblots of hog intestinal mucosal whole cell extract using two monoclonal antibodies directed to the 1,25-$(OH)_2D_3$ receptor. A: Coomassie-blue-stained gels of the extract; B: two-dimensional immunoblot using the antibody IVG8C11; arrows represent the highest molecular weight species detected. There are also low molecular weight degradation fragments visible, which are not marked by arrows. C: a control immunoblot using an irrelevant antibody, M0PC21 and D represent an immunoblot using a different epitope group antibody XVIE6E6. Arrows denote the highest molecular weight specied detected. Note the presence of three proteins of 55,000 Da that are detected by two distinct epitope group antibodies.

molecular weight species recognized by all of the different antibodies we have produced. Of considerable importance is two-dimensional gel electrophoresis of whole hog intestinal tissue or nuclear extract to illustrate the forms of the receptor (Fig. 10). Panel A shows Coomassie-stained proteins from fresh intestinal mucosa. Panel B shows proteins detected by a radiolabeled monoclonal antibody, IVG8C11. Three forms of the receptor are detected, all with a molecular weight of about 55,000 kD. One has a pI of 6.1 and is the major protein com-

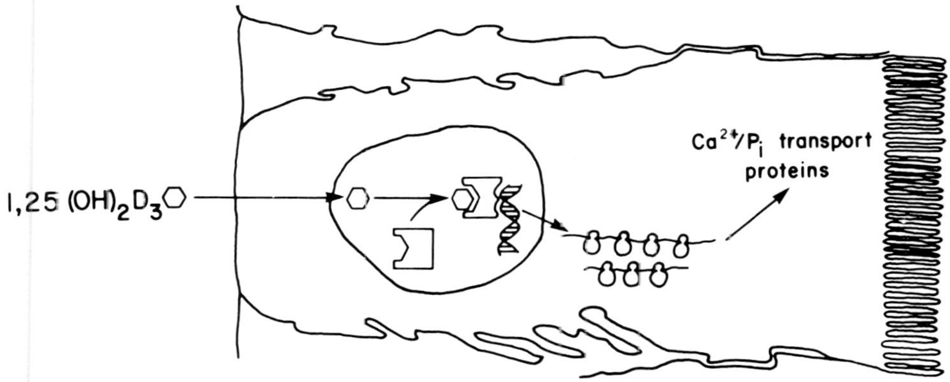

Figure 11 The expected molecular mechanism of action of 1,25-$(OH)_2D_3$ in intestinal mucosal cell in stimulating the transport of calcium and phosphorus.

ponent. There is a minor 55,000 species with a pI of 5.9 and another major spot that does not enter the electrofocusing gel from either the acid or base side and is shown on the far right side. Another monoclonal antibody in panel D provides the same information. An irrelevant antibody is illustrated in panel C of the graph, thus providing the control for the experiment carried out. The receptor for 1,25-$(OH)_2D_3$ in target tissue is heterogeneous in terms of charge but has a molecular weight of 55,000. Which of these forms is the active form of the receptor remains unknown. We have also set up a radioimmune assay for total receptor peptide and, for the first time, true regulation of 1,25-$(OH)_2D_3$ receptor can be studied.

Figure 11 illustrates the mechanism believed to operate in the small intestine in response to the hormone involving the nuclear receptor. Of considerable importance is the nature of the proteins that result from the nuclear interaction of 1,25-$(OH)_2D_3$ and its receptor. Only one protein responsive to 1,25-$(OH)_2D_3$ has been well characterized. This is the calcium binding protein originally discovered by Wasserman and Taylor (161). In mammals, this has a molecular weight of approximately 9,000. By differential hybridization, we have been able to isolate a cDNA clone of this protein as well as cDNA clones of other 1,25-$(OH)_2D_3$-regulated genes (162,163). We have used the initial cDNA probe obtained from this lambda GT10 library to probe the full-length cDNA of this substance (164). We now have a full-length cDNA for this protein that is illustrated diagrammatically in Figure 12. By making specific oligionucleotides to specific regions, we have found we have been able to characterize the structure of the full-length cDNA completely. Basic information of this is provided in Figure 12 as well as the restriction enzyme map. There are 62 bases of non-

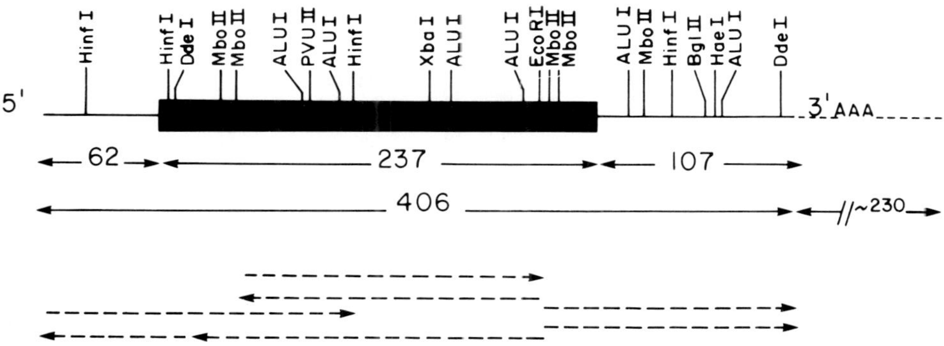

Rat Intestinal CaBP cDNA

Figure 12 Diagrammatic representation of the cDNA for rat intestinal vitamin-D-dependent calcium-binding protein. Coding region represents the 237 base pairs with noncoding regions of 62 and 107 at the 5′ and 3′ ends, respectively. There are approximately 230 adenylate bases at the 3′ end.

coding region, 237 bases of coding region, 107 bases after the stop codon, and approximately 230 polyA bases. We have used the full-length cDNA to isolate the gene from a rat lambda Charon library and find that this entire cDNA sequence is encased in a 4.1 Kb fragment of genomic DNA that includes a large 5′ upstream sequence to the gene including the regulatory regions. We are now looking for the tight-binding regions of receptor plus ligand in the calcium-binding protein gene, and we are also, by transfection experiments, hoping to isolate the regulatory regions. Thus, vitamin D hormone regulatory regions of expressed genes may soon become known with the use of this technology.

Where is the application to medicine of this information? With Normal Bell, we were able to discover a new form of vitamin-D-resistant rickets called vitamin-D-dependent rickets type II (165). This is believed to be an autosomal recessive disorder in which children present with very high blood levels of 1,25-$(OH)_2D_3$, severe rickets, and often a lack of hair (165,166). Administration of large amounts of 1,25-$(OH)_2D_3$ has little or no benefit. Thus, any portion of the machinery from receptor on to the final gene products might be defective under these circumstances. In fact, preliminary results by Marx et al. (152) have shown that one subgroup is likely to have a defective receptor. However, other kindreds of this type of D-resistant rickets are likely to have a defect in the regulatory region of a gene, or in recognition of the regulatory region, or in the structural genes that bring about the calcium transport process. This will probably be deciphered as new basic information becomes available on the vitamin D hormone.

An obvious question is: How are these patients with vitamin-D-dependent rickets type II managed? Until recently, very little could be done because a lack of responsiveness to the vitamin D hormone prevented adequate calcium absorption, adequate regulation of blood calcium and phosphorus, and hence inadequate mineralization. Balsan and her associates, however, have utilized the information that vitamin D is not required for mineralization or for synthesis of bone but is necessary for intestinal absorption of calcium and phosphorus (153). By providing calcium and phosphorus intravenously, Dr. Balsan and her associates have been able to mineralize the skeleton of these patients (153). Thus, by placing an indwelling catheter and by providing calcium and phosphorus infusions at night, it is possible that these children can be provided with much improved skeletons.

IX. POSSIBLE NONCLASSIC ACTIONS OF VITAMIN D

When Stumpf et al. carried out frozen section autoradiography using high specific activity labeled 1,25-$(OH)_2D_3$, they were able to locate nuclear localization of the vitamin D hormone at sites not previously thought to be targets of vitamin D action (78). A list of these sites is provided in Table 4. Furthermore, with the technology available for locating ligand binding receptor, many of these tissues have been found to have receptor, especially the parathyroid glands (79),

Table 4 1,25-$(OH)_2D_3$ Receptor-Containing Tissue

Tissue	Nuclear localization of 1,25-$(OH)_2D_3$	Receptor: Major	Receptor: Minor
Intestine (small)	X	X	
Kidney	X	X	
Bone	X	X	
Parathyroid gland	X	X	
Colon	X		X
Pancreas	X		X
Placenta	X		X
Brain	X		X
Pituitary	X		X
Skin	X		X
Spleen	?		?
Stomach endo cells	0		0
Lymphocytes	0		0
Activated	0		X

the islet cells of the pancreas, and of considerable interest are such sites as the keratinocytes of skin (78) and some of the bone marrow cells. These results suggested that functions of vitamin D not previously appreciated might well be found. The question of whether the vitamin D hormone plays a role in insulin secretion is currently under investigation and being intensely debated (168–171). It is likely that some function of the vitamin D hormone will be found in the islet cells, although it may be simply one of intercellular calcium regulation that may play a role in insulin secretion.

Another important finding is the existence of large amounts of receptor in 60% or more of all cancer cell lines (172). This led to the addition of the vitamin D hormone to cancer cell lines, some of which produced a stimulation of growth, and others a suppression. Most cancer cell lines, however, at high concentrations of the vitamin D hormone, show a suppression of growth and a differentiation into more benign cells (173,174). This has excited many researchers about possible therapeutic agents derived from the vitamin D system. Perhaps the most exciting discovery was provided by Suda and his colleagues (175,176), who demonstrated in both M1 promyelocytes and in human promyelocytes HL-60 that the addition of the vitamin D hormone causes these cells to become differentiated into monocytes or macrophages, as illustrated in Figure 13. Thus, the malignant promyelocyte is rendered benign by the vitamin D hormone in culture. The mechanism of this growth suppression and differentiation is unknown. Phorbol esters (TPA) can reproduce this action of the vitamin D hormone, but probably by a different mechanism. Large amounts of phorbol ester are required, whereas 10^{-9} M vitamin D hormone can produce this differentiation response (177). This response can be measured by nonspecific monocytic esterase, by measurement of phagocytosis, by the presence of an antigenic determinant on the cell surface, or by morphological change (177).

These results raise some very important basic questions. What is the role of the vitamin D hormone in normal promyelocytic differentiation? Is this the route by which the vitamin D hormone causes formation of monocytes that are precursors of osteoclasts? And, finally, can the vitamin D hormone be used in the treatment of certain acute-myelocytic-type leukemias? It is unknown whether the vitamin D hormone functions physiologically to cause differentiation of promyelocytes into macrophages that then become osteoclasts. Certainly osteoclasts are found in vitamin-D-deficient animals (178,179), which may only prove that there are many routes by which the promyelocytes can be recruited to form osteoclasts. At the present time, it seems unlikely that the vitamin D hormone can not be used to treat acute myelocytic leukemias because the calcium-elevating activity of the vitamin D hormone is so great as to cause hypercalcemia when given at the dosages required to suppress leukemic cells.

We have been very interested in the possibility that analogs of the vitamin D hormone can be prepared to show preferential activity on differentiation of

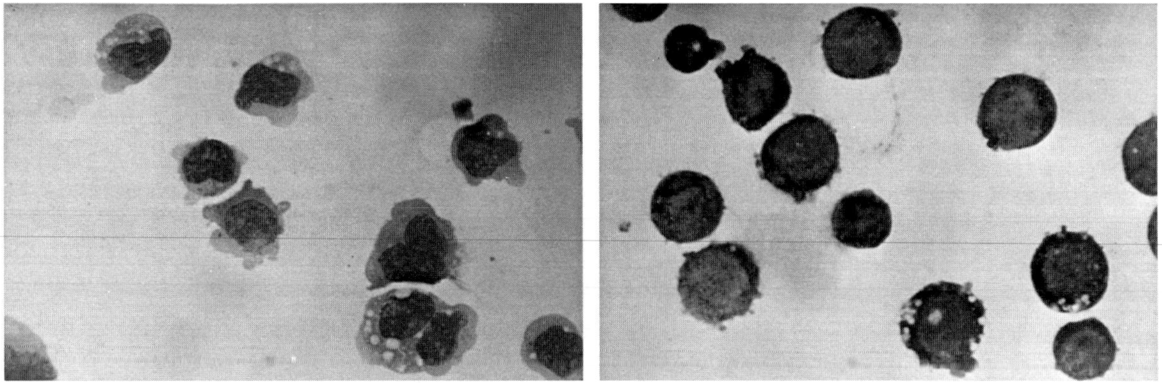

HL-60 cells treated with 100 nM 1α,25$(OH)_2D_3$ (monocytes)

HL-60 cells treated with vehicle only (ethanol) (promyelocytes)

Figure 13 1,25-$(OH)_2D_3$-induced differentiation of the promyelocyte cell line HL-60.

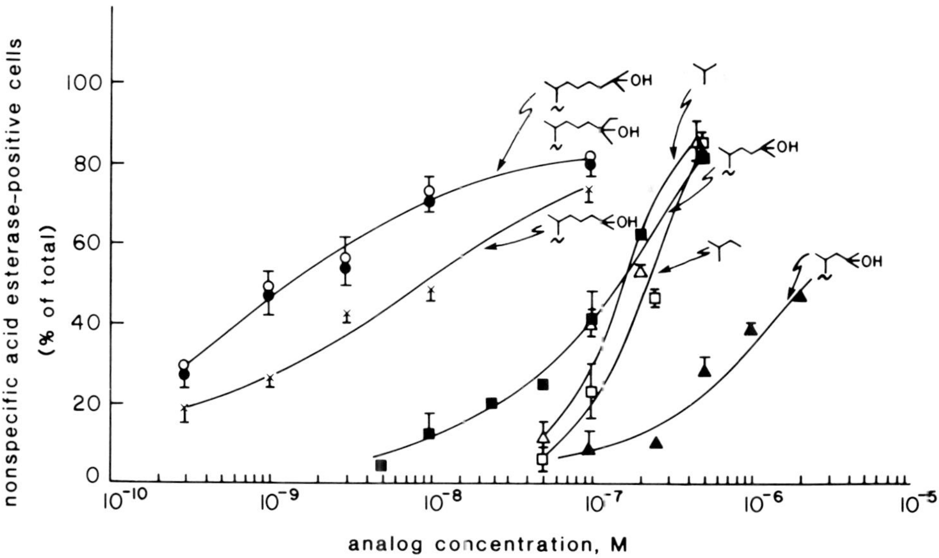

Figure 14 Log-dose–response curves denoting the effect of 1,25-$(OH)_2D_3$ and the various side chain analogs indicated in causing differentiation of HL-60 to the monocytes. Measurement of nonspecific acid esterase is the designated end point in this particular plot.

promyelocytes over its activity in elevating serum calcium levels. We have been successful in finding such analogs (177,180), as shown in Figure 14. By lengthening the side chain of 1,25-$(OH)_2D_3$ by 1 carbon or by adding another carbon to the 26-methyl, one can obtain a compound that is 10 times more active than the native hormone in causing differentiation of HL-60, whereas it either has no effect or diminishes activity in mobilizing calcium in animals. Diminishing the side-chain length reduces its effectiveness in HL-60 as long as the hydroxyl group is present. However, if one eliminates the hydroxyl, a hydrocarbon side chain of two or three carbons provides a substance that has no calcium-elevating activity in vivo but is only one-twentieth as active as 1,25-$(OH)_2D_3$ in causing HL-60 differentiation. Thus, the possibility that specific compounds tailored for action in this system can be made seems great. It also raises the question of whether the receptor in these cells might be different from that found in the small intestine or in bone. These questions cannot be answered now but may provide important information that will be of great therapeutic value. There is promise that the vitamin D system may provide important agents to be used in the treatment of certain types of malignant disease.

A final insight into possible new applications is based on the demonstration of nuclear localization of 1,25-$(OH)_2D_3$ in skin fibroblasts and keratoinocytes (78). Simpson et al. (181) and later Feldman et al. (1982) demonstrated the presence of a receptor for 1,25-$(OH)_2D_3$ in skin. A possible function of the vitamin D hormone in skin is apparent. 1,25-$(OH)_2D_3$ added to cultures of keratinocytes will cause them to differentiate and will also cause a suppression of proliferation (183).

Several groups have contributed to the finding that 1,25-$(OH)_2D_3$ may be useful in the treatment of psoriasis or contact dermatitis (183–187). Holick and his group have been very active in this area and have kindly provided information on this mode of treatment (unpublished results). By giving 1,25-$(OH)_2D_3$ systemically for 3-4 months, they documented an obvious improvement in the skin condition of psoriatic patients. Topical application of this substance is also effective in the treatment of psoriasis.

X. SUMMARY

Since its discovery in 1919, the vitamin D system has continued to provide the medical community with not only understanding of disease but also methods and compounds for their treatment. The disease rickets was resolved as a major medical problem in 1924. Other metabolic bone diseases came under treatment by vitamin D during the 1930s and 1940s. The discovery of the vitamin D endocrine system has led to the treatment of renal osteodystrophy, vitamin-D-dependency rickets, vitamin-D-resistant rickets, and hypoparathyroidism. Furthermore, the discovery that the intestinal absorption of calcium and the bone remodeling system is regulated by the vitamin D hormone has led to the possible use of the vitamin D hormone and its analogs in the treatment of a variety of osteoporotic conditions. Finally, the discovery of the vitamin D hormonal receptor in unexpected sites has led to the possible use of vitamin-D-related compounds in the treatment of certain kinds of malignancies and in skin disorders such as psoriasis and contact dermatitis.

ACKNOWLEDGMENTS

This work was supported by a Program Project Grant No. DK-14881 from the National Institutes of Health and by the Harry Steenbock Research Fund of the Wisconsin Alumni Research Foundation.

REFERENCES

1. Hess, A., ed. The history of rickets. *Rickets, Including Osteomalacia and Tetany*. Lea & Febiger, Philadelphia, 1929, pp. 22–37.

2. Whistler, D. De morbo puerli anglorum, quem patrio idiomate indigenae vocant "The Rickets" (Lugduni, Batavorum 1645). (As cited by Smerdon, G. T., Daniel Whistler and the English disease. A translation and biographical note.) *J. Hist. Med.* 5:397–415 (1950).
3. McCollum, E. V. *A History of Nutrition*. The Riverside Press, Cambridge, MA, 1957.
4. Becker, S. L. Emergence of a trace nutrient concept through animal feeding experiments. Ph.D. Thesis, University of Wisconsin-Madison, 1968.
5. Hart, E. B., McCollum, E. V., Steenbock, H., and Humphrey, G. C. Physiological effect on growth and reproduction of rations balanced from restricted sources. *Wisconsin Exp. Stat. Bull.* 17:131–205 (1911).
6. McCollum, E. V., and Davis, M. The necessity of certain lipins in the diet during growth. *J. Biol. Chem.* 15:167–175 (1913).
7. McCollum, E. V., Simmonds, N., and Pitz, W. The relation of the unidentified dietary factors, the fat-soluble A, and water-soluble B, of the diet to the growth-promoting properties of milk. *J. Biol. Chem.* 27:33–43 (1916).
8. Osborne, T. B., and Mendel, L. B. The role of vitamins in the diet. *J. Biol. Chem.* 31:149–163 (1917).
9. Mellanby, E. An experimental investigation on rickets. *Lancet* 1:407–412 (1919).
10. Mellanby, E. A. Further determination of the part played by accessory food factors in the aetiology of rickets. *J. Physiol.* 52:53 (1919).
11. McCollum, E. V., Simmonds, N., Becker, J. E., and Shipley, P. G. Studies on experimental rickets. XXI. An experimental demonstration of the existence of a vitamin which promotes calcium deposition. *Bull. Johns Hopkins Hosp.* 33:229–230 (1922).
12. Huldshinsky, K. Heilung von rachitis durch künstliche höhensonne. *Deutsch Med. Wochschr.* 45:712–713 (1919).
13. Steenbock, H. The induction of growth promoting and calcifying properties in a ration by exposure to light. *Science* 60:224–225 (1924).
14. Steenbock, H., and Black, A. Fat-soluble vitamins. XVII. The induction of growth-promoting and calcifying properties in a ration by exposure to ultraviolet light. *J. Biol. Chem.* 61:405–422 (1924).
15. Sebrell, W. H., Jr., and Harris, R. S. (eds.). *The Vitamins*. Academic Press, New York, 1954.
16. Askew, F. A., Bourdillon, R. B., Bruce, H. M., Jenkins, R. G. C., and Webster, T. A. The distillation of vitamin D. *Proc. R. Soc.* B107:76–90 (1931).
17. Windaus, A., Linsert, O., Lüttringhaus, A., and Weidlich, G. Crystalline-vitamin D_2, *Ann. Chem.* 492:226–241 (1932).
18. Windaus, A., Schenck, F., and von Werder, F. Uber das antirachitisch wirksame bestrahlungs-produkt aus 7-dehydro-cholesterin. *Hoppe-Seylers Z. Physiol. Chem.* 241:100–103 (1936).
19. Esvelt, R. P., Schnoes, H. K., and DeLuca, H. F. Vitamin D_3 from rat skins irradiated *in vitro* with ultraviolet light, *Arch. Biochem. Biophys.* 188:282–286 (1978).

20. Holick, M. F., Richtand, N. M., McNeill, S. C., Holick, S. A., Frommer, J. E., Henley, J. W., and Potts, J. T. Jr. Isolation and identification of previtamin D_3 from the skin of rats exposed to ultraviolet irradiation. *Biochemistry* 18:1003–1008 (1979).
21. Root, A. W., and Harrison, H. F. Recent advances in calcium metabolism. II. Disorders of calcium homeostasis. *J. Pediatr.* 88:177–199 (1976).
22. Velluz, J., and Amiard, G. Chimie organique—equilibre de reaction entre precalciferol et calciferol. *C. R. Soc. Biol. Paris* 228:853–855 (1949).
23. Boomsma, F., Jacobs, H. J. C., Havinga, E., and van der Gen, A. Studies on vitamin D and related compounds. XXIV. New irradiation products of previtamin D_3. *Toxisterols. Tetrahedron Lett.* 7:427–430 (1975).
24. Holick, M. F., and Clark, M. B. The photobiogenesis and metabolism of vitamin D. *Fed. Proc.* 37:2567–2574 (1978).
25. Clemens, T. L., Henderson, S. L., Adams, J. S., and Holick, M. F. Increased skin pigment reduces the capacity of skin to synthesise vitamin D_3. *Lancet* 9:74–76 (1982).
26. Slovik, D. M., Adams, J. S., Neer, R. M., Holick, M. F., and Potts, J. T. Jr. Deficient production of 1,25-dihydroxyvitamin D in elderly osteoporotic patients. *N. Engl. J. Med.* 305:372–374 (1981).
27. Holick, M. F. Photosynthesis of vitamin D in the skin: Effect of environmental and life-style variables. *Fed. Proc.* 46:1876–1880 (1987).
28. Nicolaysen, R., and Eeg-Larsen, N. The biochemistry and physiology of vitamin D. *Vitamins Hormones* 11:29–60 (1953).
29. National Academy of Sciences. *Recommended Dietary Allowances*, eighth edition. Washington, D.C., 1974, p. 56.
30. DeLuca, H. F. Mechanism of action and metabolic fate of vitamin D. *Vitamins Hormones* 25:315–367 (1967).
31. Dickson, I. R., and Kodicek, E. Effect of vitamin D deficiency on bone formation in the chick. *Biochem. J.* 182:429–435 (1979).
32. Mechanic, G. L., Toverud, S. U., Ramp, W. K., and Gonnerman, W. A. The effect of vitamin D on the structural crosslinks and maturation of chick bone collagen. *Biochim. Biophys. Acta* 383:419–425 (1975).
33. Rowe, D. W., and Kream, B. E. Regulation of collagen synthesis in fetal rat calvaria by 1,25-dihydroxyvitamin D_3. *J. Biol. Chem.* 257:8009–811 (1982).
34. Rasmussen, H., and Bordier, P. *Physiological and Cellular Basis of Metabolic Bone Disease*. Williams & Wilkins, Baltimore, 1974.
35. Rasmussen, H., and Bordier, P. Vitamin D and bone. *Metab. Bone Dis. Rel. Res.* 1:7–13 (1978).
36. de Wardener, H. E., and Eastwood, J. B. The management of renal osteodystrophy. In *Phosphate Metabolism: Advances in Experimental Medicine and Biology*. (S. G. Massry and E. Ritz, eds.). Plenum Press, New York, 1977, pp. 533–547.
37. Underwood, J. L., and DeLuca, H. F. Vitamin D is not directly necessary for bone growth and mineralization. *Am. J. Physiol.* 246:E493–E498 (1984).

38. Weinstein, R. S., Underwood, J. L., Hutson, M. S., and DeLuca, H. F. Bone histomorphometry in vitamin D-deficient rats infused with calcium and phosphorus. *Am. J. Physiol.* 246:E499–E505 (1984).
39. Holtrop, M. E., Cox, K. A., Carnes, D. L., and Holick, M. F. Effects of serum calcium and phosphorus on skeletal mineralization in vitamin D-deficient rats. *Am. J. Physiol.* 251:E234–E240 (1986).
40. DeLuca, H. F. The vitamin D system in the regulation of calcium and phosphorus metabolism. *Nutr. Rev.* 37:161–193 (1979).
41. DeLuca, H. F. The transformation of a vitamin into a hormone: The vitamin D story. In *The Harvey Lectures*, Series 75. New York, Academic Press, 1981, pp. 333–379.
42. Garabedian, M., Tanaka, Y., Holick, M. F., and DeLuca, H. F. Response of intestinal calcium transport and bone calcium mobilization to 1,25-dihydroxyvitamin D_3 in thyroparathyroidectomized rats. *Endocrinology* 94: 1022–1027 (1974).
43. Talmage, R. V., Grubb, S. A., Vander Wiel, C. J., Doppelt, S. H., and Norimatsu, H. The demand for bone calcium in maintenance of plasma calcium concentrations. *Calcif. Tiss. Res.* 22:73–91 (1978).
44. Sutton, R. A. L., and Dirks, J. H. Renal handling of calcium. *Fed. Proc.* 37: 2112–2119 (1978).
45. Yamamoto, M., Kawanobe, Y., Takahashi, H., Simazawa, E., Kimura, S., and Ogata, E. Vitamin D deficiency and renal calcium transport in the rat. *J. Clin. Invest.* 74:507–513 (1984).
46. DeLuca, H. F. Vitamin D: The vitamin and the hormone. *Fed. Proc.* 33: 2211–2219 (1974).
47. Lund, J., and DeLuca, H. F. Biologically active metabolite of vitamin D_3 from bone, liver, and blood serum. *J. Lipid Res.* 7:739–744 (1966).
48. Kodicek, E. The metabolism of vitamin D. In *Vitamin Metabolism*, Vol. XI. (W. Umbreit and H. Molitor, eds.). Pergamon Press, London, 1960, pp. 198–208.
49. Haussler, M. R., and Norman, A. W. The subcellular distribution of physiological doses of vitamin D_3. *Arch. Biochem. Biophys.* 118:145–153 (1967).
50. Blunt, J. W., DeLuca, H. F., and Schnoes, H. K. 25-Hydroxycholecalciferol. A biologically active metabolite of vitamin D_3. *Biochemistry* 7:3317–3322 (1968).
51. Madhok, T. C., and DeLuca, H. F. Characteristics of the rat liver microsomal enzyme system converting cholecalciferol into 25-hydroxycholecalciferol. Evidence for the participation of cytochrome P-450. *Biochem. J.* 184:491–499 (1979).
52. Holick, M. F., Schnoes, H. K., DeLuca, H. F., Suda, T., and Cousins, R. J. Isolation and identification of 1,25-dihydroxycholecalciferol. A metabolite of vitamin D active in intestine. *Biochemistry* 10:4799–3804 (1971).
53. Gray, R. W., Omdahl, J. L., Ghazarian, J. G., and DeLuca, H. F. 25-Hydroxycholecalciferol-1-hydroxylase: Subcellular location and properties. *J. Biol. Chem.* 247:7528–7532 (1972).

54. Ghazarian, J. G., Jefcoate, C. R., Knutson, J. C., Orme-Johnson, W. H., and DeLuca, H. F. Mitochondrial cytochrome P_{450}: A component of chick kidney 25-hydroxycholecalciferol-1α-hydroxylase. *J. Biol. Chem.* 249:3026-3033 (1974).
55. Haddad, J. G., and Stamp, T. C. B. Circulating 25-hydroxyvitamin D in man. *Am. J. Med.* 57:57–62 (1974).
56. Eisman, J. A., Shepard, R. M., and DeLuca, H. F. Determination of 25-hydroxyvitamin D_2 and 25-hydroxyvitamin D_3 in human plasma using high-pressure liquid chromatography. *Anal. Biochem.* 80:298–305 (1977).
57. Preece, M. A., Tomlinson, S., Ribot, C. A., Pietrek, J., Korn, H. T., Davies, D. M., Ford, J. A., Dunnigan, M. G., and O'Riordan, J. L. H. Studies of vitamin D deficiency in man. *Q. J. Med. New Series* 44:575–589 (1975).
58. Preece, M. A., McIntosh, W. B., Tomlinson, S., Ford, J. A., Dunnigan, M. G., and O'Riordan, J. L. H. Vitamin D deficiency among Asian immigrants to Britain. *Lancet* 1:907–910 (1973).
59. Reeve, L., Tanaka, Y., and DeLuca, H. F. Studies on the site of 1,25-dihydroxyvitamin D_3 synthesis in vivo. *J. Biol. Chem.* 258:3615–3617 (1983).
60. Shultz, T. D., Fox, J., Heath, J. III, and Kumar, R. Do tissues other than the kidney produce 1,25-dihydroxyvitamin D_3 *in vivo*? A reexamination. *Proc. Natl. Acad. Sci. USA* 80:1746–1750 (1983).
61. Howard, G. A., Turner, R. T., Sherrard, D. J., and Baylink, D. J. Human bone cells in culture metabolite 25-hydroxyvitamin D_3 to 1,25-dihydroxyvitamin D_3 and 24,25-dihydroxyvitamin D_3. *J. Biol. Chem.* 256:7738–7740 (1981).
62. Koeffler, H. P., Reichel, H., Bishop, J. E., and Norman, A. W. γ-Interferon stimulates production of 1,25-dihydroxyvitamin D_3 by normal human macrophages. *Biochem. Biophys. Res. Commun.* 127:596–603 (1985).
63. Adams, S. J., Singer, F. R., Gacad, M. A., Sharma, O. P., Hayes, M. J., Vouros, P., and Holick, M. F. Isolation and identification of 1,25-$(OH)_2D_3$ produced by cultured alveolar macrophages in sarcoidosis. *J. Clin. Endocrinol. Metab.* 60:960 (1985).
64. Shephard, R. M., Horst, R. L., Hamstra, A. J., and DeLuca, H. F. Determination of vitamin D and its metabolites in plasma from normal and anephric man. *Biochem. J.* 182:55–69 (1979).
65. Lambert, P. W., Stern, P., Avioli, R. C., Brackett, N. C., Turner, R. P., Green, A., Fu, I. Y., and Bell, N. H. Evidence for extrarenal production of 1,25-dihydroxyvitamin D_3 in man. *J. Clin. Invest.* 69:722–725 (1982).
66. Barbour, G. L., Coburn, J. W., Slatopolsky, E., Norman, A. W., and Horst, R. L. Hypercalcemia in an anephric patient with sarcoidosis: Evidence for extrarenal generation of 1,25-dihydroxyvitamin D. *N. Engl. J. Med.* 305: 440–443 (1981).
67. Zerwekh, J. E., Pak, C. Y. C., Kaplan, R. A., Mcguire, J. L., Upchurch, K., Breslau, N., and Johnson, R. Pathogenetic role of 1α,25-dihydroxyvitamin-D in sarcoidosis and absorptive hypercalciuria. Different responses to prednisolone therapy. *J. Clin. Endocrinol. Metab.* 51:381–385 (1980).

68. Stern, P. H., De Olazabal, J., and Bell, N. H. Evidence for abnormal regulation of circulating 1α,25-dihydroxyvitamin D in patients with sarcoidosis and normal calcium metabolism. *J. Clin. Invest.* 66:852–855 (1980).
69. Gray, T. K., Lester, G. E., and Lorenc, R. S. Evidence for extra-renal 1α-hydroxylation of 25-hydroxyvitamin D_3 in pregnancy. *Science* 204:1311–1313 (1979).
70. Weisman, Y., Vargas, A., Duckett, G., Reiter, E., and Root, A. Synthesis of 1,25-dihydroxyvitamin D in the nephrectomized pregnant rat. *Endocrinology* 103:1992–1998 (1978).
71. Halloran, B. P., and DeLuca, H. F. Vitamin D deficiency and reproduction in rats. *Science* 204:73–74 (1979).
72. Fraser, D. R., and Kodicek, E. Unique biosynthesis by kidney of a biologically active vitamin D metabolite. *Nature* 228:764–766 (1970).
73. DeLuca, H. F., and Steenbock, H. 1,25-Dihydroxycholecalciferol: Isolation, identification, regulation and mechanism of action. In *Endocrinology 1971*, (S. Taylor, ed.). William Heinemann Medical Books, London, 1972, pp. 452–467.
74. DeLuca, H. F. Vitamin D: New approaches to treatment of metabolic bone disease. *Nutrition M.D.*2:1 (1976).
75. DeLuca, H. F. The vitamin D hormonal system: Implications for bone diseases. *Hosp. Pract.* 15:57–63 (1980).
76. DeLuca, H. F., and Avioli, L. V. Renal osteodystrophy. In *Renal Disease*. (D. Black and N. F. Jones, eds.). Blackwell, London, 1979, pp. 766–803.
77. Slatopolsky, E., Weerts, C., Thieland, J., Horst, R., Harter, H., and Martin, K. Marked suppression of secondary hyperparathyroidism by I.V. administration of 1,25-dihydroxycholecalciferol in uremic patients. *J. Clin. Invest.* 74:2136– (1984).
78. Stumpf, W. E., Sar, M., Reid, F., Tanaka, Y., and DeLuca, H. F. Target cells for 1,25-dihydroxyvitamin D_3 in intestinal tract, stomach, kidney, skin, pituitary and parathyroid. *Science* 206:1188–1190 (1979).
79. Stumpf, W. E., Sar, M., Reid, F. A., Huang, S., Narbaitz, R., and DeLuca, H. F. Autoradiographic studies with ^3H 1,25 $(OH)_2$ vitamin D_3 and ^3H 25 (OH) vitamin D_3 in rat parathyroid glands. *Cell Tissue Res.* 221:333–338 (1981).
80. Russell, J., Lettieri, D., and Sherwood, L. M. Suppression by $1,25(OH)_2D_3$ of transcription of the pre-proparathyroid hormone gene. *Endocrinology* 119:2864-2868 (1986).
81. Chesney, R. W., Moorthy, A. V., Eisman, J. A., Jax, D. K., Mazess, R. B., and DeLuca, H. F. Increased growth after long-term oral 1α-25-vitamin D_3 in childhood renal osteodystrophy. *N. Engl. J. Med.* 298:238–242 (1978).
82. Prader, A., Illig, R., and Heierli, E. Eine besondere from der primaren vitamin D-resistenten rachitis mit hypocalcamie und autosomal-dominantem erbgang: Die hereditare pseudo-mangelrachitis. *Helv. Paediatr. Acta* 16: 452–468 (1961).
83. Fraser, D., Kooh, S. W., Kind, H. P., Holick, M. F., Tanaka, Y., and DeLuca, H. F. Pathogenesis of hereditary vitamin D dependent rickets: An inborn

error of vitamin D metabolism involving defective conversion of 25-hydroxyvitamin D to 1α,25-dihydroxyvitamin D. *N. Engl. J. Med.* 289: 817–822 (1973).

84. Scriver, C. R., Reade, T. M., DeLuca, H. F., and Hamstra, A. J. Serum 1,25-$(OH)_2$D levels in normal subjects and in patients with hereditary rickets or bone disease. *N. Engl. J. Med.* 229:976–979 (1978).

85. Shepard, R. M., and DeLuca, H. F. Plasma concentrations of vitamin D_3 and its metabolites in the rat as influenced by vitamin D_3 or 25-hydroxyvitamin D_3 intakes. *Arch. Biochem. Biophys.* 202:43–53 (1980).

86. Hughes, M. R., Baylink, D. J., Jones, P. G., and Haussler, M. R. Radioligand receptor assay for 25-hydroxyvitamin D_2/D_3 and 1α,25-dihydroxyvitamin D_2/D_3. Application to hypervitaminosis D. *J. Clin. Invest.* 58:61–70 (1976).

87. Eisman, J. A., and DeLuca, H. F. Intestinal 1,25-dihydroxyvitamin D_3 binding protein: Specificity of binding. *Steroids* 30:245–257 (1977).

88. DeLuca, H. F., and Schnoes, H. K. Vitamin D: Metabolism and mechanism of action. In *Annual Reports in Medicinal Chemistry*, Vol. 19. (D. M. Bailey, ed.). Academic Press, New York, 1984, pp. 179–190.

89. Balsan, S., Garabedian, M., Sorgniard, R., Dommergues, J. P., Courtecuisse, V., Holick, M. F., and DeLuca, H. F. Metabolites and analogs of vitamin D: Therapeutic effects in D-deficiency and "pseudo-deficiency" rickets. In *Vitamin D and Problems Related to Uremic Bone Disease*. (A. W. Norman, K. Schaefer, H. G. Grigoleit, D. von Herrath, and E. Ritz, eds.). Walter de Gruyer, Berlin, 1975, pp. 247–258.

90. Boyle, I. T., Miravet, L., Gray, R. W., Holick, M. F., and DeLuca, H. F. The response of intestinal calcium transport to 25-hydroxy and 1,25-dihydroxy vitamin D in nephrectomized rats. *Endocrinology* 90:605–608 (1972).

91. Holick, M. F., Garabedian, M., and DeLuca, H. F. 1,25-Dihydroxycholecalciferol: Metabolite of vitamin D_3 active on bone in anephric rats. *Science* 176:1146–1147 (1972).

92. DeLuca, H. F. The metabolism and function of vitamin D. In *Biochemistry of Steroid Hormones*, second edition. (Makin, H. L. J., ed.). Blackwell, Boston, 1984, pp. 71–116.

93. Holick, M. F., Schnoes, H. K., DeLuca, H. F., Gray, R. W., Boyle, I. T., and Suda, T. Isolation and identification of 24,25-dihydroxycholecalciferol: A metabolite of vitamin D_3 in the kidney. *Biochemistry* 11:4251–4255 (1972).

94. Boyle, I. T., Gray, R. W., and DeLuca, H. F. Regulation by calcium of *in vivo* synthesis of 1,25-dihydroxycholecalciferol and 21,25-dihydroxycholecalciferol. *Proc. Natl. Acad. Sci. USA* 68:2131–2134 (1971).

95. Tanaka, Y., Lorenc, R. S., and DeLuca, H. F. The role of 1,25-dihydroxyvitamin D_3 and parathyroid hormone in the regulation of chick renal 25-hydroxyvitamin D_3-24-hydroxylase. *Arch. Biochem. Biophys.* 171:521–526 (1975).

96. Tanaka, Y., and DeLuca, H. F. Rat renal 25-hydroxyvitamin D_3-1- and 24-hydroxylases: Their *in vivo* regulation. *Am. J. Physiol.* 246:E168–E173 (1984).
97. Castillo, L., Tanaka, Y., DeLuca, H. F., and Ikekawa, N. On the physiological role of 1,24,25-trihydryoxyvitamin D_3. *Miner. Electrolyte Metab.* 1:198–207 (1978).
98. Henry, H. L., and Norman, A. W. Vitamin D: Two dihydroxylated metabolites are required for normal chicken egg hatchability. *Science* 201: 835–837 (1978).
99. Norman, A. W., Leathers, V., and Bishop, J. E. Normal egg hatchability requires the simultaneous administration to the hen of 1α,25-dihydroxycholecalciferol and 24R,25-dihydroxycholecalciferol. *J. Nutr.* 113:2505–2515 (1983).
100. Norman, A. W., Henry, H. L., and Malluche, H. H. 24R,25-Dihydroxyvitamin D_3 and α1,25-dihydroxyvitamin D_3 are both indispensable for calcium and phosphorus homeostasis. *Life Sci.* 27:229–237 (1980).
101. Norman, A. W. 1,25-Dihydroxyvitamin D_3 and 24,25-dihydroxyvitamin D_3: Key components of the vitamin D endocrine system. *Contrib. Nephrol.* 18:1–11 (1980).
102. Tanaka, Y., DeLuca, H. F., Kobayashi, Y., Taguchi, T., Ikekawa, N., and Morisaki, M. Biological activity of 24,24-difluoro-25-hydroxyvitamin D_3. Effect of blocking of 24-hydroxylation on the functions of vitamin D. *J. Biol. Chem.* 254:7163–7167 (1979).
103. Jarnagin, K., Brommage, R., DeLuca, H. F., Yamada, S., and Takayama, H. 1- But not 24-hydroxylation of vitamin D is required for growth and reproduction in rats. *Am. J. Physiol.* 244:E290–E297 (1983).
104. Brommage, R., Jarnagin, K., DeLuca, H. F., Yamada, S., and Takayama, H. 1- But not 24-hydroxylation of vitamin D is required for skeletal mineralization in rats. *Am. J. Physiol.* 244:E298–E304 (1983).
105. Brommage, R., and DeLuca, H. F. Evidence that 1,25-dihydroxyvitamin D_3 is the physiologically active metabolite of vitamin D_3. *Endocrine Rev.* 6:491–511 (1985).
106. Tanaka, Y., Wichmann, J. K., DeLuca, H. F., Kobayashi, Y., and Ikekawa, N. Metabolism and binding properties of 24,24-difluoro-25-hydroxyvitamin D_3. *Arch. Biochem. Biophys.* 225:649–655 (1983).
107. Hart, L. E., Schnoes, H. K., and DeLuca, H. F. Studies on the role of 1,25-dihydroxyvitamin D in chick embryonic development. *Arch. Biochem. Biophys.* 250:426–434 (1986).
108. Hart, L. E., DeLuca, H. F., Yamada, S., and Takayama, H. Hydroxylation of carbon-24 of 25-hydroxycholecalciferol is not necessary for normal embryonic development in chickens. *J. Nutr.* 114:2059–2065 (1984).
109. Hart, L. E., and DeLuca, H. F. Effect of vitamin D_3 metabolites on calcium and phosphorus metabolism in chick embryos. *Am. J.. Physiol.* 248:E281–E285 (1985).
110. Tanaka, Y., Pahuja, D. N., Wichmann, J. K., DeLuca, H. F., Kobayashi, Y., Taguchi, T., and Ikekawa, 25-Hydroxy-26,26,27,27,27-hexafluoro-

vitamin D_3: Biological activity in the rat. *Arch. Biochem. Biophys.* 218: 134–141 (1982).

111. Nakada, M., Tanaka, Y., DeLuca, H. F., Kobayashi, Y., and Ikekawa, N. Biological activities and binding properties of 23,23-difluoro-25-hydroxyvitamin D_3 and its 1α-hydroxy derivative. *Arch. Biochem. Biophys.* 241: 173–178 (1985).
112. Tanaka, Y., DeLuca, H. F., Kobayashi, Y., and Ikekawa, N. 26,26,26,27,27,27-Hexafluoro-1,25-dihydroxyvitamin D_3: A highly potent, long-lasting analog of 1,25-dihydroxyvitamin D_3. *Arch. Biochem. Biophys.* 229:348–354 (1984).
113. Okamoto, S., Tanaka, Y., DeLuca, H. F., Kobayashi, Y., and Ikekawa, N. Biological activity of 24,24-difluoro-1,25-dihydroxyvitamin D_3. *Am. J. Physiol.* 7:E159–E163 (1983).
114. Gray, R. W., Calcas, A. E. Wilz, D. R., Lemann, J., Jr., Smith, G. A., and DeLuca, H. F. Metabolism and excretion of ^3H-1,25-$(OH)_2$-vitamin D_3 in healthy adults. *J. Clin. Endocrinol. Metab.* 46:756–765 (1978).
115. Garabedian, M., Holick, M. F., DeLuca, H. F., and Boyle, I. T. Control of 25-hydroxycholecalciferol metabolism by the parathyroid glands. *Proc. Natl. Acad. Sci. USA* 69:1673–1676 (1972).
116. Zull, J. E., and Repke, D. W. The tissue localization of tritiated parathyroid hormone in thyroparathyroidectomized rats. *J. Biol. Chem.* 247: 2195–2199 (1972).
117. Brunette, M. G., Chan, M., Ferriere, C., and Roberts, K. D. Site of 1,25-dihydroxyvitamin D_3 synthesis in the kidney. *Nature* 276:287–290 (1978).
118. Trechsel, U., Eisman, J. A., Bonjour, J. P., and Fleisch, H. Evidence for a calcium-dependent, PTH-independent regulation of plasma 1,25-dihydroxyvitamin D in rats. In *Vitamin D: Basic Research and its Clinical Application.* (A. W. Norman, K. Schaefer, D. v. Herrath, H. G. Grigoleit, J. W. Coburn, H. F. DeLuca, E. B. Mawer, and T. Suda, eds.). Walter de Gruyter, Berlin, 1979, pp. 511–513.
119. Boyle, I. T., Gray, R. W., Omdahl, J. L., and DeLuca, H. F. Calcium control of the *in vivo* biosynthesis of 1,25-dihydroxyvitamin D_3: Nicolaysen's endogenous factor. In *Endocrinology 1971.* (Taylor, S., ed.). Wm. Heinemann, London, 1972, pp. 468–476.
120. Potts, J. T. Jr. Introductory remarks. In *Parathyroid Hormone and Thyrocalcitonin (Calcitonin).* (R. V. Talmage, and L. F. Belanger, eds.). Excerpta Medica, Amsterdam, 1968, pp. 403–406.
121. Blum, J. W., Mayer, G. P., and Potts, J. T. Jr. Parathyroid hormone responses during spontaneous hypocalcemia and induced hypercalcemia in cows. *Endocrinology* 95:84–92 (1974).
122. Neer, R. M., Holick, M. F., DeLuca, H. F., and Potts, J. T. Jr. Effects of 1α-hydroxyvitamin D_3 and 1,25-dihydroxyvitamin D_3 on calcium and phosphorus metabolism in hypoparathyroidism. *Metabolism* 24:1403–1413 (1975).

123. Kooh, S. W., Fraser, D., DeLuca, H. F., Holick, M. F., Belsey, R. E., Clark, M. B., and Murray, T. M. Treatment of hypoparathyroidism and pseudohypoparathyroidism with metabolites of vitamin D: Evidence for impaired conversion of 25-hydroxyvitamin D to 1α,25-dihydroxyvitamin D. *N. Engl. J. Med.* 293:840–844 (1975).
124. Kletzien, S. W. F., Templin, V. M., Steenbock, H., and Thomas, B. H. Vitamin D and the conservation of calcium in the adult. *J. Biol. Chem.* 97: 265–280 (1932).
125. Nicolaysen, R., Eeg-Larsen, N., and Malm, O. J. Physiology of calcium metabolism. *Physiol. Rev.* 33:424–444 (1953).
126. DeLuca, H. F. The vitamin D endocrine system in health and disease. Proceedings from the Annual Meeting of the Royal College of Physicians and Surgeons of Canada, Toronto, January 29, 1977, pp. 216–225.
127. Harrison, H. E., and Harrison, H. C. Transfer of Ca^{45} across intestinal wall *in vitro* in relation to action of vitamin D and cortisol. *Am. J. Physiol.* 199:265–271 (1960).
128. Hahn, T. J. Corticosteroid-induced osteopenia. *Arch. Intern. Med.* 138: 882–885 (1978).
129. Favus, M. J., Kimberg, D. V., Millar, G. N., and Gerson, E. Effects of cortisone administration on the metabolism and localization of 25-hydroxycholecalciferol in the rat. *J. Clin. Invest.* 52:1328–1335 (1973).
130. Stumpf, W. E., Sar, M., and DeLuca, H. F. Sites of action of $1,25(OH)_2$ vitamin D_3 identified by thaw-mount autoradiography. In *Hormonal Control of Calcium Metabolism.* (D. V. Cohn, R. V. Talmage, and J. L. Matthews, eds.). Excerpta Medica, Amsterdam, 1981, pp. 222–229.
131. Raisz, L. G., Trummel, C. L., Holick, M. F., and DeLuca, H. F. 1,25-Dihydroxycholecalciferol: A potent stimulator of bone resorption in tissue culture. *Science* 175:768–769 (1972).
132. Reynolds, J. J., Holick, M. F., and DeLuca, H. F. The effects of vitamin D analogues on bone resorption. *Calcif. Tissue Res.* 15:333–339 (1974).
133. Reynolds, J. J., Holick, M. F., and DeLuca, H. F. The role of vitamin D metabolites in bone resorption. *Calcif. Tissue Res.* 12:295–301 (1973).
134. Tanaka, Y., Frank, H., and DeLuca, H. F. Biological activity of 1,25-dihydroxyvitamin D_3 in the rat. *Endocrinology* 92:417–422 (1973).
135. Frost, H. M. *Bone Dynamics in Osteoporosis and Osteomalacia.* Henry Ford Hospital Surgical Monograph Series. Charles C. Thomas, Springfield, 1966.
136. Jee, W. S. S., and Nolan, P. D. Origin of osteoclasts from diffusion of phagocytes. *Nature* 200:225–226 (1963).
137. Nilas, L., Christiansen, C., and Rodbro, P. Calcium supplementation and post-menopausal bone loss. *Br. Med. J.* 289:1093–1096 (1984).
138. Riggs, B. L., Seemone, E., Hodgson, S. F., Taves, D. R., and O'Fallon, W. M. The effect of fluoride/calcium regimen on vertebral fracture occurrence in postmenopausal osteoporosis: Comparison with conventional therapy. *N. Engl. J. Med.* 306:446–450 (1982).

139. Gallagher, J. C., Jerpbak, C. M., Jee, W. S. S., Johnson, K. A., DeLuca, H. F., and Riggs, B. L. 1,25-Dihydroxyvitamin D_3: Short- and long-term effects on bone and calcium metabolism in patients with postmenopausal osteoporosis. *Proc. Natl. Acad. Sci. USA* 79:3325–3329 (1982).
140. Christiansen, C., Christensen, M. S., Rodbro, P., Hagen, C., and Transbol, I. Effect of 1,25-dihydroxyvitamin D_3 in itself or combined with hormone treatment in preventing postmenopausal osteoporosis. *Eur. J. Clin. Invest.* 11;305–307 (1981).
141. Aloia, J., Vasawi, A., Yeh, J., Allis, K., and Cohn, S. Calcitriol in the treatment of postmenopausal osteoporosis. In *Calcium Regulation and Bone Metabolism. Basic and Clinical Aspects*, Vol. 9. (Cohn, D. V., Martin, T. J., and Muenler, P. J., eds.). Excerpta Medica, Amsterdam, 1987, pp. 113–118.
142. Bullamore, J. R., Gallagher, J. C., Wilkinson, R., and Nordin, B. E. C. Effect of age on calcium absorption. *Lancet* 2:535–537 (1970).
143. Horst, R. L., DeLuca, H. F., and Jorgensen, N. A. The effect of age on calcium absorption and accumulation of 1,25-dihydroxyvitamin D_3 in intestinal mucosa of rats. *Metab. Bone Dis. Rel. Res.* 1:29–33 (1978).
144. Gallagher, J. C., Riggs, B. L., Eisman, J., Hamstra, A., Arnaud, S. B., and DeLuca, H. F. Intestinal calcium absorption and serum vitamin D metabolites in normal subjects and osteoporotic patients. Effect of age and dietary calcium. *J. Clin. Invest.* 64:729–736 (1979).
145. Slovik, D. M., Adams, J. S., Neer, R. M., Holick, M. F., and Potts, J. T. Deficient production of 1,25-dihydroxyvitamin D in elderly osteoporotic patients. *N. Engl. J. Med.* 305:372–375 (1981).
146. Slovik, D. M., Rosenthal, D. I., Doppelt, S. H., Potts, J. T., Jr., Daly, M. A., Campbell, J. A., and Neer, R. M. Restoration of spinal bone in osteoporotic men by treatment with human parathyroid hormone (I-34) and 1,25-dihydroxyvitamin D. *J. Bone Min. Res.* 1:377–379 (1986).
147. Braumbaugh, P. F., and Haussler, M. R. Nuclear and cytoplasmic binding components for vitamin D metabolites. *Life Sci.* 16:353–362 (1975).
148. Kream, B. E., Reynolds, R. D., Knutson, J. C., Eisman, J. A., and DeLuca, H. F. Intestinal cytosol binders of 1,25-dihydroxyvitamin D_3 and 25-hydroxyvitamin D_3. *Arch. Biochem. Biophys.* 176:779–787 (1976).
149. Link, R., and DeLuca, H. F. The vitamin D receptor. In *The Receptors*, Vol. II. (P. M. Conn, ed.). Academic Press, New York, 1985, pp. 1–35.
150. Holick, M. F., Kleiner-Bassaller, A., Schnoes, H. K., Kasten, P. M., Boyle, I. T., and DeLuca, H. F. 1,24,25-Trihydroxyvitamin D_3: A metabolite of vitamin D_3 effective on intestine. *J. Biol. Chem.* 248:6691–6696 (1973).
151. Tanaka, Y., DeLuca, H. F., Schnoes, H. K., Ikekawa, N., and Kobayashi, Y. 24,24-Difluoro-1,25-dihydroxyvitamin D_3: *In vitro* production, isolation, and biological activity. *Arch. Biochem. Biophys.* 199:473–478 (1980).
152. Eil, C., Liberman, U. A., and Marx, S. J. The molecular basis for resistance to 1,25-dihydroxyvitamin D—studies in cells cultured from patients with hereditary hypocalcemic 1,25$(OH)_2D_3$-resistant rickets. In *Steroid Hor-*

mone Resistance, Vol. 196. (G. P. Chrousos, D. L. Loriaus, and M. B. Lipsett, eds.). Plenum, New York, 1986, pp. 407–422.
153. Halloran, B. P., and DeLuca, H. F. Appearance of the intestinal cytosolic receptor for 1,25-dihydroxyvitamin D_3 during neonatal development in the rat. *J. Biol. Chem.* 256:7338–7342 (1981).
154. Massaro, E., Simpson, R. U., and DeLuca, H. F. Stimulation of specific 1,25-dihydroxyvitamin D_3 binding protein in cultured postnatal rat intestine by hydrocortisone. *J. Biol. Chem.* 257:13736–13739 (1982).
155. Simpson, R. U., Hamstra, A., Kendrick, N. C., and DeLuca, H. F. Purification of the receptor for 1α,25-dihydroxyvitamin D_3 from chicken intestine. *Biochemistry* 22:2586–2594 (1983).
156. Pike, J. W., and Haussler, M. R. Purification of chicken intestinal receptor for 1,25-dihydroxyvitamin D. *Proc. Natl. Acad. Sci. USA* 76:5485–5489 (1979).
157. Dame, M. C., Pierce, E. A., and DeLuca, H. F. Identification of the porcine intestinal 1,25-dihydroxyvitamin D_3 receptor on sodium dodecyl sulfate-polyacylamide gels by renaturation and immunoblotting. *Proc. Natl. Acad. Sci. USA* 82:7825–7829 (1985).
158. Dame, M. C., Pierce, E. A., Prahl, J. M., Hayes, C. E., and DeLuca, H. F. Monoclonal antibodies to the porcine intestinal receptor for 1,25-dihydroxyvitamin D_3: Interaction with distinct receptor domains. *Biochemistry* 25:4523–4534 (1986).
159. McDonnell, D. P., Mangelsdorf, D. J., Pike, J. W., Haussler, M. R., and O'Malley, B. W. Molecular cloning of complementary DNA encoding the avian receptor for vitamin D. *Science* 235:1214–1217 (1987).
160. Pierce, E. A., Dame, M. C., and DeLuca, H. F. Immunological characterization of the porcine 1,25-dihydroxyvitamin D receptor. The Endocrine Society, p. 54 (Abstract 94).
161. Wasserman, R. H., and Taylor, A. N. Vitamin D_3-induced calcium-binding protein in chick intestinal mucosa. *Science* 152:791–793 (1966).
162. Kessler, M. A., and DeLuca, H. F. The action of 1α,25-dihydroxyvitamin D_3 on rat small intestine: Changes in translatable mRNA species. *Arch. Biochem. Biophys.* 236:17–25 (1985).
163. Kessler, M. A., Lamm, L., Jarnagin, K., and DeLuca, H. F. 1,25-Dihydroxyvitamin D_3 stimulated mRNAs in rat small intestine. *Arch. Biochem. Biophys.* 251:403–412 (1986).
164. Darwish, H. M., Krisinger, J., Strom, M., and DeLuca, H. F. Molecular cloning of the cDNA and chromosomal gene for vitamin D-dependent calcium-binding protein of rat intestine. *Proc. Natl. Acad. Sci. USA*, 84: 6108–6111.
165. Bell, N. H., Hamstra, A. J., and DeLuca, H. F. Vitamin D-dependent rickets Type II: Resistance of target organs to 1,25-dihydroxyvitamin D. *N. Engl. J. Med.* 298:996–999 (1978).
166. Rosen, J. F., Fleischman, A. R., Finberg, L., and DeLuca, H. F. A new type of rickets: Unresponsiveness of bone and intestine to high levels of endogenously synthesized 1,25-dihydroxyvitamin D_3. American Pediatric Society (abstract) (1978).

167. Balsan, S., Garabedian, M., Larchet, M., Groski, A. M., Cournot, G., Tau, C., Bordeau, A., Silve, C., and Ricour, C. Long-term nocturnal calcium infusions can cure rickets and promote normal mineralization in hereditary resistance to 1,25-dihydroxyvitamin D. *J. Clin. Invest.* 77:1661–1666 (1986).
168. Chertow, B. S., Sivitz, W. I., Baranetsky, N. G., Clark, S. A., Waite, A., and DeLuca, H. F. Cellular mechanisms of insulin release. The effects of vitamin D deficiency and repletion on rat insulin secretion. *Endocrinology* 113:1511–1518 (1983).
169. Kadowaki, S., and Norman, A. W. Demonstration that the vitamin D metabolite 1,25$(OH)_2$-vitamin D_3 and not 24R,25$(OH)_2$-vitamin D_3 is essential for normal insulin secretion in the perfused rat pancreas. *Diabetes* 34:315–320 (1985).
170. Kadowaki, S., and Norman, A. W. Time course study of insulin secretion after 1,25-dihydroxyvitamin D_3 administration. *Endocrinology* 117:1765–1771 (1985).
171. Kadowaki, S., and Norman, A. W. Dietary vitamin D is essential for normal insulin secretion from the perfused rat pancreas. *J. Clin. Invest.* 73: 759–766 (1984).
172. Frampton, R. J., Suva, L. J., Eisman, J. A., Findlay, D. M., Moore, G. E., Moseley, J. M., and Martin, T. J. Presence of 1,25-dihydroxyvitamin D_3 receptors in established human cancer cell lines in culture. *Cancer Res.* 42:1116–1119 (1982).
173. Eisman, J. A., MacIntyre, I., Martin, T. J., Frampton, R. J., and King, R. J. Normal and malignant breast tissue is a target organ for 1,25-$(OH)_2$ vitamin D. *Clin. Endocrinol.* 13:267–272 (1980).
174. Frampton, R. J., Omond, S. A., and Eisman, J. A. Inhibition of human cancer cell growth by 1,25-dihydroxyvitamin D_3 metabolites. *Cancer Res.* 43:4443–4447 (1983).
175. Abe, E., Miyaura, C., Sakagami, H., Takeda, M., Konno, K., Yamazaki, T., Yoshiki, S., and Suda, T. Differentiation of mouse myeloid leukemia cells induced by 1α,25-dihydroxyvitamin D_3. *Proc. Natl. Acad. Sci. USA* 78:7990–4994 (1981).
176. Tanaka, H., Abe, E., Miyaura, C., Kurbayashi, T., Konno, K., Nishii, Y., and Suda, T. 1α,25-Dihydroxycholecalciferol and a human myeloid leukaemia cell line (HL-60). The presence of a cytosol receptor and induction of differentiation. *Biochem. J.* 204:713–719 (1982).
177. Ostrem, V. K., Tanaka, Y., Prahl, J., and DeLuca, H. F. 24- and 26-Homo-1,25-dihydroxyvitamin D_3: Preferential activity in inducing differentiation of human leukemia cells HL-60 *in vitro*. *Proc. Natl. Acad. Sci. USA* 84: 2610–2614 (1987).
178. Miller, S. C., Halloran, B. P., DeLuca, H. F., and Jee, W. S. S. Role of vitamin D in maternal skeletal changes during pregnancy and lactation: A histomorphometric study. *Calcif. Tissue Int.* 34:245–252 (1982).

179. Holtrop, M. F., Cox, K. A., Clark, M. B., Holick, M. F., and Anast, C. S. 1,25-Dihydroxycholecalciferol stimulates osteoclasts in rat bones in the absence of parathyroid hormone. *Endocrinology* 108:2293–2301 (1981).

180. Ostrem, V. K., Lau, W. F., Lee, S. H., Perlman, K., Prahl, J., Schnoes, H. K., DeLuca, H. F., and Ikekawa, N. Induction of monocytic differentiation of HL-60 cells by 1,25-dihydroxyvitamin D analogs. *J. Biol. Chem.* 262:14164–14171 (1987).

181. Simpson, R. U., and DeLuca, H. F. Characterization of a receptor-like protein for 1,25-dihydroxyvitamin D_3 in rat skin. *Proc. Natl. Acad. Sci. USA* 77:5822–5826 (1980).

182. Feldman, D., Chen, T., Hirst, M., Colston, K., Karasek, M., and Cone, C. Demonstration of 1,25-dihydroxyvitamin D_3 receptors in human skin biopsies. *J. Clin. Endocrinol. Metab.* 51:1463–1465 (1980).

183. Smith, E. L., Walworth, N. C., and Holick, M. F. Effect of 1α,25-dihydroxyvitamin D_3 on the morphologic and biochemical differentiation of cultured human epidermal keratinocytes grown in serum-free conditions. *J. Invest. Dermatol.* 86:709–711 (1986).

184. Takamoto, S., Onishi, T., Morimoto, S., Imanaka, S., Yukawa, S., Kozuka, T., Kitano, Y., Seino, Y., and Kumahara, Y. Effect of 1α-hydroxycholecalciferol on psoriasis vulgaris: A pilot study. *Calcif. Tissue Int.* 39:370–364 (1986).

185. Staberg, B., Oxholm, A. S., Klemp, P., and Christiansen, C. Abnormal vitamin D metabolism in patients with psoriasis. *Acta Dermato-Venereol.* 67: 65–70 (1987).

186. Morimoto, S., Yoshikawa, K., Kozuka, T., Kitano, Y., Imanaka, S., Fukuo, K., Koh, E., Onishi, T., and Kumahara, Y. Treatment of psoriasis vulgaris by oral administration of 1α-hydroxyvitamin D_3 —Open-design study. *Calcif. Tissue Int.* 39:209–215 (1986).

187. Morimoto, S., Onishi, T., Imanaka, S., Yukawa, H., Kozuka, T., Kitano, Y., Yoshikawa, K., and Kumahara, Y. Topical administration of 1,25-dihydroxyvitamin D_3 for psoriasis: Report of five cases. *Calcif. Tissue Int.* 38:119–125 (1986).

2

The Metabolism of Vitamin D and the Renal Handling of Calcium and Phosphate

Russell W. Chesney and Israel Zelikovic

College of Medicine, University of Tennessee, Memphis, Memphis, Tennessee

I. RECENT DEVELOPMENTS IN VITAMIN D METABOLISM

The appreciation some 20 years ago that vitamin D_3 is further metabolized to produce several metabolites with physiological functions has led to a flurry of activity that has continued to this day (1). The scheme of the conversion of 7-dehydrocholesterol in the skin to pre-vitamin D_3 under the influence of ultraviolet B rays at 288 nm, the further thermal conversion to vitamin D_3, its hepatic microsomal hydroxylation at the 25 carbon of the steroid molecule, and finally the renal conversion to the active metabolite, 1,α,25-dihydroxyvitamin D_3 under the influence of hypocalcemia, hypophosphatemia, and elevated circulating parathyroid hormone levels is now fully accepted as the mechanism producing the most potent and rapidly acting metabolite of vitamin D (2). That the area of bone and mineral metabolism has undergone an explosion in knowledge over these two decades and that a therapeutic approach to many of the major metabolic bone disorders now has a more logical basis cannot be doubted. Thus, we focus here on newer developments in the area of vitamin D metabolism and indicate the possible implications of these recent studies.

Upon exposure to ultraviolet radiation, 7-dehydrocholesterol in mammalian skin is photoisomerized to pre-vitamin D_3. This compound is thermally converted to vitamin D_3, which, in turn, is transported into the circulation by a 52 kD vitamin-D-binding protein (3). Until recently, it had been assumed that only one pro-vitamin D, 7-dehydrocholesterol, was in skin. However, by reverse-phase high-performance liquid chromatography of lipid extracts of skin, a 24 dehydro-pro-vitamin D_3 can be separated from 7-dehydrocholesterol. This compound accounts for 22% of total pro-vitamin D content (4). This second pre-vitamin D also undergoes ultraviolet photolysis. Preliminary evidence suggests that this compound is found in the skin of reptiles, amphibians, birds, aquatic mammals, and humans. It has also been shown that 24 dehydrovitamin D_3 has biological activity, but to a lesser degree than vitamin D_3 (5). Whether this compound will be of biological importance remains to be established.

Vitamin D and many of its metabolites are tightly bound to vitamin-D-binding protein (DBP), which has also been called group-specific (Gc)-globulin (6). A high association constant (Ka) exists between DBP and vitamin D metabolites, particularly 25-hydroxyvitamin D (25 [OH] D). However, this Ka is variable and thus a "free 25(OH)D index" is difficult to determine (6,7). By the use of a Scatchard plot however, one can determine such an index and only at very high endogenous 25(OH)D values do inaccuracies exist. The utility of this assay system is shown by the fact that only 2 of 68 patients with normal 25(OH)D levels have a low free 25(OH)D index, whereas patients with low 25(OH)D values, with anticonvulsant-induced osteomalacia, and on hemodialysis have low indexes and patients with high 25(OH)D levels have a high index (6).

Vitamin-D-binding protein has unusual biological properties: it binds actin with a high affinity and links immunoglobulins bound on B-lymphocytes to actin (8). The group-specific component circulates at 20–50 mg/dl; at least 84 separate Gc alleles have been detected. To indicate further the universality of DBP, its N-terminal amino acid sequence aligns with several sequences or pre-proalbumin and human pre-α-fetoprotein. Thus, although this protein clearly functions as a transporter of vitamin D (since it binds 99% of circulating 25 [OH] D) (6,7), its biological activities and its role as a genetic marker will likely be subject to greater scrutiny in the future.

After vitamin D-DBP is transported to the liver, it releases vitamin D for its initial hydroxylation. An ontogeny of hepatic 25 hydroxylation has recently been reported (9,12). Changes in carbon-25 (C-25) hydroxylation of the vitamin D molecule could be the result of reduced transfer of vitamin D_3 from DBP into the hepatocyte, where this enzymatic step occurs. However, fetal rat liver can take up tracer doses of $[^3H]$ vitamin D_3 at a level even higher than that found in the first 2 weeks postpartum (9). Between 14 and 21 days, rat liver takes up vitamin D_3 at a capacity equal to that found in adult liver. It is noteworthy that weaning occurs between the second and third week of life in the rat and that gut receptors for 1,25-dihydroxyvitamin D_3 ($1{,}25\,[OH]_2D_3$) first appear at the same time (13). The production of 25(OH)D is a property of fetal

(10) and neonatal liver (11,12), but there is evidence for a maturational delay in the full expression of vitamin D-25 hydroxylase activity (10–12). In the rat, C-25 hydroxylation parallels the increase in microsomal P-450-specific content and reaches a peak on the third day postpartum (10). In humans, the efficiency of hepatic conversion is directly correlated with gestational age (11). Following vitamin D_2 administration, 25(OH)D_2 values rise only after several weeks of age (12). The rat studies are potentially important since they indicate that only at or near weaning is the intrahepatic concentration of substrate (vitamin D_3) sufficient to permit full 25(OH)D synthesis. A synchronization of vitamin D movement into the liver (9), appearance of the intestinal receptor for 1,25(OH)$_2$D (13), the need for 1,25(OH)$_2$D to promote intestinal calcium absorption (14), increases in the circulating levels of 25(OH)D (15) and of 1,25(OH)$_2$$D_3$ (16), and the ingestion of solid food is evident.

New evidence suggests that other factors may influence the synthesis of 25(OH)D. White subjects maintain significantly higher plasma concentrations of vitamin D_3 and 25(OH)D than do black subjects (17). Since maternal vitamin D stores influence fetal vitamin D status, the black infant appears to be more likely to develop vitamin D deficiency, which is then apparent after delivery. White mothers have greater milk vitamin D activity than do black mothers, which may account for the greater incidence of vitamin D deficiency in black breastfed infants than in similarly fed white infants (18). The production of pro-vitamin D_3 and vitamin D_3 in pigmented skin is limited compared to nonpigmented skin (19). Hence, a variety of factors coincide to prevent full hepatic C-25 hydroxylation in the black infant.

One organ that is fully capable of 1,25(OH)$_2$D synthesis is the placenta (1); decidua (20) and receptors for 1,25(OH)$_2$D are present in the placenta (21). It has recently been shown that the placenta can also produce 24,25 di-hydroxyvitamin D_3 (24,25[OH]$_2$$D_3$) and that treatment of pregnant rats with human chorionic gonadotropin will increase the concentrations both of 25(OH)D and 24,25(OH)$_2$D in the placenta (22). However, gonadotropin did not influence either fetal levels or values of these metabolites in nonpregnant animals. Whether this placental hormone influences 1,25(OH)$_2$D synthesis has not been established.

The transport of 25(OH)D bound to DBP to the kidney is the step prior to the action of the two principal renal vitamin D metabolizing enzymes: 25(OH)D-1α hydroxylase and 25(OH)D-(24R)-hydroxylase (23). The activities of both enzymes are under tight ionic and hormonal control and a reciprocal change exists in the activities of these enzymes (1,2,24). During periods of hypocalcemia, hypophosphatemia, and hypovitaminosis D, 25(OH)D-(24R)-hydroxylase activity is absent (2). After treatment with 1,25(OH)$_2$D, levels of (24R) hydroxylase are increased (23). Both enzymes require molecular O_2, which is incorporated at the C_1 or C_{24} position in the steroid molecule; reduced NADP, which can arise from

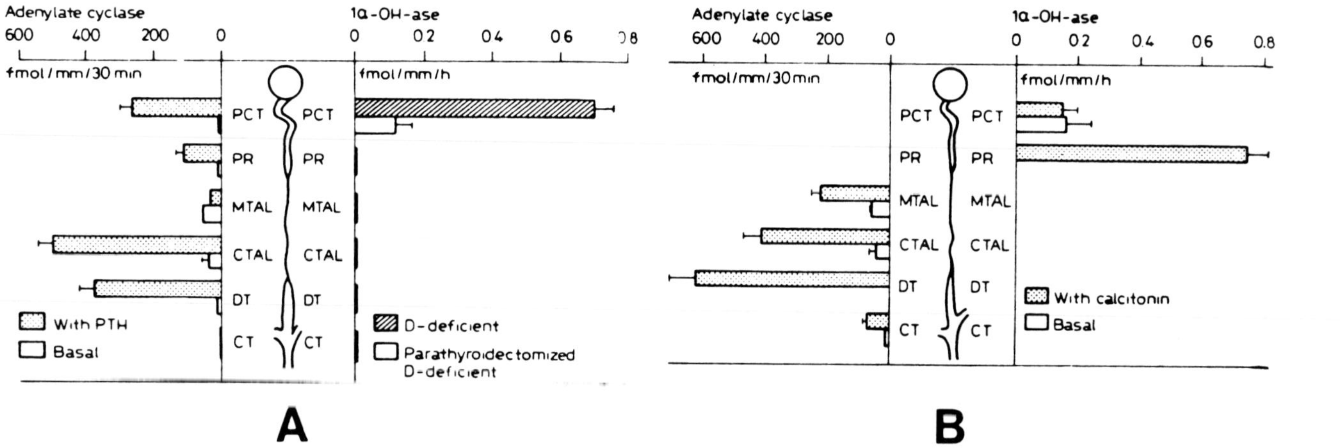

Figure 1 A. Distribution of PTH-sensitive adenylate cyclase and 1 α hydroxylase activity. B. Calcitonin-sensitive adenylate cyclase and 1 α hydroxylase activity in the rat nephron. PCT, proximal convoluted tubules; PR, pars recta or straight tubules; MTAL and CTAL, medullary and cortical thick ascending limbs of Henle; DT, distal convoluted tubules; CT, collecting tubules (adapted from Ref. 23 with permission).

mitochondrial succinate; malate or isocitrate oxidation, and both are cytochrome P-450 dependent monooxygenase. It now appears that 1α-hydroxylase activity is localized in both the proximal convoluted and proximal straight tubules with parathyroid hormone (PTH)-stimulated adenylate cyclase activity enhancing hydroxylase in the convoluted tubule and calcitonin in the straight tubule (23). Enzyme activity in the convoluted tubule falls after thyroparathyroidectomy and again rises after PTH or cAMP administration (Fig. 1). Evidence suggests that 1α-hydroxylase activity in the straight tubule is not detected in the absence of calcitonin. Studies using microdissected single nephron segments confirm the presence of these two distinctive 1α-hydroxylase systems. The convoluted tubule enzyme is stimulated by PTH via cAMP and fully activated in vitamin D deficiency. The straight tubule enzyme is insensitive to PTH and cAMP, latent in vitamin D deficiency, and stimulated by calcitonin in a cAMP-independent fashion (23). The possible reason for this calcitonin-stimulated enzyme activity is that the fetus, with its hypercalcemic milieu, has suppressed PTH levels and thus requires another mechanism for $1{,}25(OH)_2D$ production (23).

Studies of the subcellular location of the enzyme show that the 1α-hydroxylase in the mitochondria of rat proximal tubule is inhibited by metapyrone and carbon monoxide, indicating the involvement of cytochrome P-450 (25). In chick kidneys, a mitochondrial ferrodoxin will support the 1α-hydroxylation of 25(OH)D in the presence of bovine adrenodoxin reductase (26). When bovine renal cells are grown in culture, the generation of oxygen-derived free radicals and/or lipid perioxidation can suppress activity of both 1α-hydroxylase and 24R hydroxylase (27). Antioxidants added to the culture medium will reduce the decline in enzyme activity. Other factors, such as dietary calcium restriction, will alter $1{,}25(OH)_2D$ production (28). At either a low calcium intake (0.6%) or markedly reduced intake (0.02%), enzyme activity was higher in male than in female rats along with higher tubule cAMP levels. L-Epinephrine levels also increased $1{,}25(OH)_2$ production, which was blocked by the α_2-receptor antagonist, yohimbine. This greater capacity for $1{,}25(OH)_2D$ production may account for the higher circulating values of $1{,}25(OH)_2D$ and greater calcium absorption in male animals. Recent advances now permit investigators to pinpoint the mechanisms controlling this enzymatic reaction in vitamin-D-replete mammalian kidney (23,25,27–30). This is important, since the control steps and alterations in disease can now be more clearly understood.

It is now apparent that omission of malate, the source of mitochondrial reducing equivalents, will block both 1α-hydroxylase activity and the degradation of previously formed $1{,}25(OH)_2D$ (30). Changes in hydrogen ion concentration also can reduce enzyme activity (23): the activity is reduced in vitamin-D-deficient rats and chicks given NH_4Cl acutely. After 16 days of NH_4Cl treatment, enzyme activity is normal when rat proximal convoluted tubules are evaluated in vitro (31). Studies in children indicate that chronic metabolic acidosis due to renal tubular acidosis types I and II does not lower circulating $1,25(OH)_2D$ values (32), but that a hypophosphatemic stimulus, which should increase enzyme activity, does not increase metabolite concentrations (33).

Ample evidence exists that 1α-hydroxylase activity is abnormal in X-linked hypophosphatemia in both humans and the mouse model (34–36). In these hypophosphatemic subjects and mice, hypophosphatemia does not augment enzyme activity as anticipated, and the rise in circulating $1,25(OH)_2D$ values that occurs with dietary phosphate restriction does not occur in animals or human subjects with the hypophosphatemic allele (35–37). Furthermore, $1,25(OH)_2D$ levels do rise after PTH infusion or hypocalcemia in the X-linked hypophosphatemic mouse (38,39), so the most plausible explanation for an abnormal response to phosphate depletion is a resetting of the threshold for phosphate in the renal tubule (38). To complicate the issue further, 1α-hydroxylase levels actually rise following a high-calcium, high-phosphate diet in the mouse (37) which is completely opposite to the findings in healthy mice or other mammalian species. It is clear that deranged control of 1α-hydroxylase activity exists in this disorder and in its animal model.

An important consideration in all studies of 1α-hydroxylase activity, $1,25(OH)_2D$ receptor studies, studies of $1,25(OH)_2D$ biological function, and clinical studies using this metabolite is the measurement of circulating values of this renal metabolite. The gold standard is the Eisman assay (40). This technique uses lipid extraction, a series of chromatographic separations, high pressure liquid chromatography (HPLC), and competitive binding radioassay using cytosolic preparations of the $1,25(OH)_2D$ receptor derived from vitamin-D-deficient chick intestine. Newer techniques have arisen that primarily use other cell types that display the receptor, including cultured rat osteosarcoma cell lines (41,42), calf thymus (43), or human breast carcinoma cell lines (43). These methods have two advantages: first, serum samples can be separated using a short, disposable, sialic acid column; and, second, the receptor in these cell lines is more specific for $1,25(OH)_2D$ than is the vitamin-D-deficient chick intestinal receptor (40–43). Thus, $1,25(OH)_2D$ levels can actually be measured without HPLC (42,43). This metabolite can also be measured by mass spectrometry–gas chromatography. Finally, other metabolites, such as $25(OH)D_2$ and $25(OH)D_3$, have been measured using protein binding assays, but can be accurately determined by HPLC (44).

As with any steroid hormone, $1,25(OH)_2D_3$ must combine with a high-affinity intracellular receptor that mediates hormone response by initiating transcription of a gene or genes with mRNA translation. Active investigation in this area has resulted in considerable recent progress, which is summarized below. Receptors for $1,25(OH)_2D_3$ are polypeptides present in miniscule amounts in target cells that selectively bind this vitamin D metabolite over all other forms of the vitamin and display an equilibrium dissociation constant for

$1,25(OH)_2D$ of 10^{-10}-10^{-15} M (21). Receptors sediment at 3.3-3.7S and have a molecular weight ranging from 5.2 to 6.0 kD. Receptor activity has been found in a variety of tissues, including intestine, bone, and kidney, where they are found in the greatest concentration, which is not surprising since these are the traditional sites of the biological action of vitamin D. However, receptors are also present in parathyroid gland, pituitary, parotid, thymus, pancreas, muscle, leukocytes, skin, testes, ovary, uterus, placenta, yolk sac, and breast, as well as a variety of malignant cells (21,45-47). The meaning of receptors at these sites is unclear, but has evoked provocative theories concerning a wider role for the biological action of $1,25(OH)_2D$. An interesting finding is that receptor density increases with development in many tissues (13,20,21,46-48).

Within the cell, the location of the receptor is uncertain. It is clearly within the nucleus when it is in its unoccupied form and may be also in the cytoplasm when it is occupied with $1,25(OH)_2D$ (21). The receptor has different domains, some of which bind $1,25(OH)_2D$ and some of which bind DNA, chromatin, and nuclei. The receptor interacts with both single- and double-standard DNA and with RNA, but will preferentially combine with double-standard DNA (21). In its occupied form, binding to DNA is enhanced, but the $1,25(OH)_2D$ binding sites and the DNA binding site are distinctive, since trypsin or proteolysis can remove the DNA binding site without influencing $1,25(OH)_2D$ binding. Following $1,25(OH)_2D$ binding a hormone-dependent phosphorylation of receptor occurs, which is consistent with the idea that the hormone induces a conformational change that permits phosphorylation and potentially functional activation (49).

Defects in receptor number or binding characteristics have been identified in vitamin-D-deficiency rickets type II, where the defect could include reduced receptor density, abnormal DNA-binding, or abnormal $1,25(OH)_2D_3$ binding (50). This defect is discussed in Chapter 7 and will not be discussed further here. Decreased nuclear uptake of $1,25(OH)_2D$ by duodenal mucosa in the X-linked hypophosphatemic mouse has also been described in which there is a reduction in the number of binding sites per cell (51); this reduced density of receptor may account for the need for very high levels of vitamin D or of $1,25(OH)_2D$ in treating children with this disorder (52).

Following binding of hormone to receptor a variety of biological changes occur: 25 hydroxyvitamin D-(24R)-hydroxylase is induced, intestinal calcium transport increases, bone-related proteins appear to increase (including collagens, vitamin-K-dependent osteocalcin, and alkaline phosphatase), cell differentiation ensues, and there is suppression of malignant phenotypes in certain cell lines (1,21,53). Several of these changes will be discussed, since they are germane to an understanding of vitamin D action. The role of $1,25(OH)_2D$ in the regulation of PTH secretion has recently been shown to involve reversible reduction of preproPTH messenger RNA (54). Suppression of mRNA is specific for the precursor of PTH and is dose dependent. Several vitamin D metabolites demonstrate this action but $1,25(OH)_2D$ suppresses mRNA at 2–3 orders of magnitude lower. Further, in the absence of $1,25(OH)_2D$, as is encountered clinically in uremic patients, the set point for calcium suppression of PTH secretion is shifted to the right and higher extracellular calcium concentrations are needed to reverse secondary hyperparathyroidism (55). The inability of $1,25(OH)_2D$ to induce the synthesis of 24R-hydroxylase in skin fibroblasts cultured from certain patients with vitamin-D-dependency rickets type II indicates a defect in high-affinity $1,25(OH)_2D$ bindint to its receptor (56).

Perhaps the best-established effect of $1,25(OH)_2D$ is upon intestinal calcium absorption, where active calcium uptake follows hormone binding to a receptor in target cells in the duodenum and remaining small bowel (21). The messenger RNA for cholecalcin or calbindin (the 9 kD calcium-binding protein) arises within 1 hr after exposure of rat intestine to $1,25(OH)_2D_3$ (57). By using a sensitive two-dimensional gel electrophoresis technique, the message for the 9 kD calbindin (or cholecalcin) can be detected in 12 min (58). A 28 kD calbindin is found in kidney; in mouse kidney it appears along with the 9 kD calbindin (59). The relation of this rapid expression of messenger RNA after hormone exposure to active calcium transport remains to be established, but the time course of action is reasonable in terms of a role for calbindin. Nonetheless, the genomic product(s) of $1,25(OH)_2D$-receptor–DNA interaction are uncertain at this time.

The induction of calbindin also depends on the intracellular calcium concentration. The calcium channel blocker, verapamil, blocks $1,25(OH)_2D$-induced calbindin synthesis in embryonic chick duodenum grown in tissue culture, but this effect can be overcome with dexamethasone. These results indicate that calcium has a regulatory role in the intestinal calcium absorptive mechanism (60).

Additional characteristics of hormone action on the intestine include a stimulation of Na^+ entry across the brush border surface by augmenting the rate (Vmax) of Na^+/H^+ exchange (61). As is well recognized, $1,25(OH)_2D$ increases intestinal calcium and phosphorus absorption (1,2,16,62), but its effects on magnesium are less clear. In some animals, this metabolite increases intestinal magnesium absorption but only when they are ingesting a low-calcium, low-magnesium diet (62). Despite the powerful influence of $1,25(OH)_2D$ on active intestinal calcium transport, its intramuscular administration to adult men does not alter the circadian rhythm for calcium normally present (63). This study points out the differences between enteral and parenteral exposure to $1,25(OH)_2D$: parenteral hormone is free to bind to receptors other than within the enterocyte. Intestinal absorption of $1,25(OH)_2D$ is greater than that of 25(OH)D or vitamin D, but only a small portion of administered $1,25(OH)_2D$ appears in thoracic diet lymph and intestinal homogenates contain radiolabeled vitamin (64,65).

Additional properties of 1,25$(OH)_2$D in the intestine include a stimulation of Na^+ entry across the brush border surface by enhancing the rate (Vmax) of Na^+/H^+ exchange (61), an augmentation of the synthesis of membrane-bound actin and alkaline phosphatase (66), and an increase in membrane-related lipid turnover, which may increase intestinal calcium transport (67). Recent evidence also suggests that aluminum may compromise the ability of intestinal cells to respond to 1,25$(OH)_2D_3$ (68).

Several tumor cell lines have receptors for 1,25$(OH)_2$D. In a myeloid leukemia cell line (HL60), this hormone will suppress cell growth and induce differentiation into mature granulocytes (69). Why should neoplastic tissue express 1,25$(OH)_2D_3$ receptors? Some cell lines expressing receptor, such as a cultured human breast cancer cell line (MCF-7), can resorb bone in cell culture (70). In an osteogenic sarcoma cell line, 1,25$(OH)_2D_3$ receptor occupancy precedes the induction of alkaline phosphatase (71). Hormone can also slow down the growth of malignant melanoma cells grown in culture (72) and, by contrast, increase the growth of a human breast cell line (73). What is the meaning of these effects on cell growth?

Several tumor cell lines with monocyte and myeloid features can be grown in tissue culture. These lines respond to chemical inducers (such as the phorbol esters), to physiological metabolites (such as glucocorticoids), and to factors such as retinoic acid by differentiation and or maturation. Induced maturation has been examined in three cell lines: murine myeloid leukemia (M1), human histiocytic lymphoma (U937), and human promyelocytic leukemia (HL-60). Each of these cell lines can be induced to differentiate in tissue culture upon addition of 1,25$(OH)_2D_3$ (74,75), has a receptor for 1,25$(OH)_2D_3$ (74,76,77), and is induced by 1,25$(OH)_2D_3$ in preference to other vitamin D metabolites by 1–4 orders of magnitude (69–77). Cells can be induced to differentiate into monocytes, macrophages, and granulocytes (74,77) and differentiation occurs during the G_1 phase of the cell cycle (77). Cells can also be induced to express the C_3 receptor, phagocytosis, NBT reduction, the F_C receptor, and to express antibody-dependent cellular cytotoxicity (killer cell activity) (74,78). Finally, 1,25$(OH)_2D_3$ can interact with T and B lymphocytes to block proliferation and interleukin II cannot overcome this inhibitory effect (79,80); this inhibition occurs in the G_1 phase of the cell cycle (79). The influence of 1,25$(OH)_2$D on myeloid and lymphocytic cells is of great interest because this hormone is perceived as being primarily involved with calcium homeostasis. The potential role of vitamin D compounds in regulating cell growth and in inducing maturation may represent a "steroid effect," since vitamin D compounds are steroid hormones. However, many of these effects of 1,25$(OH)_2$D occur at a concentration perhaps 100-fold lower than the most potent glucocorticoid, dexamethasone (74). Thus, a fundamental role for 1,25$(OH)_2$D in cellular growth and differentiation may emerge over the next several years.

Other effects of $1,25(OH)_2D_3$ have been suggested in relation to receptors in sites other than the intestine. Some of these effects help to maintain normal extracellular calcium concentrations. Increased bone resorption to elevate extracellular calcium levels is an important property of $1,25(OH)_2D_3$ (81,82). This can occur in the presence or absence of PTH and generally involves increased osteoclastic activity (82). Chronic infusion of $1,25(OH)_2D$ will actually increase osteoclastic-induced resorption more than mineral apposition rate (83). Hormone-induced bone resorption can be blocked by diphosphonates (81), the high mineral content of the medium (84), and the presence of fractures (85).

Vitamin D_3 can also increase insulin secretion, but the impaired insulin secretion in vitamin-D-deficient rats is more likely due to hypocalcemia (86); nonetheless, receptors for $1,25(OH)_2D_3$ are present in pancreas (1).

Effects not related to calcium homeostasis include a $1,25(OH)_2D_3$ induction of S-adenoxylmethionine decarboxylase in chick intestine (87), a positive influence on primary antibody formation by mice immunized with sheep red cells (88), and a change in renal brush border membrane phospholipid composition with the appearance of more phosphatidyl choline (89). Finally, $1,25(OH)_2D_3$ in concert with γ-interferon can help regulate C-myc oncogene expression in human HL-60 cells (90). The importance of these "non-calcium-related" events awaits further investigation.

II. RENAL HANDLING OF CALCIUM

The body homeostasis of calcium is largely regulated at the level of the intestine (1), with the renal handling of calcium being far less important than the degree of intestinal calcium absorption. However, without a means of reabsorbing the amounts of calcium appearing in the glomerular ultrafiltrate, massive urinary calcium losses would ensue and hypercalciuria, nephrocalcinosis, and nephrolithiasis would develop.

Plasma-ionized calcium and calcium complexed with various anions—a fraction that forms 0.6 of the total plasma concentration of calcium—is freely filterable. The fraction of calcium bound to plasma protein is nonfiltered (91). Ninety-eight percent of the filtered calcium is reabsorbed in the renal tubule: 50% in the proximal convoluted tubule, 20% in the thick ascending limb of Henle, 10% in the distal convoluted tubule, and the rest in the granular portion of the cortical collecting duct (92). The mechanisms of calcium transport along the nephron have not been fully elucidated. However, some recent studies reviewed in this chapter shed more light on the mechanisms of calcium reabsorption at each of the nephron segments.

Passive paracellular, as well as active transcellular, transport mechanisms are responsible for calcium reabsorption in the S_1 and S_2 segments of the proximal convoluted tubule (93), although the relative role of each of these mechanisms

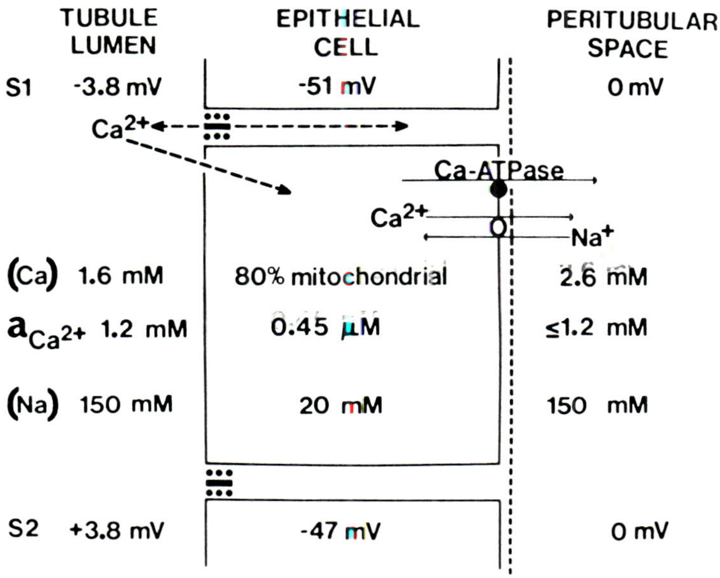

Figure 2 Possible mechanisms of calcium transport across S_1 and S_2 superficial proximal tubules. Broken arrows indicate possible pathways for passive movement and solid arrows indicate possible active transport steps. (Ca), total chemical calcium concentration; ($^aCa^{2+}$), Ca^{2+} activity; (Na), sodium concentration; (Ca-ATPase), high-affinity Ca-Mg-ATPase (adapted from Ref. 93 with permission).

in calcium transport is controversial (94). Paracellular calcium diffusion from the tubular lumen to the peritubular space in the proximal convoluted tubule is driven by solvent drag produced by a high rate of fluid reabsorption (95), a favorable ionized calcium concentration gradient (93,96), a high permeability for calcium in this nephron segment (92), and, in the S_2 segment, a lumen-positive transepithelial voltage (93) (Fig. 2). Indeed, a recent microperfusion study (97) demonstrated a predominantly passive Ca transport in the S_2 segment of the proximal tubule.

Two energy-requiring active transport systems for calcium are located in the proximal peritubular cell membrane: Na^-/Ca^{2+} exchange system (98–100) and Ca^{2+}-stimulated ATPase (100–102). In both mechanisms, calcium diffuses passively across the apical cell membrane into the cytoplasm, down both an electrical potential and a chemical concentration gradient, and then is actively "pumped out" to the peritubular space against a large electrochemical gradient by the above-mentioned systems (93). The Na^+/Ca^{2+} antiporter, which derives its energy from the Na^+-K^+-ATPase system, is a high-affinity, low-capacity system (99) and operates by means of three Na+ ions per one Ca^{2+} ion carrier complex (98,100). The Na+/Ca^{2+} antiporter has a key role in maintaining the low intracellular Ca^{2+} activity (0.1 μm) that is crucial for the physiological function of many organ systems including renal tubular cells (103a,104), a subject that is beyond the scope of this chapter. The Ca^{2+}-dependent ATPase is a high-affinity, low-capacity Mg^{2+}- and calmodulin-dependent system (102). The same enzyme also possesses a low-affinity, high-capacity component that may operate when cystolic Ca^{2+} activity is high (103a). Recently, a different, Mg^{2+}- and calmodulin-independent, 1,25$(OH)_2$-vitamin-D-sensitive, Ca^{2+}-stimulated ATPase has been demonstrated in basolateral membranes of rat kidney cortex (105,106), the exact role of which remains to be established. Controversy exists as to whether the Na+/Ca^{2+} exchange system (107) or the Ca^{2+}-dependent ATPase (99,108) has the primary role in active Ca^{2+} transport across proximal tubular cells.

The S_3 segment of the proximal tubule as well as the thin limb of Henle have minor roles in calcium transport (93,109). Disagreement exists as to the mechanism, whether passive or active, by which calcium is reabsorbed in the thick ascending limb (TAL) of Henle (110–112). It may well be that calcium transport in the cortical TAL is active while it is passive in the medullary segment, driven by the lumen-positive transepithelial voltage (93). While there is no evidence of Na+/Ca^{2+} exchange in the TAL of Henle, the role of the high-affinity Ca^{2+}–Mg^{2+}-ATPase demonstrated in this nephron segment (101) remains to be determined.

The distal nephron is the site of fine regulation of urinary calcium excretion (93,113). Ca^{2+} absorption in this nephron segment is active because it occurs against both large chemical concentration and electrical potential gradients (93,94). High-affinity Ca^{2+}–Mg^{2+}–ATPase (101) and vitamin-D-dependent calcium-binding protein (114) found in distal tubular cells may participate in active calcium transport in this nephron segment. Recently, a role for Na+/Ca^{2+} exchange in the distal tubule has also been suggested (115). Under normal conditions significant calcium transport is absent in the collecting duct (94).

A. Factors Regulating Renal Handling of Calcium

Parathyroid hormone probably decreases calcium reabsorption in the proximal tubule but enhances it across the cortical TAL of Henle and the distal tubule, so that the net effect is hypocalciuric (93,94). The effect of PTH is mediated by cyclic AMP (116) and recent studies have demonstrated that the hormone increases Na+/Ca^{2+} exchange activity in the basolateral membrane of tubular cells (100,117,188). Other proposed mechanisms for enhancement of calcium reabsorption by PTH are increased apical influx of calcium due to stimulation of phosphorylation of the brush border membrane (119) and alteration in the permeability properties of calcium channels in the intercellular tight junctions (93).

Calcitonin generally stimulates calcium reabsorption in the tubule segments that contain calcitonin-sensitive adenylate cyclase, namely, the TAL of Henle and distal convoluted tubule (116,120). However, its exact mechanism of action is unknown.

In the vitamin-D-depleted state, vitamin D appears to increase tubular calcium reabsorption (94). However, decreased as well as enhanced calcium reabsorption have been reported in response to 1,25$(OH)_2$ vitamin D administration (94,121, 122). The effect of vitamin D metabolites on renal transport of calcium is complex and depends on the status of Ca, phosphate, PTH, vitamin D, and other hormones. The localization of vitamin-D-dependent Ca-binding protein exclusively in distal convoluted tubule and the connecting duct (114) suggests that this nephron segment is the primary site of vitamin D action in the kidney.

Chronic glucocorticoid excess is associated with hypercalciuria due to negative net bone balance (94). Other hormones that increase urinary calcium excretion are mineralocorticoids, growth hormone, thyroid hormone, glucagon, catecholamines, adrenocorticotropic hormone (ADH), and angiotensin (91,94). The diabetic state as well as glucose and insulin administration result in hypercalciuria secondary to an alteration in renal tubular electrolyte transport (92,123).

Furosemide, through its inhibition of chloride reabsorption in the TAL of Henle, decreases simultaneously the lumen-positive transepithelial voltage and calcium absorption in this nephron segment (124). Thiazide diuretics and amiloride dissociate Na+ and Ca+ transport and are hypocalciuric. Thiazides increase calcium reabsorption, probably in the proximal tubule as a result of chronic volume depletion (94) while amiloride reduces calcium backflow in the late distal tubule and the cortical collecting duct secondary to a decrease in lumen-negative transepithelial voltage (125). Recently, an increased rate of Na+/Ca^{2+} exchange across the peritubular membrane of the distal tubular cells has been proposed as responsible for the hypocalciuric effect of thiazides and amiloride (115).

Hypercalcemia and hypermagnesemia result in hypercalciuria, not necessarily due to PTH suppression (94). Phosphate loading is associated with decreased urinary calcium excretion whereas phosphate depletion results in hypercalciuria (91). Metabolic acidosis leads to hypercalciuria while alkalosis enhances calcium reabsorption. Anions such as sulfate and citrate, which form luminal complexes with calcium, reduce tubular calcium reabsorption. Expansion of extracellular volume enhances calcium excretion (94).

Advanced renal failure results in high fractional excretion of calcium secondary to depressed proximal and Henle's loop fractional calcium reabsorption (126).

Spontaneously hypertensive rats have abnormal calcium metabolism, which includes hypocalcemia, elevated PTH levels, and hypercalciuria (127,128), the exact mechanism of which remains to be clarified.

III. RENAL HANDLING OF PHOSPHATE

Phosphate is an important chemical with multiple biological functions; maintaining its body pools within physiological range is of crucial importance. In contrast to calcium, body homeostasis of phosphate is regulated mainly by the kidney with the intestine having only a minor role (129).

Inorganic plasma phosphate exists in one of two forms: monovalent ($H_2PO_4^-$) or divalent (HPO_4^{2-}). Since the pKa of the phosphoric acid buffering system is 6.8, the ratio of divalent/monovalent form in physiological pH of 7.4 is 4:1 (91). About 90% of the plasma phosphate is ultrafilterable, with 10% remaining in the blood as proteinbound and complexed phosphate (mainly with calcium and magnesium) (129).

With normal dietary intake and intact parathyroid glands, 80–95% of the filtered phosphate is reabsorbed in the renal tubules: 70% in the S_1 segments of the proximal tubule and 5–10% in the distal tubule and the collecting ducts (130). In addition to the segmental heterogeneity in phosphate reabsorption along the proximal tubule, there is also a nephron heterogeneity: different phosphate transport characteristics between superficial and deeper juxtamedullary nephrons (131,132).

Phosphate transport in the proximal tubule is active (130,133) and consists of two steps. The first step is an active Na+-gradient-dependent uptake of phosphate from the tubular lumen across the apical or brush border membrane (BBM) into the cell against an electrical and a chemical concentration gradient (98,130,134). The Na+ gradient necessary for this process is maintained by active extrusion of Na+ from the cell by Na+–K+–ATPase located in the basolateral membrane (BLM). The second step is a Na+-independent passive facilitated diffusion of phosphate across the BLM into the peritubular fluid, which is driven by a concentration and an electrical gradient (98,130).

The Na/Pi cotransport across the BBM always operates to transport two Na+ ions with one molecule of either HPO_4^{2-} (electroneutral transport) or $H_2PO_4^-$ (electrogenic transport) depending on luminal pH (135,136). Recent efforts to isolate the Na/Pi cotransport carrier molecule from the BBM have yielded a Pi binding proteolipid named phosphorin, which might be a part of the molecule (137). The phosphate uptake across the BBM is the rate-limiting step in renal phosphate transport and is influenced by a variety of factors, as discussed later. Although, as mentioned, the phosphate transport across the BLM is generally assumed to be passive, recent studies have demonstrated in the BLM of proximal tubular cells a Na+-independent anion exchanger (common for phosphate, sulfate, and other anions) (138) and Na+-dependent phosphate transport system (139). While the first may participate in phosphate efflux from the cell, the latter may be responsible for phosphate uptake into the cell when phosphate entry across the BBM becomes restricted and insufficient for metabolic needs (136,139). While there is no evidence of phosphate transport across the loop of

Henle, significant phosphate reabsorption occurs in the distal tubule (140) and in the collecting duct (141), the mechanism of which remain to be elucidated.

A. Factors Regulating Renal Handling of Phosphate

Various hormones, drugs, and metabolic states alter the reabsorption of phosphate in the nephron (130,133). In most situations, the alteration involves a specific change in the capacity of the Na–Pi cotransport system localized in the BBM (136). Based on the rapidity of the response, the factors modulating this cotransport system have been recently classified into two categories (142):

1. Factors inducing a Vmax effect (change in number of carriers), which occurs within minutes to hours and is not prevented by inhibitors of protein synthesis. The change is achieved via a "2nd messenger," which acts by either in situ modification of existing Na–Pi cotransporter molecule (134,142) or possibly by a shift in the distribution of the cotransporter molecule between the BBM and the cytoplasm ("membrane recycling") (142,143).
2. Factors inducing a Vmax and/or Km effect (change in affinity of carrier), which occurs after 1-2 days and is prevented by inhibitors of protein synthesis. The effect involves a change in either the rate of synthesis of the Na+/Pi cotransporter molecule in rough endoplasmic reticulum (Vmax effect) or the synthesis of mRNA coding enzymes in the processing of the cotransporter molecule (Vmax, Km effect) (142).

1. *Factors Producing Rapid Changes*

Parathyroid hormone is the major hormonal regulator of renal phosphate transport (133). The phosphaturic action of PTH, which is released in response to hypocalcemia, is a result of decreased Na+/Pi cotransport across the BBM of tubular cells (130,144). It exerts its phosphaturic action in all nephron segments containing PTH-sensitive adenylate cyclase (120,145), with the exception of TAL of Henle, namely, proximal tubule, distal tubule, and early collecting duct. At the cellular level PTH binds to a specific receptor on the basolateral cell membrane, which results in activation of adenylate cyclase, which in turn converts ATP to cyclic AMP (a "2nd messenger") (130,145a). The subsequent metabolic changes responsible for the above-mentioned modification of the Na+–Pi cotransporter molecule could be cyclic AMP-dependent phosphorylation (146,147) or NAD-dependent ADP-ribosylation (148,149), which were found to be associated with specific inhibition of Na+-dependent Pi transport (Fig. 3). Other proposed mechanisms of PTH's effect on renal Pi transport are an alteration in metabolism of BBM phospholipids (150); an increase in intracellular Ca^{2+} activity, which in turn stimulates gluconeogenesis and NAD+ production or modifies cAMP levels (133); and a change in phosphatidylinositol–protein C kinase system (151,152). The phosphaturic action of PTH is modulated by dietary phosphate intake and acid–base status (133).

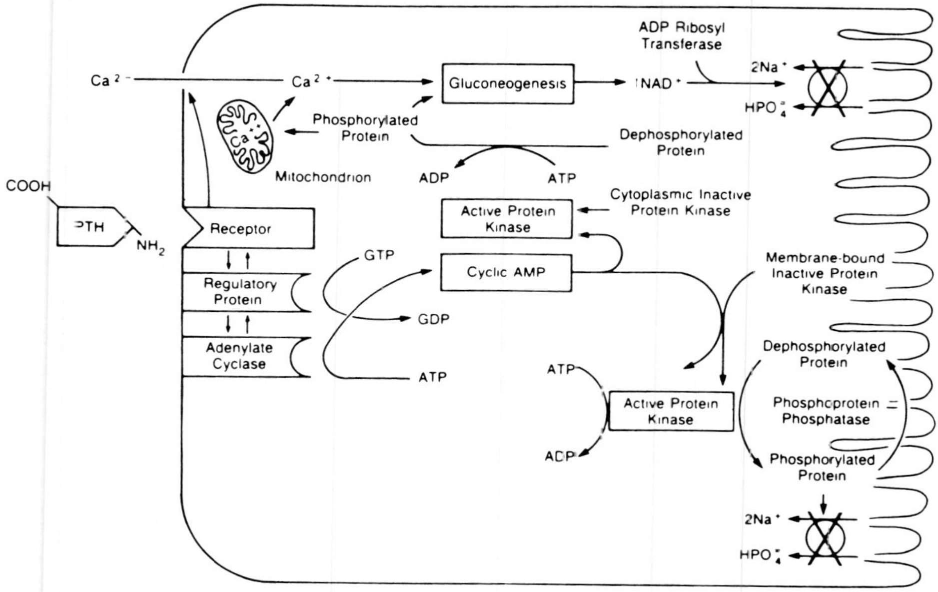

Figure 3 Schematic illustration of the mechanism of PTH-induced inhibition of proximal tubule phosphate uptake (adapted from Ref. 145a with permission).

Other hormones that produce rapid phosphaturia due to direct inhibition of Na+/Pi cotransport in the proximal tubule are calcitonin (153) and atrial natriuretic factor (154). Insulin (155) and growth hormone (156) produce rapid antiphophaturic effect secondary to direct enhancement of Na+/Pi cotransport.

Acute phosphate load results in phosphaturia. Intraluminal alkaline pH enhances phosphate uptake across the BBM while intraluminal acidosis decreases it (157,158). The pH sensitivity is mediated by a direct effect of (H+) or the Na+–Pi cotransporter system and not by changing the relative concentrations of $HPO_4{}^{2-}/H_2PO^{4-}$ (98,157). Acute hypercapnea is another factor that causes rapid phosphaturia due to change in BBM Na+/Pi cotransport (142,159).

2. Factors Producing Long-Term Changes

Dietary Phosphate Uptake. The renal tubule adjusts the reabsorption rate of phosphate to the availability and needs of phosphate (133). The response to chronic phosphate deprivation or load involves a long-term adaptive change in the Na+/Pi cotransport located in the BBM (136,160), which is independent of factors including PTH, vitamin D, plasma calcium, or acute change in phosphate load (130,133). The exact mechanism of this adaptation is unknown. The adaptation to dietary phosphate is maximal in the proximal tubule (130) and is greater in the proximal tubule of superficial rather than of deep nephrons (132, 161), but also involves the distal tubule and the collecting ducts (133).

Acid-Base Status. Renal phosphate handling is greatly influenced by the acid-base status (136). The acute effects were mentioned above. Chronic metabolic acidosis increases urinary phosphate excretion by modulating the BBM Na+/Pi cotransporter, while metabolic alkalosis increases phosphate reabsorption (130, 133).

Thyroid hormone (162) and vitamin D (163) are long-term stimulants of phosphate reabsorption. Glucocorticoids (164) are phosphaturic. Starvation results in decreased tubular phosphate reabsorption (133).

3. *Other Factors*

Extracellular fluid volume expansion results in phosphaturia. Increased concentrations of solutes cotransported with Na (glucose, amino acids, organic acids) in the tubular fluid will dissipate the Na+ gradient across the BBM and will decrease phosphate reabsorption (165).

Calcium is an important modulator of tubular phosphate transport. The serum-calcium-dependent PTH activity and the importance of intracellular Ca^{2+} concentration in renal phosphate transport have already been mentioned. A recent microperfusion study has demonstrated a direct stimulatory effect of intraluminal Ca^{2+} on the Na+-Pi cotransporter in the proximal tubule (166).

Recently, a blunted phosphaturic response to PTH has been demonstrated in immature rats (167). This may contribute to the maintenance of the physiologically important positive phosphate balance characteristic of early life.

ACKNOWLEDGMENT

This work was supported in part by grants from the NIDDK-AM37223 and a fellowship grant to Dr. Zelikovic from the National Kidney Foundation.

REFERENCES

1. Brommage, R., and DeLuca, H. F. Evidence that 1,25 dihdyroxyvitamin D_3 is the physiologically active metabolite of vitamin D_3. *Endocr. Rev. 6*:491–511 (1985).
2. Fraser, D. R. Regulation of the metabolism of vitamin D. *Physiol. Rev. 60*: 551–613 (1980).
3. Holick, M. F. The photobiology of vitamin D_3 in man. In: *Vitamin D: Basic and Clinical Aspects*. (R. Kumar, ed.). Martinus Nijhoff, Boston, 1984, pp. 197–216.
4. Holick, S. A., St. Lezin, M., Young, D., Malikal, S., and Holick, M. F. Isolation and identification of 24-dehydroprovitamin D_3 and its photolysis to

24-dehydroprevitamin D_3 in mammalian skin. *J. Biol. Chem. 260*:12181–12184 (1985).
5. Onisko, B. L., Schnoes, H. K., DeLuca, H. S., and Gover, R. S. Metabolism and binding activity of 25-fluorcholecalciferol, 24 dehydrocholecalciferol and 25-dehydrocholecalciferol in the rat. *Biochemistry 182*:1–9 (1979).
6. Woloszczuk, W. Determination of vitamin D binding protein by Scatchard analysis and estimation of a free 25 hydroxy-vitamin D index. *Clin. Chim. Acta 145*:27–35 (1985).
7. Bouillon, R., Van Baelen, H., and DeMoor, P. Comparative study of the affinity of the serum vitamin D-binding protein. *J. Steroid Biochem. 13*:1029–1034 (1980).
8. Schoentgen, F., Metc Boutigue, M.-H., Jolles, J., Constans, J., and Jolles, P. Homology between human vitamin D-binding protein (group specific component), α-fetoprotein and serum albumin. *FEBS Lett. 185*:47–50 (1985).
9. Martial, J., Plourde, V., and Gascon-Barre, M. Sequestration of ^{3}H-vitamin D_3 by the fetal and neonatal rat liver. *Biol. Neonate 48*:21–28 (1985).
10. Plourde, V., Haddad, P., and Gascon-Barre, M. Microsomal C-25 hydroxylation of [^{3}H]-vitamin D_3 by the fetal and neonatal rat liver. *Pediatr. Res. 19*:1206–1209 (1985).
11. Hollis, B. W., and Pittard, W. B. Evidence for a maturational change in the ability to convert vitamin D to 25-hydroxyvitamin D in neonate. *Pediatr. Res. 20*:412A (1986).
12. Hillman, L. S., Hollis, B., Salmons, S., Martin, L., Slatopolsky, E., McAlister, W., and Haddad, J. Absorption, dosage and effect on mineral homeostasis of 25-hydroxycholecalciferol in premature infants: Comparison with 400 and 800 IV vitamin D supplementation. *J. Pediatr. 106*:981–987 (1985).
13. Halloran, B. P., and DeLuca, H. F. Appearance of the intestinal cystolic receptor for 1,25-dihydroxy vitamin D_3 during neonatal development in the rat. *J. Biol. Chem. 256*:7338–7342 (1981).
14. Dostal, L. A. and Toverud, S. U. Effect of vitamin D_3 on duodenal calcium absorption in vivo during early development. *Am. J. Physiol. 246*:G528–G534 (1984).
15. Mendelsohn, M., and Haddad, J. G. Postnatal fall and rise of circulating 25-hydroxyvitamin D in the rat. *J. Lab. Clin. Med. 86*:32–37 (1975).
16. Halloran, B. P., and DeLuca, H. F. Calcium transport in small intestine during early development: Role of vitamin D. *Am. J. Physiol. 239*:G473–G479 (1980).
17. Hollis, B. W., and Pittard, W. B. Evaluation of the total fetomaternal vitamin D relationships at term: Evidence for racial differences. *J. Clin. Endocrinol. Metab. 59*:652–637 (1984).
18. Specker, B. L., Tsang, R. C., and Hollis, B. W. Effect of race and diet on human milk vitamin D and 25-hydroxyvitamin D. *Am. J. Dis. Child. 139*:1134–1137 (1985).

19. Clemens, T. L., Henderson, S. L., Adams, J. S., and Holick, M. F. Increased skin pigment reduces the capacity of skin to synthesize vitamin D_3. *Lancet 2*:8263–8265 (1982).
20. Whitsett, J. A., Ho, M., Tsang, R. C., Norman, E. J., and Adams, K. G. Synthesis of 1,25-dihydroxyvitamin D by human placenta *in vitro*. *J. Clin. Endocrinol. Metab. 53*:484–488 (1981).
21. Pike, J. W. Intracellular receptors mediate the biologic action of 1,25-dihydroxyvitamin D_3. *Nutr. Rev. 43*:161–168 (1985).
22. Kidroni, G., Hochner-Celnikier, D., Har-Nir, R., Menczel, J., Cohen, L., Palti, Z., and Ron, M. Increased placental concentrations of 25 hydroxyvitamin D_3 and 24,25 dihydroxyvitamin D_3 in pregnant rats treated with human chorionic gonadotropin. *Biochem. Int. 9*:335–342 (1984).
23. Kawashima, H., and Kurokawa, K. Unique hormonal regulation of vitamin D metabolism in the mammalian kidney. *Miner. Electrolyte Metab. 9*:227–235 (1983).
24. Rosen, J. F., and Chesney, R. W. Circulating calcitriol concentrations in health and disease. *J. Pediatr. 103*:1–19 (1983).
25. Paulson, S. K., and DeLuca, H. F. Subcellular location and properties of rat renal 25-hydroxyvitamin D_3-1-α-hydroxylase. *J. Biol. Chem. 290*:11488–11492 (1985).
26. DeLuca, H. F., and Schnoes, H. K. Vitamin D: Recent advances. *Annu. Rev. Biochem. 52*:411–439 (1983).
27. Crivello, J. F. Bovine renal mitochondrial vitamin D_3 hydroxylases: Regulation of *in vitro* activities by inhibitors and antioxidants. *Endocrinology 117*:447–456 (1985).
28. Langman, C. B., Favus, M. J., Bushinsky, D. A., and Coe, F. L. Effects of dietary calcium restriction on 1,25-dihydroxyvitamin D_3 net synthesis by rat proximal tubules. *J. Lab. Clin. Med. 106*:286–292 (1985).
29. Tanaka, Y., and DeLuca, H. F. Measurement of mammalian 25 hydroxyvitamin D_3-24R and 1 α hydroxylase. *Proc. Natl. Acad. Sci. (USA) 78*:196–199 (1981).
30. Delvin, E. E., and Dussault, M. Kinetics of kidney mitochondrial 25-hydroxycholecalciferol-1α-hydroxylase in vitamin D-repleated weanling guinea pigs. *Arch. Biochem. Biophys. 240*:337–344 (1985).
31. Kawashima, H., Kraut, J. A., and Kurokawa, K. Metabolic acidosis suppresses 25 hydroxyvitamin D_3-1 α hydroxylase in rat kidney: Distinct site and mechanism of action. *J. Clin. Invest. 70*:135–140 (1982).
32. Chesney, R. W., Kaplan, B. S., Phelps, M., and DeLuca, H. F. Renal tubular acidosis does not alter circulating values of calcitriol. *J. Pediatr. 104*:51–55 (1984).
33. Portale, A., Halloran, D. P., Harris, S. T., and Morris, R. C. Metabolic acidosis decreases the serum concentration of $1,25(OH)_2 D$ in phosphate restricted normal men. *J. Bone Miner. Res. 1*:379A (Suppl) (1986).
34. Chesney, R. W., Mazess, R. B., Rose, P., Hamstra, A. J., and DeLuca, H. F. Supranormal 25-hydroxyvitamin D and subnormal 1,25-dihydroxyvitamin D: Their role in X-linked hypophosphatemic rickets. *Am. J. Dis. Child. 134*:140–143 (1980).

35. Meyer, R. A., Gray, R. W., and Meyer, M. H. Abnormal vitamin D metabolism in the X-linked hypophosphatemic mouse. *Endocrinology 107*:1577–1581 (1980).
36. Lobaugh, B., and Drezner, M. K. Abnormal regulation of renal 25-hydroxyvitamin D-1-hydroxylase activity in the X-linked hypophosphatemic mouse. *J. Clin. Invest. 71*:400–403 (1983).
37. Yamakoa, K., Seino, Y., Satomura, K., Tanaka, Y., Yabuuchi, H., and Haussler, M. R. Abnormal relationship between serum phosphate concentration and renal 25-hydroxycholecalciferol-1-alpha-hydroxylase activity in X-linked hypophosphatemic mice. *Miner. Electrolyte Metab. 12*:194–198 (1986).
38. Tenenhouse, H. S. Metabolism of 25-hydroxyvitamin D_3 in renal slices from the X-linked hypophosphatemic (Hyp) mouse: Abnormal response to fall in all calcium. *Cell Calcium 5*:43–55 (1984).
39. Meyer, R. A., Grey, R. W., Roos, B. A., and Kiebzak, G. M. Increased plasma 1,25 dihydroxyvitamin D after low calcium challenge in X-linked hypopohsophatemic mice. *Endocrinology 111*:174–178 (1982).
40. Eisman, J. A., Hamstra, A. J., Kream, B. E., and DeLuca, H. F. A sensitive, precise and convenient method for determination of 1,25-dihydroxyvitamin D in human plasma. *Arch. Biochem. Biophys. 176*:235–243 (1976).
41. Manolagas, S. C., Culler, F. L., Howard, J. E., Brickman, A. S., and Deltos, L. J. The cytoreceptor assay for 1,25-dihydroxyvitamin D and its application to clinical studies. *J. Clin. Endocrinol. Metab. 56*:751–760 (1983).
42. Nicholson, G. C., Kent, J. C., Gutteridge, D. H., and Retallack, R. W. Estimation of 1,25 dihydroxyvitamin D by cytoreceptor and competitive protein binding assays without high pressure liquid chromatography. *Clin. Endocrinol. 22*:597–609 (1985).
43. Reinhardt, T. A., Horst, R. L., Orf, J. W., and Hollis, B. W. A microassay for 1,25-dihydroxyvitamin D not requiring high performance liquid chromatography: Application to clinical studies. *J. Clin. Endocrinol. Metab. 58*: 91–98 (1984).
44. Bruton, J., Wray, H. L., Dawson, E., and Butler, V. 25 Hydroxyvitamin D_2 and 25 hydroxyvitamin D_3 as measured by liquid chromatography and by competitive protein binding. *Clin. Chem. 31*:783–784 (1985).
45. Simpson, R. V., Thomas, G. A., and Arnold, A. J. Identification of 1,25-dihydroxyvitamin D_3 receptors and activities in muscle. *J. Biol. Chem. 260*: 882–891 (1985).
46. Levy, F. O., Eikvar, L., Jutte, N. H. P. M., Cervenka, J., and Yoganathan, T., and Hansson, V. Appearance of rat testicular receptor for calcitriol (1, 25 dihydroxyvitamin D_3) during development. *J. Steroid Biochem. 23*:51–56 (1985).
47. Stumf, W. E., Sar, M., Narbaitz, R., Huang, S., and DeLuca, H. F. Autoradiographic localization of 1,25 dihydroxyvitamin D_3 in rat placenta and yolk sac. *Hormone Res. 18*:215–220 (1983).
48. Kim, Y. S., Clark, S. A., Stumpf, W. E., and DeLuca, H. F. Nuclear uptake of 1,25 dihydroxyvitamin D_3 in developing rodent teeth: An autoradiographic study. *Anat. Rec. 212*:301–306 (1985).

49. Pike, J. W., and Sleator, N. M. Hormone-dependent phosphorylation of the 1,25 dihydroxyvitamin D_3 receptor in mouse fibroblasts. *Biochem. Biophys. Res. Commun. 131*:378–385 (1985).
50. Pike, J. W., Dokoh, S., Haussler, M. R., Liberman, V. A., Marx, S. J., and Eil, C. Vitamin D_3-resistant fibroblasts have immunoassayable 1,25-dihydroxyvitamin D_3 receptors. *Science 224*:879–881 (1984).
51. Yamamoto, T., Seino, Y., Yamaoka, K., and Yabunchi, H. Decreased nuclear uptake of 1,25 dihydroxyvitamin D_3 by duodenal mucosal cells in the X-linked hypophosphatemic mouse. *Endocrinology 117*:2252–2255 (1985).
52. Chesney, R. W., and Dabbagh, S. Renal tubular defects of calcium and phosphorus. In: *Pediatric Nephrology* (M. A. Holliday, R. Vernier, and T. M. Barrett, eds.). Williams & Wilkins, Baltimore, 1986.
53. Price, P. A., and Baukol, S. A. 1,25-Dihydroxyvitamin D_3 increases serum levels of the vitamin K-dependent bone protein. *Biochem. Biophys. Res. Commun. 99*:928–934 (1981).
54. Silver, J., Russell, J., and Sherwood, L. M. Regulation by vitamin D metabolites of messenger ribonucleic acid for preproparathyroid hormone in isolated bovine parathyroid cells. *Proc. Natl. Acad. Sci. (USA) 82*:4270–4273 (1985).
55. Brown, E. M., Wilson, R. E., Eastman, R. C., Pallolta, J., and Marymick, S. P. Abnormal regulation of parathyroid hormone release by calcium in secondary hyperparathyroidism due to chronic renal failure. *J. Clin. Endocrinol. Metab. 54*:172–179 (1982).
56. Feldman, D., Chen, T., Cone, C., Hirst, M., Shani, S., Benderli, A., and Hochberg, Z. Vitamin D resistant rickets with alopecia: Cultured skin fibroblasts exhibit defective cytoplasmic receptors and unresponsiveness to $1{,}25(OH)_2D_3$. *J. Clin. Endocrinol. Metab. 55*:1020–1022 (1982).
57. Perrett, C., Desplan, C., and Thomasset, M. Cholecalcin (a 9K DA cholecalciferol-induced calcium-binding protein) messenger RNA: Distribution and induction by calcitriol in the rat digestive tract. *Eur. J. Biochem. 150*: 211–217 (1985).
58. Bishop, C. E., Kendrick, N. C., Darne, M. C., and DeLuca, H. F. 1 α 25 Dihydroxyvitamin D-induced modification of a cytosolic protein in embryonic chick intestine. *J. Biol. Chem. 260*:5209–5212 (1985).
59. Rhoten, W. B., Bruns, M. E., and Christakos, S. Presence and localization of two vitamin D-dependent calcium binding proteins in kidneys of higher vertebrates. *Endocrinology 117*:674–683 (1985).
60. Corradino, R. A. Effects of verapamil and dexamethasone on the 1,25-dihydroxyvitamin D_3-mediated calcium absorptive mechanism in the organ-cultured embryonic duck duodenum. *Biochem. Pharmacol. 34*:1971–1974 (1985).
61. Fuchs, R., Graf, J., and Peterlik, M. Effects of 1α,25-dihydroxycholecalciferol on sodium-ion translocation across chick intestinal brush-border membrane. *Biochem. J. 230*:441–449 (1985).
62. Schnider, K. M., Parkinson, G. B., Houston, J. C., and Leaver, D. D. 1,25 dihydroxyvitamin D_3 increases plasma magnesium and calcium in sheep fed liquid diets low in calcium and magnesium. *Aust. Vet. J. 62*:82–85 (1985).

63. Markowitz, M. E., Rosen, J. F., and Mizruchi, M. Effects of 1,25 dihydroxyvitamin D_3 administration on circadian mineral rhythms in humans. *Calcif. Tissue Int. 37*:351–356 (1985).
64. Sitrin, M. D., Pollack, K. L., and Bolt, M. J. G. Intestinal absorption of 1,25-dihydroxyvitamin D_3 in the rat. *Am. J. Physiol. 248*:G718–G725 (1985).
65. McDonald, G. B., Kin-Hng, W. L., Schy, A. L., Wergedal, J. E., and Baylink, D. J. Intestinal metabolism and portal venous transport of 1,25$(OH)_2D_3$, 25$(OH)D_3$ and vitamin D_3 in the rat. *Am. J. Physiol. 248*:G633–638 (1985).
66. Lawson, D. E. M. Some observations on the connection of 1,25 dihydroxyvitamin D with intestinal protein synthesis and Ca absorption. In *Vitamin D* (R. Kumar, ed.). Martinus Nijhoff, Boston, 1984, pp. 303–324.
67. Matsumoto, T., Fontaine, O., and Rasmussen, H. Effect of 1,25-dihydroxyvitamin D_3 on phospholipid metabolism in chick duodenal mucosal cell. *J. Biol. Chem. 256*:3354–3360 (1981).
68. Henry, H. L., and Norman, A. L. Interactions between aluminum and the actions and metabolism of vitamin D_3 in the chick. *Calcif. Tissue Int. 37*: 484–490 (1985).
69. Miyaura, C., Abe, E., Kuribayshi, T., Tanaka, H., Konno, K., Nishu, Y., and Suda, T. 1,25-dihydroxyvitamin D_3 induces differentiation of human myeloid leukemia cells. *Biochem. Biophys. Res. Commun. 102*:937–943 (1981).
70. Eisman, J. A., Martin, T. J., MacIntyre, F., Frampton, R. J., Mosley, J. M., and Whitehead, R. 1,25-dihydroxyvitamin D_3 receptor in a cultured human breast cancer cell line (MCF7 cells). *Biochem. Biophys. Res. Commun. 93*: 9–15 (1980).
71. Manolagas, S. C., Haussler, M. R., and Deftos, L. J. 1,25-Dihydroxyvitamin D_3 receptor-like macromolecule in rat osteogenic sarcoma cell line. *J. Biol. Chem. 255*:4414–4417 (1980).
72. Colston, K., Colston, M. J., and Feldman, D. 1,25-Dihydroxyvitamin D_3 and malignant melanoma: The presence of receptors and inhibition of cell growth in culture. *Endocrinology 108*:1083–1086 (1981).
73. Freake, H. C., Marcocei, C., Iwasaki, J., and MacIntyre, I. 1,25-Dihydroxyvitamin D_3 specifically binds to a human breast cancer cell line (T47D) and stimulates growth. *Biochem. Biophys. Res. Commun. 101*:1131–1138 (1981).
74. Suda, T., Abe, E., Miyaura, C., Tanaka, H., Shuna, Y., and Kuribayashi, T. Vitamin D in the differentiation of myeloid leukemia cells. In: *Vitamin D* (R. Kumar, ed.). Martinus Nijhoff, Boston, 1984, pp. 343–363.
75. Dodd, R. C., Cohen, M. S., Newman, S. L., and Gray, T. K. Vitamin D metabolites change phenotype of monoblastic U937 cells. *Proc. Natl. Acad. Sci. USA 80*:7538–7541 (1983).
76. Manglesdorf, D. J., Koeffler, H. P., Donaldson, C. A., Pike, J. W., and Haussler, M. R. 1,25-Dihydroxyvitamin D_3-induced differentiation in a human promyelocytic leukemia cell line (HL-60): Receptor-mediated maturation to macrophage-like cells. *J. Cell Biol. 93*:391–400 (1984).

77. Studzinski, G. P., Ghandal, A. K., and Brelvi, Z. S. Cell cycle sensitivity of HL-60 cells to the differentiation-inducing effects of 1α-25-dihydroxyvitamin D_3. *Cancer Res. 45*:3898–3905 (1985).
78. Espevik, T. 1,25 Dihydroxyvitamin D_3-differentiated human promyelocytic leukemia cells (HL-60) can kill antibody-coated tumor cells (K562). *Scan. J. Immunol. 22*:105–109 (1985).
79. Rigby, W. F. C., Noell, R. J., Krause, K., and Fanger, M. W. The effects of 1,25-dihydroxyvitamin D_3 on human T lymphocyte activation and proliferation: A cell cycle analysis. *J. Immunol. 13S*:2279–2286 (1985).
80. Matsui, T., Nakao, Y., Koizumi, T., Nakagawa, T., and Fujita, T. 1,25-Dihydroxyvitamin D_3 regulates proliferation of activated T-lymphocyte subsets. *Life Sci. 37*:95–101 (1985).
81. Marie, P. J., Hott, M., and Garba, M. T. Inhibition by aminohydroxypropylidene biphosphionate (AHPrBP) of 1,25$(OH)_2$ vitamin D_3-induced stimulated bone turnover in the mouse. *Calcif. Tissue Int. 37*:268–275 (1985).
82. Holtrop, M. E., Cox, K. A., Clark, M. B., Holick, M. F., and Anast, C. S. 1,25-Dihydroxycholecalciferol stimulates osteoclasts in rat bones in the absence of parathyroid hormone. *Endocrinology 108*:2293–2301 (1981).
83. Marie, P. J., Hott, M., and Garba, M. T. Contrasting effects of 1,25 dihydroxyvitamin D_3 on bone matrix and mineral oppositional rates in the mouse. *Metabolism 34*:777–783 (1985).
84. Mahgoub, A. Effects of calcium and (inorganic) phosphate on bone resorption produced by vitamin D_3 metabolites in vitro. *Endocrinol. Res. 11*:27–37 (1983).
85. Carr, E. A., Jr., Carroll, M., Montes, M., and Zielezny, M. Uptake of technetium-99m methylene diphosphonate by fractured and osteoporotic bone after a pulse dose of vitamin D_3. *J. Nucl. Med. 26*:385–389 (1985).
86. Tawaka, Y., Seino, Y., Ishida, M., Yamaoka, K., Satomura, K., Yabuchi, H., Seino, Y., and Imura, H. Effect of 1,25-dihydroxyvitamin D_3 in insulin secretion: Direct or mediated? *Endocrinology 118*:1971–1976 (1986).
87. Steeves, R. M., and Lawson, D. E. M. Effect of 1,25-dihydroxyvitamin D on S-adenosylmethionine decarboxylase in chick intestine. *Biochim. Biophys. Acta 841*:292–298 (1985).
88. Komori, T., Nakano, T., Ohsugi, Y., and Sugawara, Y. The effect of 1α-hydroxyvitamin D_3 in primary antibody formation in mice. *Immunopharmacology 9*:141–146 (1985).
89. Tsutsumi, M., Alvarez, V., Avioli, L. V., and Hruska, K. A. Effect of 1,25-dihydroxyvitamin D_3 on phospholipid composition of rat renal brush border membrane. *Am. J. Physiol. 249*:F117–F123 (1985).
90. Matsui, T., Takahashi, R., Mihara, K., Nakagawa, T., Koizumi, T., Nakao, Y., Sugiyama, T., and Fujita, T. Cooperative regulation of C-mye expression in differentiation of human promyelocytic leukemia induced by recombinant γ-interferon and 1,25-dihydroxyvitamin D_3. *Cancer Res. 45*: 4366–4371 (1985).
91. Lang, F. Renal handling of calcium and phosphate. *Klin. Wochenschr. 58*: 985–1003 (1980).

92. Suki, W. N., and Rouse, D. Mechanisms of calcium transport. *Miner. Electrolyte Metab. 5*:175–182 (1981).
93. Bourdeau, J. E. Renal handling of calcium. In: *Divalent Ion Homeostasis.* (B. M. Brenner and J. H. Stein, eds.). Churchill Livingstone, New York, 1983, pp. 1–31.
94. Sutton, R. A. L., and Dirks, J. H. Calcium and magnesium: Renal handling and disorders of metabolism. In: *The Kidney* (B. M. Brenner and F. C. Rector, eds.). W. B. Saunders, Philadelphia, 1986, pp. 551–618.
95. Schafer, J. A. Salt and water absorption in the proximal tubule. *Physiologist 25*:95–103 (1982).
96. Bomsztyk, K., and Wright, F. S. Contribution of diffusion to transport of calcium by renal proximal tubule. *Clin. Res. 30*:443A (1982).
97. Ng, R. C. K., Rouse, D., and Suki, W. N. Calcium transport in the rabbit superficial proximal convoluted tubule. *J. Clin. Invest. 74*:834–842 (1984).
98. Schafer, J. A., and Kevin, L. K. Membrane transport. Mechanisms coupling the transport of ions in the nephron. In: *Contemporary Nephrology* (S. Klahr and S. G. Massry, eds.). Plenum, New York, 1985, pp. 1–59.
99. Van Heeswijk, M. P. E., Geertsen, J. A. M., and Van Os, C. H. Kinetic properties of the ATP dependent Ca+ pump and the Na+/Ca+ exchange system in basolateral membranes from rat kidney cortex. *J. Membr. Biol. 79*:19–31 (1984).
100. Scoble, J. E., Mills, S., and Hruska, K. A. Calcium transport in canine renal basolateral membrane vesicles: Effects of parathyroid hormone. *J. Clin. Invest. 75*:1096–1105 (1985).
101. Doucet, A., and Katz, A. I. High-affinity Ca-Mg-ATPase along the rabbit nephron. *Am. J. Physiol. 242*:F346–F352 (1982).
102. Gimaj, P., Zurini, M., Murer, H., and Carafoli, E. Ca^{++}-transporting ATPase of rat kidney basal lateral plasma membranes. *Prog. Clin. Biol. Res. 164*:407–415 (1984).
103. Viera, A., Nachbin, L., deDios Abad, E., Goldfeld, M., Meyer-Fernandez, J. R., and de Moraes, L. Comparison between calcium transport and adenosine triphosphatase activity in membrane vesicles derived from rabbit kidney proximal tubules. *J. Biol. Chem. 261*:4247–4255 (1986).
103a. Windhager, E. E., and Taylor, A. Regulatory role of intracellular calcium ions in epithelial Na transport. *Annu. Rev. Physiol. 45*:519–532 (1983).
104. Lorenzen, M., Lee, C. O., and Windhager, E. E. Cystolic Ca^{++} and Na^{+} activities in perfused proximal tubules of necturns kidney. *Am. J. Physiol. 247*:F93–F102 (1984).
105. Ghijsen, W., Gmaj, P., and Murer, H. Ca^{++}-stimulated, Mg^{++}-independent ATP hydrolysis and the high affinity Ca^{++}-pumping ATPase: Two different activities in rat kidney basolateral membranes. *Biochim. Biophys. Acta 778*:481–488 (1984).
106. Tsuhamoto, Y., Suki, W. N., Liang, T., and Sacktor, B. Ca^{++}-dependent ATPase in the basolateral membrane of rat kidney cortex. *J. Biol. Chem. 261*:2718–2724 (1986).

107. Gmaj, P., Murer, H., and Kinne, R. Calcium ion transport across plasma membranes isolated from rat kidney cortex. *Biochem. J. 178*:549–557 (1979).
108. Borle, A. B. Effect of sodium on cellular calcium transport in rat kidney. *J. Membr. Biol. 66*:183–191 (1982).
109. Rouse, D., Ng, R. C. K., and Suki, W. N. Calcium transport in the pars recta and thin descending limb of Henle of the rabbit, perfused *in vitro. J. Clin. Invest. 65*:37–42 (1980).
110. Burg, M. B. Thick ascending limb of Henle's loop. *Kidney Int. 22*:454–464 (1982).
111. Ng, R. C. K., Peraino, R. A., and Suki, W. N. Divalent cation transport in isolated tubules. *Kidney Int. 22*:492–497 (1982).
112. Greger, R. Ion transport mechanisms in thick ascending limb of Henle's loop of mammalian nephron. *Physiol. Rev. 65*:760–797 (1985).
113. Costanzo, L. S., and Windhager, E. E. Effects of PTH, ADH and cyclic AMP on distal tubular Ca and Na reabsorption. *Am. J. Physiol. 239*: F478–F485 (1980).
114. Taylor, A. N., McIntosh, J. E., and Bourdeau, J. E. Immunocytochemical localization of vitamin D dependent calcium binding protein in renal tubules of rabbit, rat and chick. *Kidney Int. 21*:765–773 (1982).
115. Costanzo, L. S. Comparison of calcium and sodium transport in early and late rat distal tubules: Effect of amiloride. *Am. J. Physiol. 246*:F937–F945 (1984).
116. Morel, F., and Daucet, A. Hormonal control of kidney functions at the cell level. *Physiol. Rev. 66*:377–468 (1986).
117. Jayakumar, A., Cheng, L., Liang, C. T., and Sacktor, B. Sodium gradient dependent calcium uptake in renal basolateral membrane vesicles: Effect of parathyroid hormones. *J. Biol. Chem. 259*:10827–10833 (1984).
118. Hanai, H., Ishida, M., Liang, C. T., and Sacktor, B. Parathyroid hormone increases sodium/calcium exchange activity in renal cells and the blunting of the response in aging. *J. Biol. Chem. 261*:5419–5425 (1986).
119. Khalifa, S., Mills, S., and Hruska, K. A. Stimulation of calcium uptake by parathyroid hormone in renal brush border membrane vesicles: Relationship to membrane phosphorylation. *J. Biol. Chem. 258*:14400–14406 (1983).
120. Morel, F. Sites of hormone action in the mammalian nephron. *Am. J. Physiol. 240*:F159–F164 (1981).
121. Yamamoto, M., Kawanobe, Y., and Ogata, E. *In vivo* renal cotransport in vitamin D deficient rats. Abstracts of the VIII International Conference on Calcium Regulating Hormones, Kobe, Japan, 1983, p. 123.
122. Burnatowska, M. A., Harris, C. A., Sutton, R. A. L., and Seely, J. F. Effects of vitamin D on renal handling of calcium, magnesium and phosphate in the hamster. *Kidney Int. 27*:864–870 (1985).
123. Hough, S., Russell, J. E., Teitelbaum, S. L., and Avioli, L. V. Calcium homeostasis in chronic streptozotocin induced diabetes mellitus in the rat. *Am. J. Physiol. 242*:E451–E456 (1982).

124. Bourdeau, J.E., Buss, S. L., and Vurek, G. G. Inhibition of calcium absorption in the cortical thick ascending limb of Henle's loop by furosemide. *J. Pharmacol. Exp. Ther. 221*:815–819 (1982).
125. Bourdeau, J. E., and Hellstrom-Stein, R. J. Voltage dependent calcium movement across the cortical collecting duct. *Am. J. Physiol. 242*:F285–F292 (1982).
126. Wong, N. L. M., Quamme, G. A., Dirks, J. H., and Sutton, R. A. L. Divalent ion transport in dogs with experimental chronic renal failure. *Can. J. Physiol. Pharmacol. 60*:1296–1302 (1982).
127. McCarron, D. A., Yung, N. N., Ugoretz, B. A., and Krutzik, S. Disturbances of calcium metabolism in the spontaneously hypertensive rat. *Hypertension 3* Suppl. I:I162–I167 (1981).
128. Wright, G. L., and Rankin, G. O. Concentrations of ionic and total calcium in four models of hypertension. *Am. J. Physiol. 243*:H365–H370 (1982).
129. Chesney, R. W., and Dabbagh, S. Renal handling of calcium, phosphate, and magnesium and disorders of calcium and magnesium. In: *Pediatric Nephrology* (M. A. Holliday, R. Vernier, and T. M. Barrett, eds.). Williams & Wilkins, Baltimore, 1986.
130. Knox, F. B., and A. Haramati. Renal handling of phosphate. In: *Divalent Ion Homeostasis* (B. M. Brenner and J. H. Stein, eds.). Churchill Livingstone, New York, 1983, pp. 33–51.
131. Haramati, A. Tubular capacity for phosphate reabsorption in superficial and deep nephrons. *Am. J. Physiol. 248*:F729–F733 (1985).
132. Turner, S. T., and Dousa, T. P. Phosphate transport by brush border membranes from superficial and juxtamedullary cortex. *Kidney Int. 27*:879–885 (1985).
133. Mizgala, L. M., and Quamme, G. A. Renal handling of phosphate. *Physiol. Rev. 65*:431–466 (1985).
134. Hammerman, M. R., and Schwab, S. J. Phosphate transport in the kidney. Studies with isolated membrane vesicles. *Prog. Clin. Biol. Res. 168*:325–330 (1984).
135. Burchkhardt, G., Stern, H., and Murer, H. The influence of pH on phosphate transport into rat renal brush border membrane vesicles. *Pflügers Arch. 390*:191–197 (1981).
136. Gmaj, P., and Murer, H. Cellular mechanisms of inorganic phosphate transport in kidney. *Physiol. Rev. 66*:36–70 (1986).
137. Kessler, R. J., and Vaughn, D. A. Divalent metal is required for both phosphate transport and phosphate binding to phosphorin, a proteolipid isolated from brush border membrane vesicles. *J. Biol. Chem. 259*:9059–9063 (1984).
138. Löw, I., Friedrich, T., and Burckhurdt, G. Properties of an anion exchanger in rat renal basolateral membrane vesicles. *Am. J. Physiol. 246*: F334–F342 (1984).
139. Schwab, S. J., Klahr, S., and Hammerman, M. R. Na^+ gradient-dependent Pi uptake in basolateral membrane vesicles from dog kidney. *Am. J. Physiol. 246*:F663–F669 (1984).

140. Haramati, A., and Knox, F. B. Is phosphate reabsorbed by the distal nephron? *Miner. Electrolyte Metab.* *6*:165–173 (1981).
141. Shareghi, G. R., and Agus, Z. S. Phosphate transport in the light segment of the rabbit corticol collecting tubule. *Am. J. Physiol.* *242*:F379–F384 (1982).
142. Kempson, S. A., and Dousa, T. P. Current concepts of regulation of phosphate transport in renal proximal tubules. *Biochem. Pharmacol.* *35*:721–726 (1986).
143. Stanton, B. A. Regulation of ion transport in epithelium: Role of membrane recruitment from cytoplasmic vesicles. *Lab. Invest.* *51*:255–257 (1984).
144. Hammerman, M. R., Kare, I. E., and Hruska, K. A. Regulation of canine renal vesicle Pi transport by growth hormone and parathyroid hormone. *Biochim. Biophys. Acta* *603*:322–335 (1980).
145. Chabardes, D., Gagnon-Brunette, M., Imbert-Teboul, M., Grontchare, O., Montejout, M., Clique, A., and Morel, F. Adenylate cyclase responsiveness to hormones in various portions of the human nephron. *J. Clin. Invest.* *65*:439–448 (1980).
145a. Knochel, J. P., and Jacobson, H. R. Renal handling of phosphorus, clinical hypophosphatemia, and phosphorus deficiency. In: *The Kidney* (B. M. Brenner and F. C. Rector, eds.). W. B. Saunders, Philadelphia, 1986, pp. 619–662.
146. Hammerman, M. R., and Hruska, K. A. Cyclic AMP-dependent protein phosphorylation in canine renal brush border membrane vesicles is associated with decreased phosphate transport. *J. Biol. Chem.* *257*:992–999 (1982).
147. Hammerman, M. R., Hansen, V. A., and Morrisey, J. J. Cyclic AMP-dependent protein phosphorylation and dephosphorylation alter phosphate transport in canine renal brush border vesicles. *Biochim. Biophys. Acta* *755*:10–16 (1983).
148. Haramati, A., and Knox, F. G. Tubular capacity of phosphate transport in phosphate deprived rats: Effects of nicotineamid and PTH. *Am. J. Physiol.* *244*:F178–F184 (1983).
149. Kempson, S. A., Turner, S. T., Yusufi, A. N. K., and Dousa, T. S. Actions of NDA+ on renal brush border transport of phosphate *in vivo* and *in vitro*. *Am. J. Physiol.* *249*:F948–F955 (1985).
150. Brown, E. M. Regulation of the synthesis, metabolism and actions of parathyroid hormone. In: *Divalent Ion Homeostasis* (B. M. Brenner and J. H. Stein, eds.). Churchill Livingstone, New York, 1983, pp. 151–188.
151. Barret, P. Q., Zawalich, K., and Rasmussen, H. Protein kinase C activity in renal microvillus membranes. *Biochem. Biophys. Res. Commun.* *128*:494–505 (1985).
152. Kinoshita, Y., Fukose, M., Yamatani, T., Hishikawa, R., and Fujita, T. Phorbol esters stimulate phosphate accumulation synergistically with A23187 in cultured renal tubular cells. *Biochem. Biophys. Res. Commun.* *136*:177–182 (1986).

153. Berndt, T. J., and Knox, F. G. Proximal tubule site of inhibition of phosphate reabsorption by calcitonin. *Am. J. Physiol. 246*:F927–F930 (1984).
154. Hammond, T. G., Yusufi, A. N. K., Knox, F. G., and Sousa, T. P. Administration of atrial nutriuretic factor inhibits sodium-coupled transport in proximal tubules. *J. Clin. Invest. 75*:1983–1989 (1985).
155. Hammerman, M. R., Rogers, S., Hansen, V. A., Govin, J. R. III. Insulin stimulates Pi transport in brush border vesicles from proximal tubular segments. *Am. J. Physiol. 247*:E616–E624 (1984).
156. Hammerman, M. R., Karl, I. E., and Hruska, K. A. Regulation of canine renal vesicle Pi transport by growth hormone and parathyroid hormone. *Biochim. Biophys. Acta 603*:322–335 (1980).
157. Cheng, L., and Sacktor, B. Sodium gradient-dependent phosphate transport in renal brush border membrane vesicles. *J. Biol. Chem. 256*:1556–1564 (1981).
158. Quamme, G. A., and Wong, N. L. M. Phosphate transport in the proximal convoluted tubule: effect of intraluminal pH. *Am. J. Physiol. 246*:F323–F333 (1984).
159. Haramati, A., and Nienhuis, D. Renal handling of phosphate during acute respiratory acidosis and alkalosis. *Am. J. Physiol. 247*:F596–F601 (1984).
160. Cheng, L., Liang, C. T., and Sacktor, B. Phosphate uptake by renal membrane vesicles of rabbits adapted to high and low phosphorus diets. *Am. J. Physiol. 245*:F175–F180 (1983).
161. Haramati, A., Haas, J. A., and Knox, F. G. Adaptation of deep and superficial nephrons to changes in dietary phosphate intake. *Am. J. Physiol. 244*:F265–F269 (1983).
162. Yusufi, A. N. K., Murayama, N., Keller, M. J., and Dousa, T. P. Medullary effect of thyroid hormone on uptake of phosphate and other solutes across luminal brush border membrane of kidney cortex. *Endocrinology 116*:2438–2449 (1985).
163. Kurnik, B. R. C., and Hruska, K. A. Effects of 1,25-dihydroxycholecalciferol on phosphate transport in vitamin D-dependent rats. *Am. J. Physiol. 247*:F177–F182 (1984).
164. Poujeol, I., and Vandewalle, A. Phosphate uptake by proximal cells isolated from rabbit kidney: Role of dexamethasone. *Am. J. Physiol. 249*: F74–F83 (1985).
165. Barrett, P. Q., and Aronson, P. S. Glucose and alanine inhibition of phosphate transport in microvillus membrane vesicles. *Am. J. Physiol. 242*: F126–F131 (1982).
166. Rouse, D., and Suki, W. N. Modulation of phosphate absorption by calcium in the rabbit proximal convoluted tubule. *J. Clin. Invest. 76*:630–636 (1985).
167. Webster, S. K., and Haramati, A. Developmental changes in the phosphaturic response to parathyroid hormone in the rat. *Am. J. Physiol. 249*: F251–F255 (1985).

3

The Circadian Rhythms of Calcium, Phosphate, and Calcium-Regulating Hormones in Human Blood

Morri E. Markowitz and John F. Rosen

Montefiore Medical Center and Albert Einstein College of Medicine, New York, New York

I. INTRODUCTION

Many factors influence the interpretation of biochemical data. Time is one such factor. The blood concentrations of many hormones and minerals undergo cyclical variations in humans (1,2). Understanding the timing of such events helps in understanding basic physiological processes, in establishing normal ranges for clinical purposes, and in guiding therapeutic efforts to correct pathological states.

A nomenclature has evolved to describe rhythmic changes in biological functions of varying periods: A circadian rhythm is one of 24 hr duration; an ultradian rhythm is shorter, and an infradian rhythm is longer.

Data that we and others have developed indicate that the concentrations of the blood minerals calcium and phosphate vary with circadian rhythmicity in humans.

II. METHODS

Early attempts to define the fluctuations in levels of these bone minerals were hampered by infrequent sampling or were limited to assessment of the changes in serum total calcium levels. To avoid such pitfalls we developed a protocol that has been in use in all of our circadian mineral studies and that serves as a model for those interested in pursuing this area of research (2–4).

For normative studies, healthy young adult and adolescent males and regularly menstruating adult women were enrolled. None had histories of excessive calcium or vitamin D intake, recent fractures, or unusual life styles. All had approximately 7–8 hr of sleep nightly. To adapt to the clinical research center facilities, they were admitted the night prior to blood sampling. The following morning, generally before 8 A.M., an indwelling venous catheter was placed in a forearm. This catheter was used for painless blood sampling every 30 min for the duration of the study. Between samples it was kept patent by infusion of 5% dextrose with one-quarter normal saline and 5000 units of heparin/L at 5 ml/hr. An elaborate multistopcock and reservoir syringe system prevented dilution of the blood samples. In an average 24 hr study, about 1 unit of blood was withdrawn.

Samples for ionized calcium (Ca_i) concentrations were obtained anaerobically in heparinized syringes, sealed airtight, and kept on ice for 1 hr before being run on either a Noval Biomedical NOVA II or Radiometer Cal. A second sample was obtained at the same time point for later determination of serum total calcium (Ca_t) by atomic absorption spectrophotometry, and inorganic phosphate (Pi) by autoanalyzer. In addition, studies of time-dependent fluctuations in the calcium-regulating hormones parathyroid hormone (PTH), 1,25-dihydroxyvitamin D (1,25-D), and the calcium-binding, bone-derived protein osteocalcin (OC) were performed using appropriate radioimmunoassays (1,25-D was measured by a competitive binding radioassay) (5–7).

The shortest period of blood sampling was 24 hr (48 samples). At each time point, the mean of the values from all the subject in an experiment was calculated and plotted for each variable. In an average trial, six subjects were sufficient to generate a stable mean pattern. This pattern was then subjected to mean or median smoothing to eliminate minor nonrhythmic fluctuations. Power polynomial regressions of the variable against time were then performed to create a mathematical representation or idealized model of the circadian rhythm. The correlation between the raw mean data and the model determined the "goodness of fit" of the model, that is, how well the model represented the actual data (8). The correlations between the model and each individual subject's 24 hr data were then calculated to determine if there were any outliers.

A second method of statistical analyses used spectral analyses (9). In this type of time series data analysis, a string of related data points, such as an individual subject's Ca_i measurements over time, would be examined mathematically to determine if a sine wave or waves could be fit to the data. If so, this would indicate a regularly oscillating rhythm with an easily determinable period. The advantage of this method of analyses is that rhythms not readily apparent in the raw data can be separated from nonrhythmic noise. In addition, the related nature of data obtained sequentially from the same group of individuals is taken into account statistically.

III. CIRCADIAN MINERAL PATTERNS

A third-order polynomial fit the mean Ca_i data. The Ca_i pattern can be described as U-shaped with a morning peak at ~ 10 A.M. and trough ~ 8 P.M. (Fig. 1). The peak trough difference was 0.3 mg/dl. All of our normative groups studied to date (this experiment has been repeated in over 30 subjects) have demonstrated this pattern (2,3). Our findings have been confirmed by others (10). In addition, an investigation in postmenopausal women by Perry et al. found a similar pattern but with an apparent time or phase shift (11). Individuals may vary greatly from the group-derived model. This interindividual variability is true for all circadian mineral rhythms.

In contrast to what might be expected, the Cat pattern was distinct and not predictable from the Ca_i rhythm (Fig. 2). The same mathematical process was used to develop the Cat model. A skewed W-shaped curve was observed with a major midday peak followed by decline and then a minor peak in the late after-

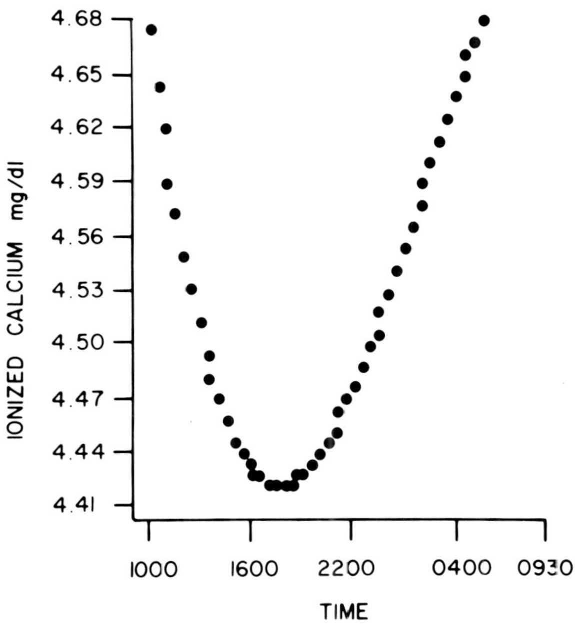

Figure 1 Model of circadian Ca_i concentration variations derived from healthy young adult male subjects (from Ref. 2).

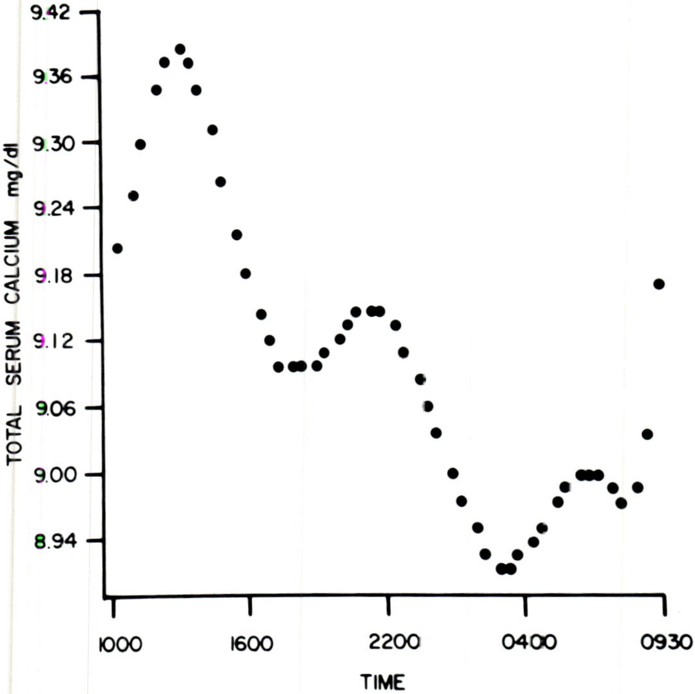

Figure 2 Model of circadian Ca_t concentration variations derived from healthy young adult male subjects (from Ref. 2).

noon. Nocturnal levels of Ca_t were depressed, rising steeply during the period before awakening. The correlation between the Ca_i and Ca_t patterns was not significant. Our findings of the Ca_t rhythm replicated that of Jubiz and others (12-14).

Data for Pi, developed in a similar manner, were fit by an eighth-order polynomial with a correlation between the raw mean data and the model of 0.95. This pattern was M-shaped (Fig. 3). A late morning trough was followed by peaks at 4 P.M. and 4 A.M. The peak-trough difference was 1.2 mg/dl in adults. However, teenagers had higher mean Pi concentrations, with much wider excursions during the 24 hr period (Fig. 4). The M shape of the curve was maintained in the adolescents.

Others have described nocturnal elevations in PTH, possibly in relation to sleep stages (12-16). We have been able to confirm the nighttime rise in our own subjects (17). Furthermore, there was an earlier increase in PTH levels discernible in the mean data, at about 4 P.M. No composite circadian rhythm of 1,25-D

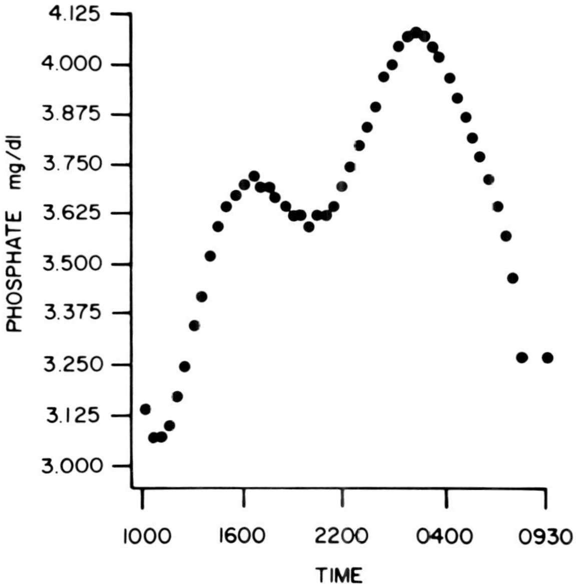

Figure 3 Model of circadian Pi concentration variations derived from healthy adult young male subjects (from Ref. 2).

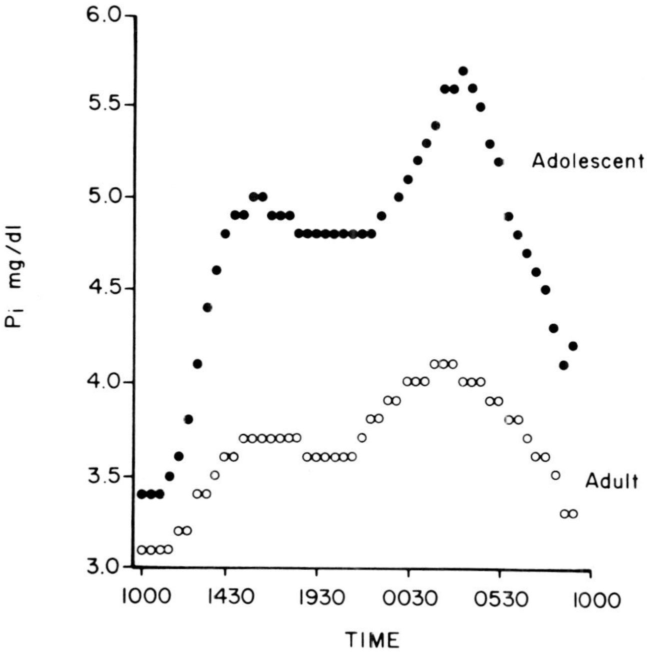

Figure 4 Comparison of adult and adolescent circadian Pi rhythms (from Ref. 3).

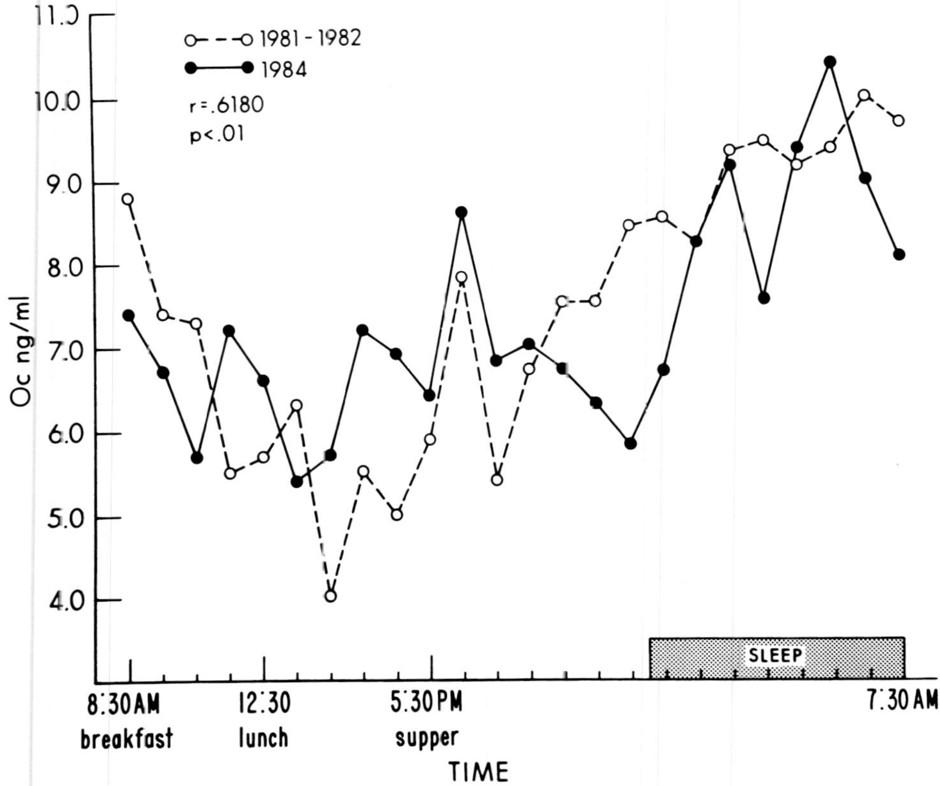

Figure 5 Mean 24 hr variations in serum OC concentrations in a group of four healthy adult males. The subjects were recalled 2 years later and the 24 hr studies were repeated.

levels could be confirmed (18,19); this hormone's levels remained fairly constant during 24 hr periods.

Serum concentrations of OC, the second most common protein found in bone, undergo rhythmic variations (20) (Fig. 5). The affinity of OC for Ca_i is well described but its precise function remains unknown. A sine wave curve roughly describes this rhythm, with a trough occurring in the late morning and nocturnal levels higher than day levels. Serum OC levels increase after 1,25-D administration under various conditions (21,22). After a 2.0 μg intravenous injection of 1,25-D was given at 8:00 A.M. to healthy adult male volunteers, the morning decline in OC levels was blunted (23). The entire curve was shifted upward; nocturnal levels remained higher than daytime values.

IV. MINERAL PATTERN INTERACTIONS

In general, the mineral patterns of Ca_i, Cat, and Pi were distinct and did not account for much of the variance in each other's patterns. The correlation between Ca_i and Cat or Pi were consistently low. Spectral analyses of the time series data derived from studies of adolescents were in agreement with this lack of a relationship between Ca_i and Cat rhythms: the ultradian rhythms of Ca_i and Cat were distinct and not overlapping (3). On the other hand, the correlation between the Cat and Pi rhythms varied with the study population but were consistently significant at the $p = 0.05$ level or better. The biological significance of this statistical relationship is not apparent, since both fasting and complete bedrest for 24 hr periods readily dissociates these two patterns.

V. MODULATORS OF MINERAL PATTERNS

A. Exogenous Factors

Circadian mineral rhythms, presumably endogenously generated, are modified by external cues. Several known modulators of Ca_i and Pi metabolism have been examined as possible modifiers of the 24 hr mineral patterns. These include age, sex, diet, and activity.

No ontogeny of the Ca_i or Cat patterns was apparent in studies of adolescent and adult males (3). Postmenopausal women had phase-shifted Ca_i rhythms; peak levels were reached in the late evening/early morning hours (11). The peak-trough amplitude in the older women was not different from that in the male groups. In contrast, the variation in amplitude of the teenage Pi rhythms was considerably greater than in the adult subjects (3). Increased Pi concentrations are observed during states of high growth hormone output such as during peak growth periods and in acromegaly (3). In fact, measuring serum Pi levels has been one way to assess the effectiveness of therapy in hypopituitary dwarfism treated with growth hormone (24). The shape of the Pi curve, however, was not different in the two groups.

Jubiz et al. fasted several subjects during 24 hr periods (12). This maneuver flattened the Pi curve without changing the Cat or PTH patterns. Different dietary regimens were probably used during the various investigations of the circadian Pi pattern performed in different laboratories, yet when blood is sampled with sufficient frequency very similar Pi patterns appear (12,14,15). This implies that if food intake is an important factor in determining the Pi pattern, there must be a broad tolerance to the content of the diet that will still result in the normal Pi rhythm. The effect of fasting or altering the diet on the Ca_i pattern has not been examined.

Several groups have postulated that the decline in Cat during the nocturnal period reflects fluctuations in its serum binding proteins (12,13). Jubiz further suggests that the decline in the latter is related to changes in the intravascular volume associated with changes in body position (12). To test this hypothesis he maintained two subjects at bed rest for 24 hr periods. During this period, both Cat and serum albumin concentrations failed to fall during the night. At the same time, the Pi and PTH patterns were maintained. The effects of bed rest on the Ca_i rhythm, which is theoretically unrelated to serum protein concentrations, should be minimal. This has not been tested.

B. Endogenous Factors

The sleep-wake cycle is determined by endogenous pacemakers that are reset daily by external cues such as daylight. A model wherein two pacemakers control many circadian functions has been described (25). After an acute reversal of the normal sleep-wake timing, for example by traveling across many time zones and adjusting activities to the new time, the functions regulated by these two pacemakers can be dissociated temporarily. Growth hormone secretion is strongly tied to the sleep cycle; the sleep-related peaks in serum growth hormone concentrations are observed at the new sleep time. In contrast, aspects of the body temperature rhythm persist at the old sleeptime for at least several days. We have acutely reversed the sleep-wake cycles of five adult men by delaying sleep for a 12 hr period (26). We observed a rapid (by the second postreversal day) shift in the Ca_i and Pi patterns to the new sleep-wake time. The Cat pattern did not shift. To our knowledge, this is the first, albeit indirect, evidence for a role of the central nervous system in the regulation of circadian mineral rhythms.

A more immediate effect on the mineral patterns would be expected by changes in the Ca-regulating hormones PTH and 1,25-D. We and others have failed to define a circadian rhythm in 1,25-D levels (18,19). Only small fluctuations, smaller in amplitude than variability in the assay, were observed. In contrast, all groups have found significant diurnal variations in PTH levels (5,12–15). The most common PTH pattern described is one in which PTH levels rise nocturnally. This rise appears to coincide with the nocturnal increases in Pi and the fall in Cat. In addition, one study observed nocturnal falls in the Ca_i concentrations as well (14). In our own study, performed in nine healthy adult men, a more complex interrelationship was defined (17). Again, the high PTH/Pi and PTH/Cat correlations were seen ($r = 0.79$ and $r = -0.74$, respectively, at concurrent time points). A more moderate correlation between PTH and Ca_i levels was found when the 24-hr time series were matched at concurrent time points ($r = 0.53$). When either the PTH or Ca_i time series was lagged by up to 12 hr and the cross-spectral analyses were calculated, a bidirectional relationship was found: changes in PTH levels preceded changes in Ca_i concentrations that occurred in the same direction by about 4 hr, and changes in Ca_i concentrations were followed 2 hr later by changes in PTH levels in the opposite direction. No such bidirectional interrelationship was observed between PTH and either of the other two mineral measures.

VI. EFFECTS OF DISEASE STATES ON MINERAL PATTERNS

Circadian mineral rhythms have been assessed in both hypo- and hyperparathyroid patients. In a group of four PTH-deficient children treated with 1,25-D, normal Ca_i patterns could be discerned in the two children receiving split daily doses of the hormone (27). One of these children remained hypocalcemic throughout the 24 hr period despite a normal pattern. The remaining two children, each of whom received their total hormone replacement as a single morning dose, were normocalcemic but without a U-shaped pattern (27). This observation implies that PTH is not a necessary factor for maintaining the circadian Ca_i rhythm, and that a normal Ca_i rhythm is not a necessary concomitant of a normocalcemic state.

Both Sinha and Locascio, but not Jubiz, found nocturnal elevations in PTH levels persisting in hyperparathyroid patients (12–14). All groups observed an upwardly shifted but normally shaped Cat curve. Twenty-four hour variations in Pi also persisted (12). Only Locascio measured Ca_i in hyperparathyoid patients and by a technique that required adjustment of pH (14). Nevertheless, the shape of the Ca_i curve was comparable in euparathyroid and hyperparathyroid patients. Again, the entire curve was shifted upward (mean Ca_i increased) in the hyperparathyroid patients.

Taken together, these limited data support the concept that PTH is a modulator of the circadian Ca_i rhythm but that it is neither essential to sustain it, nor, in excess states, likely to alter its shape.

VII. SUMMARY

We and others have defined circadian rhythms in the blood concentrations of Ca_i, Cat, and Pi. All three mineral patterns are distinct and neither the Cat nor Pi pattern is a predictor of the Ca_i rhythm. Many factors modulate these rhythms, including patient's age, sex, food intake, and activity. A complex interrelationship exists between PTH and Ca_i levels over 24 hr periods; changes in one variable affect the other with a lag time of 2–4 hr. Limited evidence suggests a role for the CNS in the maintenance of these rhythms. The physiological role of these rhythms is unknown.

The magnitude of the peak-trough differences in amplitude of the rhythms in conditions of health and disease lead us to recommend that a fixed time of day be set for drawing routine samples, and that the interpretation of blood sample analyses be referenced to the timing of sample drawing.

REFERENCES

1. Moore-Ede, M. C., Sulzman, F. M., and Fuller, C. A. *The Clocks That Time Us, Physiology of the Circadian Timing System*. Harvard University Press, Cambridge, 1982.
2. Markowitz, M. E., Rotkin, L., and Rosen, J. F. Circadian rhythms of blood minerals in humans. *Science* 213:672 (1981).
3. Markowitz, M. E., Rosen, J. F., Laximinarajan, S., and Mizruchi, M. Circadian rhythms of blood minerals during adolescence. *Pediatr. Res.* 18:456 (1984).
4. Markowitz, M. E., Rosen, J. F., and Mizruchi, M. Circadian variations in serum zinc concentrations: Correlation with blood ionized calcium, serum total calcium and phosphate in humans. *Am. J. Clin. Nutr.* 41:689 (1985).
5. Arnaud, C. D., Tsau, H. S., and Littledike, T. Radioimmunoassay of human parathyroid hormone in serum. *J. Clin. Invest.* 50:21 (1971).
6. Shepard, R. M., Horst, R. L., Hamstra, A. J., and DeLuca, H. F. Determination of vitamin D and its metabolites in plasma from normal and anephric man. *Biochem. J.* 182:55 (1979).
7. Gundberg, C. M., Lian, J. B., and Gallop, P. M. Measurement of y-carboxyglutamate and circulating osteocalcin in normal children and adults. *Clin. Chim. Acta* 128:1 (1983).
8. Armore, S. J. *Statistical Analyses and Inference*. Wiley, New York, 1967.
9. Gottman, J. M. *Time-Series Analysis: A Comprehensive Introduction for Social Scientists*. Cambridge University Press, Cambridge, 1981.
10. Ishida, M., Seino, Y., Yamaoka, K., Tanaka, Y., Satomura, K., Kurose, Y., and Yabunchi, H. The circadian rhythms of blood ionized calcium in humans. *Scand. J. Clin. Lab. Invest.* 43(suppl 165):83 (1983).
11. Perry, H. M., Province, M. A., Droke, D. M., Kim, G. S., Shaheb, S., and Avioli, L. V. Diurnal variation of serum calcium and phosphorus in postmenopausal women. *Calcif. Tissue Int.* 38:115 (1986).
12. Jubiz, W., Canterbury, J. M., Reiss, E., and Tyler, F. H. Circadian rhythm in serum parathyroid hormone concentration in human subjects: correlation with serum calcium, phosphate, albumin, and growth hormone levels. *J. Clin. Invest.* 51:2040 (1972).
13. Sinha, T. K., Miller, S., Fleming, J., Kkhairi, R., Edmondson, J., Johnston, C. C., and Bell, N. H. Demonstration of a diurnal variation in serum parathyroid hormone in primary and secondary hyperparathyroidism. *J. Clin. Endocrinol. Metab.* 41:1009 (1975).
14. LoCascio, V., Cominacini, L., Adami, S., Galvanini, G., Davoli, A., and Scuro, L. A. Relationship of total and ionized serum calcium circadian variations in normal and hyperparathyroid subjects. *Horm. Metab. Res.* 14:442 (1982).
15. Radjaipour, M., Kindtner, E., Rosler, H., and Eggstein, M. Circadiane Rhythmik der Konzentrationen von Parathyrin und Calcitonin im Serum. *J. Clin. Chem. Clin. Biochem.* 24:175 (1986).

16. Kripke, D. F., Lavie, P., Parker, D., Huey, L., and Deftos, L. J. Plasma parathyroid hormone and calcium are related to sleep stage cycles. *J. Clin. Endocrinol. Metab.* 47:1021 (1978).
17. Markowitz, M. E., Arnaud, S., Rosen, J. F., Thorpy, M., and Laximinarayan, S. Temporal interrelationships between the circadian rhythms of serum parathyroid hormone and calcium concentrations. *J. Clin. Endocrinol. Metab.* 67:1068 (1988).
18. Halloran, B. P., Protale, A. A., Castro, M., Morris, R. C., and Goldsmith, R. S. Serum concentration of 1,25-dihydroxyvitamin D in the human: Diurnal variation. *J. Clin. Endocrinol. Metab.* 60:1104 (1985).
19. Markowitz, M. E., Rosen, J. F., Holick, M. F., Hannifan, N., Endres, D. B., Time-related variations in serum 1,25-$(OH)_2$ vitamin D concentrations in humans. Proceedings of the Sixth Workshop on Vitamin D, Merano, Italy, 1985.
20. Gundberg, C. M., Markowitz, M. E., Mizruchi, M., and Rosen, J. F. Osteocalcin in human serum: a circadian rhythm. *J. Clin. Endocrinol. Metab.* 60:736 (1985).
21. Gundberg, C. M., Cole, D. E. C., Lian, J. B., Reade, T. M., and Gallop, P. M. Serum osteocalcin in the treatment of inherited rickets with 1,25-dihydroxyvitamin D_3. *J. Clin. Endocrinol. Metab.* 56:1063 (1983).
22. Greig, F., Casas, J., and Castells, S., Plasma Osteocalcin: Before and during treatment of various forms of rickets. *Pediatr. Res.* 20:329a, 1986.
23. Markowitz, M. E., Gundberg, C. M., and Rosen, J. F. The circadian rhythm of serum osteocalcin concentrations: Effects of 1,25-dihydroxyviatmin D administration. *Calcif. Tissue Int.* 40:179 (1987).
24. Gertner, J. M., Horst, R. L., Broadus, A. E., Rasmussen, H., and Genel, M. Parathyroid function and vitamin-D metabolism during human growth hormone replacement. *J. Clin. Endocrinol. Metab.* 49:185 (1979).
25. Wagner, D. R., and Weitzman, E. D. Neuroendocrine secretion and biological rhythms in man. *Psychiatr. Clin. North Am.* 3:223 (1980).
26. Markowitz, M. E., Rosen, J. F., Gundberg, C., and Thorpy, M. Regulation of circadian mineral patterns: effects of sleep–wake reversal. *J. Bone Min. Res.* 2 (suppl 1):504 (1987).
27. Markowitz, M. E., Rosen, J. F., Smith, C. L., and DeLuca, H. F. 24-hour mineral homeostasis and sterol levels in 1,25-dihydroxyvitamin-D treated hypoparathyroid children. In: Cohn, D., Mathews, L., and Talmadge, R. (eds.). *Endocrinology of Calcium Regulating Hormones.* Excerpta Medica, Amsterdam, 1981, p. 377.

4

Rickets

Irma Fiordalisi, Binita R. Shah, and Laurence Finberg

SUNY Health Science Center at Brooklyn,
Brooklyn, New York

I. BONE

Bone is a restless tissue composed of a microfibrillar network of collagen, mucopolysaccharides, and noncollagen protein (all of which form the matrix of bone) impregnated by apatite minerals, the crystalline phase of bone. The collagen of bone matrix is made almost entirely of type I collagen molecules. Unlike the type I collagen of other connective tissue, bone matrix collagen normally calcifies. This distinctive feature is likely facilitated by the highly organized intra- and intermolecular cross-linkages of collagen helices and by the polyelectrolyte chondroitin sulfate, which is the principal mucopolysaccharide of bone matrix. Chondroitin sulfate surrounds the collagen fibrils and complexes with noncollagen protein in the matrix.

The matrix network of collagen, mucopolysaccharide, and noncollagen protein is controlled and maintained by bone cells. These include fibroblasts, chondroblasts, osteoblasts, osteocytes, and osteoclasts. Osteocytes are matured osteoblasts; they help to maintain the integrity of the surrounding matrix. Osteoclasts are large, multinucleate, parathyroid-hormone-responsive cells important in bone resorption. The fibroblasts, chondroblasts, and osteoblasts all produce collagen; the latter two cell types are rich in alkaline phosphatase and, with increasing activity, spill this enzyme in seeming anticipation of mineralization.

Apatite minerals have the general formula $Ca_{10}(PO_4)_6(A^-)_2$ where A^- is an anion; bone salt is principally calcium hydroxyapatite ($C_{10}(PO_4)_6(OH)_2$). The precise stimulus for nucleation and precipitation of calcium hydroxyapatite is incompletely understood; hormonal regulation and osteoblast activities have both been implicated as direct stimuli. The composition of bone salt, however, also depends either directly or indirectly on the local electrolyte environment of the crystal, making the ionic composition of the local extracellular fluid a critical determinant of the quality and quantity of bone mineral. Linear growth is achieved by orderly, progressive mineralization of the metaphyseal ends of long bones; bone additionally serves as the body's reservoir of phosphate, calcium, and magnesium, providing an accessible pool of minerals for the maintenance of normal homeostasis of these ions (1-3).

II. TYPES OF RICKETS

Rickets is the inadequate mineralization of bone in a growing animal that results in excessive amounts of unmineralized matrix or osteoid. The cartilage-bone junction of rachitic bone consists of a disorganized mass of cartilaginous tissue, blood vessels, and uncalcified chondroosteoid trabeculae. Deficient mineralization of bone after cessation of linear growth is called osteomalacia. Excess accumulation of osteoid is the definitive histologic feature of both disorders. Extracellular fluid concentrations of calcium and inorganic phosphate are among the critical biochemical factors needed for calcification, and a deficiency of either will result in rickets. Hence, rickets may be classified into two major groups (Table 1). The disorders in which there is a primary abnormality of calcium homeostasis as well as a disturbance of phosphate metabolism make up the first group. Included are the vitamin D deficiency states, the rare circumstance of dietary calcium deficiency, and disorders of end-organ unresponsiveness to vitamin D. Hypocalcemia may occur in each of these disorders but may be compensated by induction of secondary hyperparathyroidism. Hypophosphatemia occurs in this group due to impaired absorption of phosphate from the gut and impaired renal tubular reabsorption of phosphate. This is due to an effective deficiency of 1,25 dihydroxyvitamin D ($1{,}25(OH)_2D$) and/or the phosphaturic and hypophosphatemic effects of secondary hyperparathyroidism generated in response to the primary insult, a low serum calcium level. In the second group, the primary abnormality is one of phosphate homeostasis. In this group, hypocalcemia and secondary hyperparathyroidism are not a feature and hypophosphatemia results from either a primary phosphate loss via the kidney or, less commonly, inadequate intake or absorption of phosphate. It is important to appreciate that hypophosphatemia is therefore a feature of rickets in both groups.

Besides these two major groups, there are two additional types of rickets for which there is no known disturbance of either phosphate or calcium metabolism:

Table 1 Classification of Rickets

Disturbances of Calcium and Phosphate Homeostasis
Sunlight deficiency
Dietary vitamin D deficiency
Vitamin D malabsorption
Liver disease
Drug-related enzyme induction, especially anticonvulsants
Deficiency of 25-OH-vitamin D 1-α-hydroxylase (vitamin-D-dependent, type I rickets)
End-organ unresponsiveness to 1,25$(OH)_2$ vitamin D (vitamin-D-dependent, type II rickets)
Renal osteodystrophy
Dietary calcium deficiency
Disturbances of Phosphate Homeostasis
Renal tubular disease with phosphate loss
Familial hypophosphatemia
Fanconi's syndrome
Renal tubular acidosis, especially distal type
Oncogenous rickets
Low phosphate intake
Dietary phosphate deficiency
Phosphate malabsorption (aluminum hydroxide chelation of phosphate in the gut)
No known disturbance of calcium or phosphate homeostasis
Hypophosphatasia
Metaphyseal dysostosis (Schmid type)

hypophosphatasia, a congenital deficiency of alkaline phosphatase; and metaphyseal dysostosis (Schmid type).

The typical biochemical findings in various varieties of rickets are listed in Table 2. Normal values of serum calcium are constant beyond the first week of life. However, it is important to note that the normal serum inorganic phosphorus concentration varies with age (Table 3) (3). In addition, if a blood sample is hemolyzed before analysis or obtained shortly after a high-phosphate meal, the laboratory result may be misleadingly altered, making fasting determinations necessary.

Rickets is diagnosed radiographically by a single anteroposterior view of the metaphyseal end of an actively growing long bone. In most infants and in children, the knee is most suitable (Fig. 1a). This reveals the characteristic radiographic changes of an increased zone of unmineralized osteoid seen as a lucent zone separating epiphysis from metaphysis, along with variable degrees of

Table 2 Clinical Varieties of Rickets

Disorders of Calcium and Phosphorus Homeostasis	Ca^{2+}	PO_4^{3-}	Alkaline Phosphatase	Parathyroid Hormone	25-OH-D	$1,25(OH)_2D$	Urine Amino Acids
Vitamin D deficiency							
Nutritional	N or ↓	↓	↑	↑	↓	↓, N or ↑	↑
Malabsorption	N or ↓	↓	↑	↑	↓	↓, N or ↑	↑
Hepatic disease	↓ or N	↓	↑	↑	↓	↓	↑
Drug enzyme inducers	N or ↓	↓	↑	↑	↓	↓ or N	↑
VDDR, type 1	↓	↓ or N	↑	↑	N or ↑	↓	↑
VDDR, type 2	↓	N or ↓	↑	↑	N	↑	Usually ↑
Renal osteodystrophy	↓ or N	↑ or N	↑	↑	N	↓	↑
Dietary calcium deficiency	↓ or N	N or ↓	↑	↑	N	↑	No information
Disorders of phosphorus homeostasis							
Familial hypophosphatemia	N	↓	↑	N or mildly ↑	N	↓ or "N"*	N
Oncogenous	N	↓	↑	N	N	↓	N or ↑
Fanconi's syndrome	N	↓	↑	N	N	N or ↓	Usually ↑
Nutritional	N or ↑	↓	↑	N	N	↑	N
Malabsorption	N or ↑	↓	↑	N	N	↑	N

N, normal; ↓, decreased or low-normal; ↑, increased or high-normal "N", normal numerically, but inappropriately low in the presence of hypophosphatemia.

Table 3 Variation in Serum Inorganic Phosphorus Concentration With Age

Age	Average serum phosphorus concentration (mg/dl)
Premature infants	7.9 ± 0.28
Full-term newborns	6.1 ± 0.33
1–10 years	4.6 ± 0.16
Adults	3.5 ± 0.19

Source: Ref. 3.

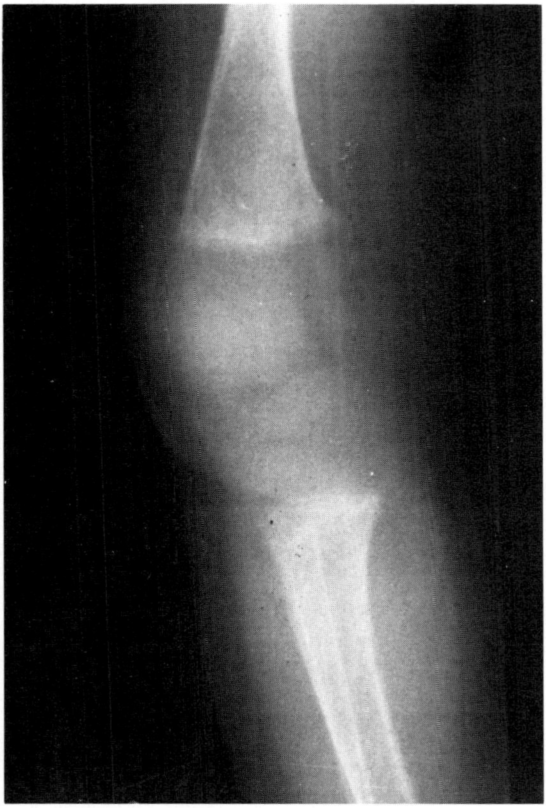

Figure 1a Nutritional vitamin-D-deficient rickets. Serial anteroposterior views of the knee in a 5-month-old boy. Above, pretreatment. Note osteopenia and metaphyseal irregularity or fraying. Ossification centers usually visible at birth are not mineralized. Radiolucent osteoid is present where the metaphyses and epiphyses would normally appear.

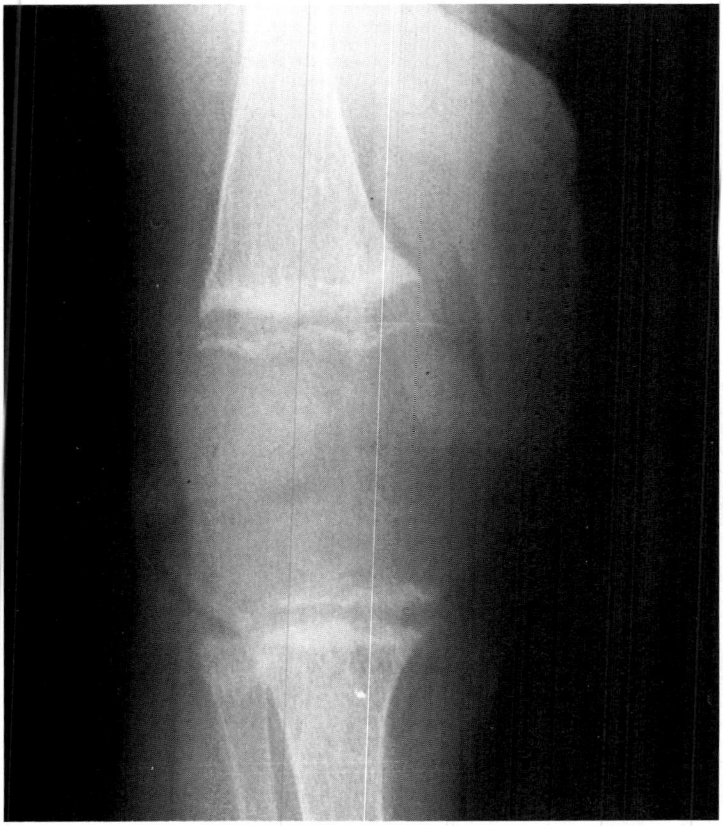

Figure 1b One week after treatment. The provisional zone of calcification is now visible.

"cupping," "fraying," and cortical spurs. Cupping is a concave deformity of the end of the bone shaft, seen best at the ends of long bones that are normally flat, such as the ulna and fibula, but even bones that have slightly convex ends (distal radius, tibia, distal femur) may develop cupping. Fraying describes the ragged rachitic metaphysis. Disorganized, linear projections protrude from the metaphysis into the radiolucent osteoid, giving the metaphysis a shaggy appearance. Cortical spurs are projections of unmineralized matrix that stem from the perichondrial-periosteal tissue and straddle the proliferative cartilage. These findings, along with biochemical evidence of rickets, confirm the diagnosis. The first radiographic sign of healing of rickets is mineralization of the provisional zone of calcification of the metaphysis (Fig. 1b, c).

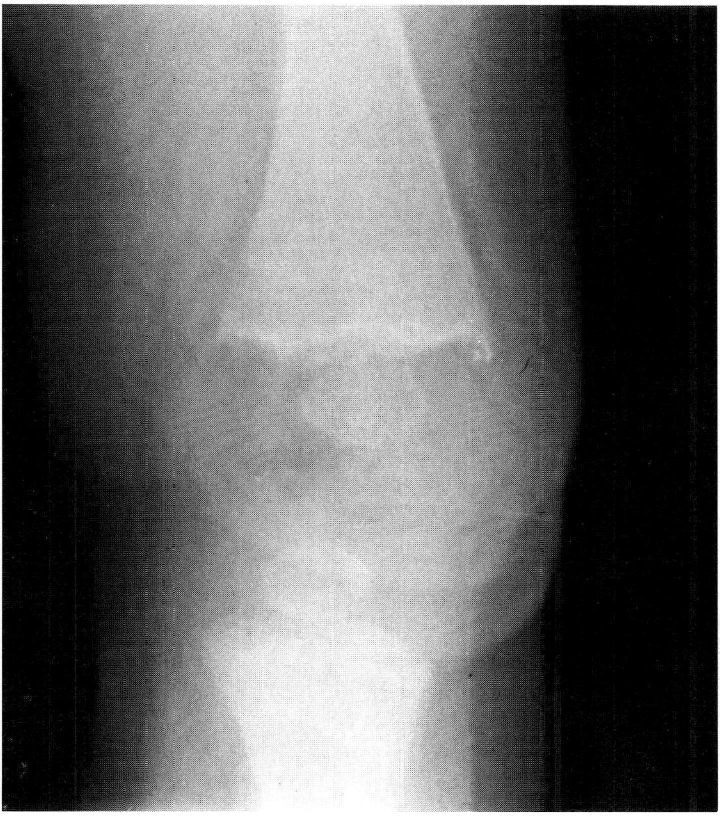

Figure 1c Four weeks after treatment. Epiphyses now visible and further ossification of the metaphysis has occurred.

III. DISTURBANCES OF CALCIUM AND PHOSPHATE HOMEOSTASIS

A. Sunlight and Dietary Vitamin D Deficiency

Nutritional vitamin D deficiency becomes clinically important only when "sunshine deficiency" due to inadequate skin exposure to sunlight precludes sufficient cutaneous activation of 7-dehydrocholesterol. Dark skin, colder climates, abundant clothing, and industrial polution are all potential barriers to endogenous vitamin D sufficiency, making certain populations dependent on nutritional sources of vitamin D. Factors predisposing to dietary deficiency include exclusive breast feeding without vitamin D supplements, dietary faddism, and strict vegetarianism. Dietary deficiency of calcium or phosphorus occuring in early infancy also results in nutritional rickets. Animal milks including human milk, contain little vitamin D. Human milk is also relatively low in phosphorus, but its calcium to phosphorus ratio of 2:1 promotes maximum calcium absorption from the intestinal tract and mineralizes the skeleton well in full-term infants, provided they are also receiving sunlight or vitamin D (400 U/day). Very-low-birthweight infants may develop rickets from phosphate and calcium deficiency even with adequate vitamin D intake (4). Clinically evident skeletal deformities are caused by widened metaphyseal–epiphyseal junctions due to accumulated osteoid and are seen only after several months of vitamin D deficiency. Typically, florid rickets appears toward the end of the first and during the second year of life. Infants born to mothers with vitamin-D-deficiency osteomalacia, however, may develop rickets within 2–3 months if fed mother's unsupplemented milk. Vitamin D deficiency rickets is rare in late childhood. Craniotabes, palpable enlargement of the costochondral junctions ("rachitic rosary"), enlargement of the wrists, and a "double" tibial maleolus (Marfan's sign) felt at the ankle constitute early evidence of skeletal changes. With advanced rickets, delayed closure of the anterior fontanelle, caput quadratum, delayed tooth eruption with enamel hypoplasia, pigeon chest deformity with Harrison's groove, kyphoscoliosis, and pelvic deformity may occur. Deformities of the extremities from twisting, muscle pull, and weight bearing occur because shafts of long bones are softened and flexible from osteoid deposition. These include genu varum (bow legs) or genu valgum (knock knees). Rachitic dwarfism is the end result of deformities of the pelvis, spine, and extremities. Potbelly and muscle weakness with hypotonia are other features. Tetany or convulsion secondary to hypocalcemia may be the first symptom of vitamin D deficiency. The diagnosis of rickets is confirmed biochemically and radiographically.

The earliest effect of vitamin D deficiency is hypocalcemia due to decreased intestinal absorption of calcium and reduced release of calcium from bone, which, in turn stimulates parathyroid hormone (PTH) secretion. Secondary hyperparathyroidism usually normalizes the serum calcium levels (by mobilizing calcium and phosphorus from bone), but also exacerbates hypophosphatemia by inhibiting tubular reabsorption of phosphate. Alkaline phosphatase overflows into plasma with increasing osteoblastic activity providing, in most instances, the first clue to abnormal bone metabolism. Secondary hyperparathyroidism also causes generalized aminoaciduria, increased urinary cyclic AMP excretion, and bone resorption. 25-Hydroxyvitamin D (25-OH-D) is the major circulating form of vitamin D in humans and a reduced plasma concentration is a characteristic finding of vitamin-D-deficiency rickets, while the serum concentration of 1,25-dihydroxyvitamin D (1,25$(OH)_2$D) can be in the normal range, low, or elevated (5–8). Hypophosphatemia and a high PTH level are important stimulants for 1-α-hydroxylase leading to increased production of

$1,25(OH)_2D$ in the renal tubule. Even though $1,25(OH)_2D$ concentration is normal or high, it is not sufficient to promote intestinal absorption of calcium and phosphorus and therefore heal rickets. The distal femur and proximal tibia, the most rapidly growing bone regions in infants, make the knee roentgenogram the most useful study to confirm the diagnosis. Roentgenograms show metaphyseal demineralization with coarse trabeculae, widening, fraying, and cupping. An increased zone of unmineralized osteoid separates the metaphysis and epiphysis; unmineralized osteoid in the subperiosteal region is seen in the diaphysis. Evidence of secondary hyperparathyroidism is best appreciated by thinning of the cortices of the small bones of the hand and erosion of the lateral ends of the clavicles.

Vitamin-D-deficiency rickets is optimally treated with administraion of vitamin D. Various preparations available include ergocalciferol, cholecalciferol, ergocalciferol in propylene glycol (Drisdol), dihydrotachysterol (DHT), 25-hydroxyvitamin D_3 (calcidiol), and 1,25 dihydroxyvitamin D_3 (calcitriol). A few thousand units of vitamin D administered daily over a period of months will heal rickets. However, rapid healing can be accomplished by administration of a much larger dose in a single day. In one such method, 600,000 U of ergocalciferol (or cholecalciferol) is given by mouth in six divided doses (100,000 U/dose given every 2 hr). Parenteral administration has no advantage over oral administration unless malabsorption is present. Calcitriol and DHT are not recommended because of their short half-lives. Vitamin D is efficiently stored in body lipid and muscle tissue and, with a large dose given in a single day, continued conversion to its active metabolite occurs over many weeks and heals rickets. Drisdol liquid is not recommended when high doses are used because of its vehicle, propylene glycol. Single-day, high-dose therapy (stosstherapy) avoids the problem of poor compliance and minimizes the induction of hypocalcemia. When lower doses of vitamin D are given in spurts, intestinal absorption of calcium increases suddenly and calcium and phosphate rapidly precipitate in bone, resulting in a transient drop in serum calcium levels. A large depot of vitamin D will prevent this sudden decline, and allow for a more constant level of the vitamin D hormone ($1,25(OH)_2D$) (3). In addition, the response to single, high-dose therapy is virtually diagnostic since patients with nutritional vitamin-D-deficiency rickets will show sustained biochemical improvement, with a rise in serum phosphorus concentration in about 4 days and radiographic evidence of healing in 7–10 days (Fig. 1), a response that is not seen in other varieties of rickets (see Table 3 in Chapter 6). Failure to respond to this form of therapy suggests another diagnosis.

Prevention is the ideal management for this disease and has been largely accomplished by vitamin D supplementation of infant formulas, cow's milk, and certain dairy products. Early identification of those at risk (dark-skinned urban dwellers, vegans, breastfed infants, and food faddists) and provision of approximately 400 U per day of vitamin D will prevent rickets.

Case Presentation

A 19-month-old black girl was brought to the emergency room with a history of fever and several episodes of twitching of both upper extremities of 1 day's duration. Birth history and past medical history were unremarkable. Dietary history included ingestion of infant formula until 8 months of age after which she refused to drink milk, but ate occasional dairy products and a nonvegetarian diet. She received no vitamin supplements. Her pertinent physical findings included knobby prominences of both wrists and ankles and genu varum. Her weight, length, and head circumference were at the 35th, 25th, and 50th percentiles, respectively. She had carpopedal spasm with a positive Chvostek's sign. Serum calcium level was 6.7 mg/dl (normal, 8.5–10.5), phosphorus 4.0 mg/dl (normal average 4.6 ± 0.16) alkaline phosphatase 1114 U/L (normal, 109–265) with normal serum concentrations of albumin and magnesium. Serum 25-OH-D level was 9 ng/ml (normal, 10–58), 1,25$(OH)_2$D was 112 pg/ml (normal, 50 ± 5.5) and iPTH was 985 pg/ml (normal 50–330/Ca 8.8–10.4 mg dl). She had generalized urinary aminoaciduria. Rickets was confirmed radiographically. Emergency management consisted of intravenous administration of calcium gluconate 10% (100 mg/kg), which resulted in rapid resolution of carpopedal spasm. Dietary modification was then instituted to ensure daily intake of milk and dairy products. She was treated in a single day with a large dose of ergocalciferol (600,000 U by mouth), followed by biochemical and radiographic healing of rickets.

Rachitic tetany due to hypocalcemia is often precipitated either during acute infection with liberation of intracellular phosphate from tissue catabolism, or following a high-phosphate feeding that increases the extracellular fluid (ECF) concentration of phosphorus rapidly. This leads to rapid utilization of calcium and phosphorus from ECF for bone mineralization. Hypocalcemic tetany is more likely to occur in the young infant with early stages of rickets than in the older child with long-standing rickets (3).

B. Malabsorptive Rickets

Any condition that causes fat malabsorption may cause vitamin D deficiency in an individual who must rely on dietary sources of the vitamin. Calcium malabsorption may also occur, especially when intestinal disease is present with pancreatic lipase normal. This results in formation of calcium long-chain fatty acid complexes (calcium soaps), leaving calcium unavailable for absorption. Gluten enteropathy (celiac disease), extrahepatic biliary atresia, and short bowel syndromes are among the more common malabsorptive states in infants and children. It is interesting that rickets is rare in children with cystic fibrosis, possibly because enzyme replacement therapy somehow facilitates vitamin D absorption more effectively than the absorption of other fat-soluble vitamins

(3). Patients' clinical conditions are similar to those with simple dietary vitamin D deficiency. Treatment involves correcting the underlying disorder if possible; otherwise, patients require a high intake of vitamin D (usually 10–20 times the usual daily allowance of 400 U per day) with titration of the dosage to maintain serum 25-OH-D in the normal range. If 25-OH-D levels are normal and hypocalcemia or normocalcemia with secondary hyperparathyroidism persists, formation of calcium soaps in the gut should be considered, long-chain fatty acids in the diet should be minimized, and consumption of calcium-rich foods encouraged.

C. Rickets in Liver Disease

Hepatocellular disease impairs 25-hydroxylation of vitamin D, resulting in the clinical picture of vitamin D deficiency. Likewise patients with biliary atresia and fat malabsorption may fail to absorb sufficient dietary vitamin D. These patients most commonly present with hypocalcemic tetany or convulsions. Measurement of serum alkaline phosphatase is generally not useful for diagnosis since levels of the hepatic form of the enzyme are already elevated and fractionation is not widely available. Serum 25-OH-D levels are decreased. Bone roentgenograms show osteopenia and rachitic changes. The latter may be less obvious than in simple nutritional vitamin D deficiency, since patients with chronic liver disease often have poor growth. Patients are best treated with 25-OH-vitamin D_3 (calcidiol) starting with 40–60 μg/day followed by monitoring of serum calcium, phosphorus, and 25-OH-D levels. Dosage is adjusted to normalize serum 25-OH-D and achieve healing of bone (9,10).

D. Drug-Related Enzyme-Induction Rickets

Liver enzymes (the mixed oxidases of the cytochrome P-450 system) that oxidize vitamin D metabolites to water-soluble, more rapidly excreted compounds, may be induced by anticonvulsant drugs. Children on chronic anticonvulsant therapy, particularly phenytoin, phenobarbital, and primidone, may become vitamin D deficient. The deficiency is usually mild but may be severe especially in institutionalized children. Limited exposure to sunlight and dietary sources of vitamin inadequate to compensate for enzyme induction are important factors; chronicity of anticonvulsant therapy and use of multiple drugs are associated with the greatest risk for rickets. The clinical presentation and treatment are similar to those of nutritional vitamin D deficiency. Alkaline phosphatase itself may be induced by anticonvulsants and elevated serum levels may represent an increased hepatic fraction; thus serum 25-OH-D levels are the most reflective measures of adequate vitamin D status in these patients. Prevention is accomplished by ensuring adequate dietary vitamin D and monitoring those at risk. An additional 1,000–3,000 U of vitamin D per week may be required for prevention (3,11).

E. Vitamin-D-Dependent Rickets

The syndrome of vitamin D dependency was first described when it was noted that certain rachitic patients would heal when given very large doses of vitamin D but would relapse when therapy was withdrawn, an apparent "dependency" on vitamin D. It is now clear that such patients have a heterogenous group of disorders; until classic terminology is replaced, however, these misnomers persist in the literature. Two types of vitamin-D-dependent rickets (VDDR) are recognized:

1. *VDDR Type I: Pseudo-vitamin-D-deficiency rickets*

This disorder, inherited as an autosomal recessive trait, is secondary to deficiency or absence of 1-hydroxylating enzyme that converts 25-OH-D to $1{,}25(OH)_2D$ in the renal tubule. Affected children present with clinical and radiological features of advanced vitamin-D-deficiency rickets despite adequate intake of vitamin D that ordinarily would prevent rickets. Severe hypocalcemia, hypophosphatemia, elevated alkaline phosphatase levels, secondary hyperparathyroidism, and generalized aminoaciduria are characteristic findings. Unlike vitamin-D-deficiency rickets, serum 25-OH-D concentrations are either normal or elevated while serum $1{,}25(OH)_2D$ concentrations are very low. The profound hypocalcemia in this disorder illustrates the refractoriness to PTH of vitamin-D-depleted subjects. Patients typically present in infancy with tetany or convulsion. In some patients, serum phosphorus, urinary phosphate, and cyclic AMP excretion is normal in the face of secondary hyperparathyroidism. Patients also fail to demonstrate a phosphaturic response to an acute PTH infusion. Treatment with calcitriol corrects all biochemical abnormalities (12). This is difficult to explain although correction of hypocalcemia may be a factor since serum calcium concentration plays a role in renal tubular response to PTH in phosphorus handling.

The preferred therapy is calcitriol, the missing metabolite. The required dosage varies among patients: most do well with physiological replacement (0.25–0.50 μg/day). Supraphysiological dosages of vitamin D_2 or D_3 or calcidiol may also be effective unless the enzyme is completely absent. Patients need close monitoring of 24 hr urinary calcium excretion to detect hypercalciuria, the first signal of vitamin D toxicity.

2. *VDDR Type 2*

This heterogeneous group of disorders involves end-organ receptor defects that result in variable degrees of unresponsiveness to $1{,}25(OH)_2D$. Inheritance appears to be autosomal recessive. Clinical varieties include patients with and without alopecia; some patients respond to pharmacological dosages of calcitriol while the condition in others remain resistant. Pathogenesis is discussed elsewhere.

F. Renal Osteodystrophy

"Renal rickets" occurs in severe chronic renal disease because of hyperphosphatemia that develops with falling glomerular filtration rates leading to hypocalcemia and secondary hyperparathyroidism, and failure of 1-hydroxylation of 25-OH-D. The parathyroid response is profound in these patients as renal failure progresses, and as hyperparathyroidism becomes ineffective in compensating for the decrease in filtered phosphate and resultant hyperphosphatemia. Vitamin D deficiency occurs simultaneously as renal tubular cells become dysfunctional. Patients often present with bone pain, pathological fractures, variable degrees of vitamin-D-deficiency rickets, and hyperparathyroid bone disease. Pathophysiology and management are discussed elsewhere.

G. Dietary Calcium Deficiency

The rare circumstance of dietary calcium deficiency without vitamin D deficiency has been reported as a cause of rickets, particularly among children from rural farming communities in southeastern Transvaal, South Africa (13–16). This population consumes a maize and vegetable diet, occasionally with meat, but essentially devoid of milk and dairy products. Calcium intake is extraordinarily low (mean, 125 mg/day) and phosphorus intake is normal. A high prevalence of hypocalcemia is reported among children in this region (17). Patients described are either hypo- or normocalcemic, hypo- or normophosphatemic, and with elevated alkaline phosphatase level, normal vitamin D status, elevated serum PTH, and normal or increased ratio of maximum tubular transport of phosphate normalized to glomerular filtration rate (TmP/GFR). The reason for normal serum phosphorus concentrations and absence of low TmP/GFR in the presence of hyperparathyroidism is not explained; it is possible that in these patients renal responsiveness to PTH is impaired while bone receptors remain relatively responsive, thus accounting for normal serum calcium levels and bone changes suggestive of hyperparathyroidism (15).

Calcium-deficiency rickets may also occur in infants given unusual diets that are unintentionally low in calcium (18). Concomitant calcium- and vitamin-D-deficiency rickets has also been reported (19).

Treatment involves the institution of an appropriate diet which includes milk and dairy products and calcium-rich foods (e.g., sardines, Swiss cheese, dandelion greens). If this is not possible, calcium supplementation to provide 800–1200 mg calcium/day is necessary.

IV. DISTURBANCES OF PHOSPHATE HOMEOSTASIS

Primary hypophosphatemia characterizes this group of rachitic disorders. These diseases are discussed in Chapter 6 on familial hypophosphatemia, which is the most common of these disturbances.

V. CONDITIONS WITH NO KNOWN DISTURBANCE OF CALCIUM OR PHOSPHATE HOMEOSTASIS

Hypophosphatasia is an autosomal recessive disorder of mineralization due to abnormally low or absent alkaline phosphatase levels. Patients have increased urinary excretion of phosphoethanolamine. In its severe form, there is complete absence of mineralization; this condition is uniformly fatal. In its milder form, rachitic changes are evident and spontaneous improvement with age may occur.

Metaphyseal dysostosis (Schmid type) is a rare disturbance of metaphyseal development. The clinical, radiographic, and histological features are similar to those in other types of rickets but no biochemical abnormality has been found. Diagnosis is made by radiographic evidence of rickets with disproportionate involvement of the proximal femoral metaphysis and normal serum calcium, phosphorus, alkaline phosphatase, parathyroid hormone, and vitamin D metabolite levels. There is no known therapy; vitamin D is contraindicated. Osteotomies, if indicated, are best postponed until growth is completed.

VI. CONDITIONS CONFUSED WITH RICKETS

Bony deformities are the hallmark of advanced rickets. While weight bearing exaggerates leg deformities, causing obvious genu valgum or varum, the other signs of classic rickets, especially in the vitamin D deficiency states, are often evident prior to weight bearing and these will aid in the clinical diagnosis. Infants or young children may present with significant bowing without a history or clinical signs suggestive of rickets. Such patients are easily evaluated radiographically, usually by a single x-ray study of one knee.

Blount's disease (tibia vara) causes bowing that may be severe and is readily diagnosed radiographically by "beaking" of the medial portion of the proximal tibial metaphysis without increased distance between the provisional zone of calcification of the metaphysis and the epiphysis. These patients have normal serum calcium, phosphorus, and alkaline phosphatase levels. On occasion, a normal toddler with exaggerated physiological bowing may be a source of concern; such problems are usually solved by careful history and physical examination. Serum chemical analyses and knee films of such patients are, of course, normal.

Primary hyperparathyroidism is rare in children. Patients are hypercalcemic and hypophosphatemic with variable skeletal changes. In growing bone, the metaphyses may become frayed and take on the radiographic appearance of rickets. Patients are distinguished by elevated serum calcium and immunoreactive parathyroid hormone (iPTH) levels. A small number of patients with pseudohypoparathyroidism, an apparent end-organ insensitivity to PTH, may demonstrate clinical and radiographic features that have been interpreted as rickets.

These patients are presumed to have bone responsiveness but renal nonresponsiveness to PTH; their bone lesions are due to the action of PTH on bone (20, 21).

REFERENCES

1. Raisz, L. G., and Kream, B. E. Regulation of bone formation. *N. Engl. J. Med.* 309:29–35 (1983).
2. Raisz, L. G., and Kream, B. E. Regulation of bone formation, *N. Engl. J. Med.* 309:83–89 (1983).
3. Harrison, H. E., and Harrison, H. C. *Disorders of Calcium and Phosphate Metabolism in Childhood and Adolescence.* (A. J. Schaffer and M. Marcowitz, eds.). W. B. Saunders, Philadelphia, 1979.
4. Rowe, J. C., and Carey, D. E. Phosphorus deficiency syndrome in very low birth weight infants. *Pediatr. Clin. North Am.* 34:997–1017 (1987).
5. Garabedian, M., Vainsel, M., Mallet, E., Guillozo, H., Toppet, M., Griamberg, R., Nguyen, T. M., and Balsan, S. Circulating vitamin D metabolite concentrations in children with nutritional rickets. *J. Pediatr.* 103:381–386 (1983).
6. Markestad, T., Halvorsen, S., Halvorsen, K. S., Aksnes, L., and Aarskog, D. Plasma concentrations of Vitamin D metabolites before and during treatment of vitamin D deficiency rickets in children. *Acta. Paediatr. Scand.* 73:225–231 (1984).
7. Papapoulos, S. E., Clemens, T. L., Fraher, L. J., Gleed, J., and O'Riordan, J. L. H. Metabolites of vitamin D in human vitamin D deficiency: Effect of vitamin D_3 or 1,25-dihydroxycholecalciferol. *Lancet* 2:612–615 (1980).
8. Chesney, R. W., Zimmerman, J., Hamstra, A., DeLuca, H. F., and Mazess, R. B. Vitamin D metabolite concentrations in vitamin D deficiency. *Am. J. Dis. Child.* 135:1025–1028 (1981).
9. Daum, F., Rosen, J. F., Roginsky, M., Cohen, M. I., and Finberg, L. 25-Hydroxycholecalciferol in the management of rickets associated with extrahepatic biliary atresia. *J. Pediatr.* 88:1041–1043 (1976).
10. Kobayashi, A., Kawai, S., Ohkubo, M., and Ohbe, Y. Serum 25-hydroxyvitamin D in hepatobiliary disease in infancy. *Arch. Dis. Child.* 54:367–370 (1979).
11. Winnacker, J. L., Yeager, H., Saunders, J. A., Russell, B., and Anast, C. S. Rickets in children receiving anticonvulsant drugs. *Am. J. Dis. Child.* 131: 286–290 (1977).
12. Delven, E. E., Glorieux, F. H., Marie, P. J., and Pettifor, J. Vitamin D-dependency: Replacement therapy with calcitriol. *J. Pediatr.* 99:26–34 (1981).
13. Pettifor, J. M., Ross, P., Wang, J., Moodley, G., and Couper-Smith, J. Rickets in children of rural origin in South Africa: Is low dietary calcium a factor? *J. Pediatr.* 92:322–324 (1978).
14. Pettifor, J. M., Ross, P., Moodley, G., and Shuenyane, E. The effect of dietary calcium supplementation on serum calcium, phosphorus and alka-

line phosphatase concentrations in a rural black population. *Am. J. Clin. Nutr.* 34:2187–2191 (1981).
15. Pettifor, J. M., Ross, P., Travers, R., Glorieux, F. H., and DeLuca, H. Dietary calcium deficiency: A syndrome associated with bone deformities and elevated serum 1,25-dihydroxy vitamin D concentrations. *Metab. Bone. Dis. Rel. Res.* 2:301–305 (1981).
16. Marie, P. J., Pettifor, J. M., Ross, P., and Glorieux, F. H. Histological osteomalacia due to dietary calcium deficiency in children. *N. Engl. J. Med.* 307: 584–588 (1982).
17. Pettifor, J. M., Ross, P., Moodley, G., and Shuenyane, E. Calcium deficiency in rural black children in South Africa—a comparison between rural and urban communities. *Am. J. Clin. Nutr.* 32:2477–2483 (1979).
18. Kooh, S. W., Fraser, D., Reilly, B. J., Hamilton, J. R., Gall, D. G., and Bell, L. Rickets due to calcium deficiency. *N. Engl. J. Med.* 297:1264–1266 (1977).
19. Frazer, D., Kooh, S. W., Reilly, B. J., Bell, L., and Duthie, D. Human rickets due to combined deficiency of calcium and vitamin D. In: *Pediatric Diseases Related to Calcium*. (H. F. DeLuca and S. Anast, eds.). Elsevier, Amsterdam, 1981, pp. 257–267.
20. Wilson, J. D., and Hadden, D. R. Pseudohypoparathyroidism presenting with rickets. *J. Clin. Endocrinol. Metab.* 51 1184–1189 (1980).
21. Dabbagh, S., Chesney, R. W., Langer, L. O., DeLuca, H. F., Gilbert, E. F., and DeWeerd, J. H. Renal nonresponsive, bone responsive pseudohypoparathyroidism: A case with normal vitamin D metabolite levels and clinical features of rickets. *Am. J. Dis. Child.* 138:1030–1033 (1984).

5

Rickets in the Newborn Period and Premature Infants

Kevin E. Halbert and Reginald C. Tsang

University of Cincinnati College of Medicine, Cincinnati, Ohio

I. INTRODUCTION

The neonate must make many adjustments to make the successful transition from an intrauterine existence to an extrauterine environment. During fetal life, bone minerals are provided via placental transfer. Once the infant is born, the gastrointestinal tract must extract the necessary nutrients from the diet to meet the needs for normal bone development. The preterm infant is placed at special risk because of decreased access to calcium (Ca) and phosphorus (P), at a time when there is very high demand for these minerals. In addition, the preterm infant is more likely to experience illnesses that will further restrict his or her attainment of adequate nutrients and minerals. Certain maternal disease states, as well as unusual dietary and/or cultural practices, can also place the infant at significant risk of rickets in the early weeks of life.

Neonatal rickets, and especially rickets of prematurity, will be reviewed here. The normal physiology of calcium homeostasis, as it pertains to the perinatal and neonatal period, will be presented briefly. Special emphasis will be placed on the problems of the preterm infant and how these conditions create an increased risk for the development of rickets. Other conditions that are more specific to the full-term infant will be discussed, along with their impact on bone development.

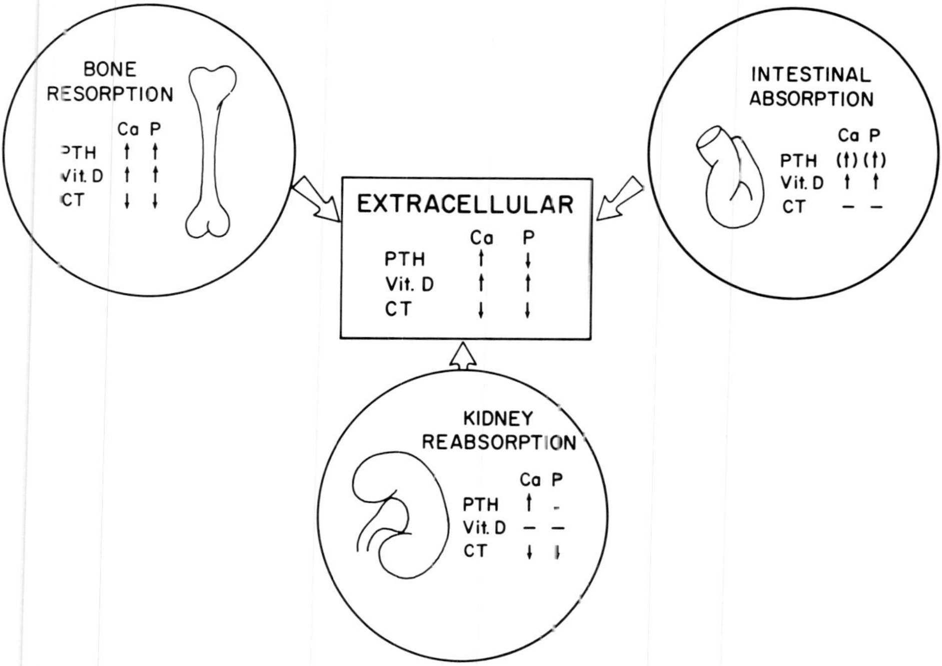

Figure 1 Calcitropic hormones and their actions on target tissues and serum Ca and P (from Tsang, R. C., Donovan, E. F., and Steichen, J. J. Calcium physiology and pathology in the neonate. *Pediatr. Clin. North Am. 23*:612, 1976, with permission).

II. PHYSIOLOGY: CALCITROPIC HORMONES

Parathyroid hormone (PTH) is released in response to a decrease in serum ionized Ca concentration (1) (Fig. 1). This peptide hormone then acts on bone to liberate Ca and P into the circulation (2,3). PTH also acts on the renal tubules to stimulate the reabsorption of Ca and decrease the tubular reabsorption of P (4,5). The result is an increase in serum Ca concentration. A coincident increase in serum P concentration, related to P released from bone, is prevented by the potent phosphaturic effect of PTH. In addition, PTH stimulates the activity of the renal 25-hydroxyvitamin D-1-alpha-hydroxylase enzyme (1 alpha-hydroxylase), resulting in increased conversion of 25-hydroxyvitamin D (25(OH)D) to 1,25-dihydroxyvitamin D ($1{,}25(OH)_2D$), the active hormonal form of vitamin D (6,7). This latter metabolite can then act on the intestinal tract to stimulate active Ca absorption (8). In the presence of hypomagnesemia, PTH secretion is impaired (9,10).

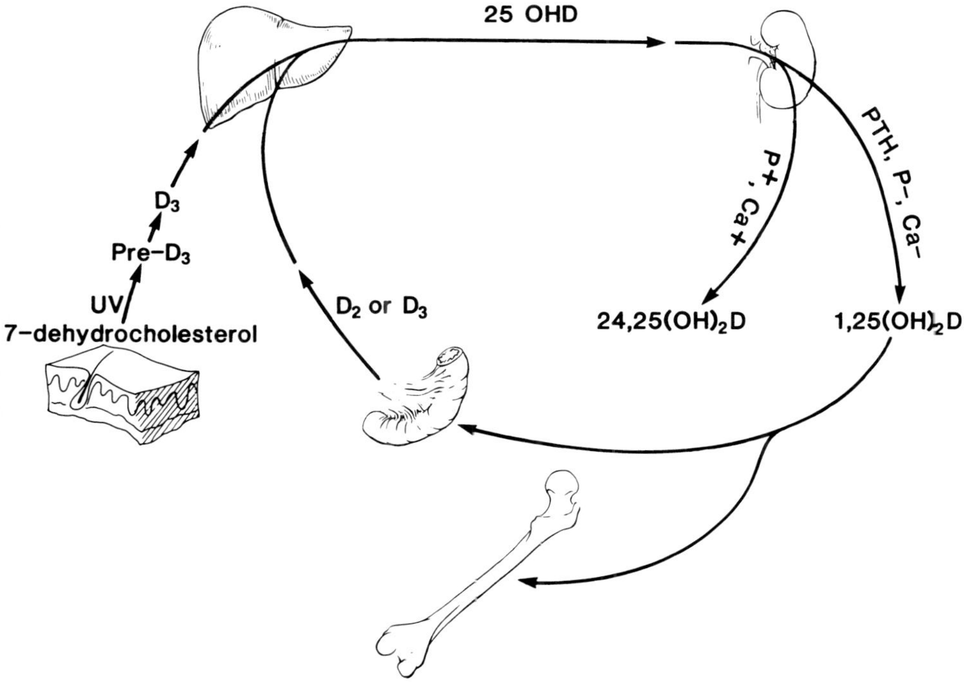

Figure 2 Vitamin D metabolism (from Tsang, R. C., Greer, F., and Steichen, J. J. Perinatal metabolism of vitamin D: Transition from fetal to neonatal life. *Clin. Perinatol. 8*:288, 1981, with permission).

Calcitonin is another peptide hormone involved in Ca homeostasis. Calcitonin is produced by the parafollicular cells of the thyroid (11,12). Elevations of serum ionized Ca, or the secretagogues glucagon and pentagastrin (13–16), will result in increased secretion of calcitonin. The principal action of calcitonin is to inhibit osteocyte and osteoclast-mediated bone resorption (17). Calcitonin also acts on the renal tubules, at a site different from PTH, to produce a decrease in tubular reabsorption of Ca and P (18,19). These actions result in a reduction of concentrations of Ca and P in serum.

Vitamin D is the third major component of the Ca-regulating system (Fig. 2). Obtained either through endogenous production in the skin through ultraviolet photoconversion of 7-dehydrocholesterol to previtamin D_3 (20), or from the diet in the form of vitamin D_2 (ergocalciferol) or vitamin D_3 (cholecalciferol), it enters the circulation where it is hydroxylated in the C-25 position in the liver to yield 25 (OH)D (21,22). This represents the principal circulating form of vitamin D and is thought to be the best marker of an individual's vitamin D status. The 25(OH)D is ultimately transported to the kidney where, in the cells of the proximal tubule, it undergoes a second hydroxylation at either the C-1 or C-24 positions to produce 1,25-dihydroxyvitamin D (1,25$(OH)_2$D) or 24,25-dihydroxyvitamin D (24,25$(OH)_2$D) (23-28). The former metabolite is the active hormonal form of vitamin D, having its actions on the gastrointestinal tract where it stimulates the active absorption of Ca and P (29-31), and on bone where, in conjunction with PTH, it can mediate bone resorption (32-35). The exact role of 24,25$(OH)_2$D has not been elucidated, but it may be involved in bone matrix formation and mineralization (36-38).

Under conditions of Ca, P, and vitamin D sufficiency, 24-hydroxylation predominates in the kidney (27,28,39,40). The renal 1 alpha-hydroxylase activity is stimulated by PTH and hypophosphatemia (6,39,41-45). In vitro, using experimental animal tissue, low Ca concentrations have been found to enhance 1 alpha-hydroxylation of 25(OH)D, but it has been difficult to show that hypocalcemia independent of PTH will stimulate this reaction in vivo (42,44,45-48).

III. RICKETS OF PREMATURITY

A. Incidence

Rickets of prematurity is a condition that has been recognized for many years. It is a disturbance of growing bone in which there is lag in mineralization such that uncalcified cartilage and bone matrix accumulate to an abnormal extent. The exact incidence of this disease is not known because of the difficulty of diagnosis and the large number of subclinical cases that remain unrecognized. Several studies have estimated that in preterm infants weighing less than 1500 g, about 30% of those surviving will show evidence of rickets (49,50). As birthweight decreases, the incidence seems to increase sharply and has been reported as high as 75% in infants weighing less than 1000 g at birth (50).

B. Causative Factors

1. Ca and P Deficiency

Maternal Disease. It is well known that certain maternal diseases can result in congenital rickets in offspring (Table 1). Maxwell, in a 1934 report, described several women in China with marked osteomalacia whose infants had both radiological and histological evidence of rickets at birth (51). From available information, it appears these women were poorly nourished, and were deficient in Ca, P, and vitamin D. Maxwell observed that a maternal product of serum Ca and P concentrations, measured each in mg/dl, of less than 20 was highly associated with the presence of rickets in the infant (51).

Congenital rickets is a rare finding in neonates. However, vitamin D deficiency in the mother still appears to be a main contributing factor in the more

Table 1 Causative Factors in Rickets of Prematurity

Ca and P deficiency
Maternal disease
Osteomalacia
Malabsorption
Pre-eclampsia
Formula and human milk feedings
Prolonged hyperalimentation
Fat malabsorption
Diuretics
Vitamin-D-related disorders
Placental transport
Ultraviolet irradiation
Race/cultural practices
Dietary vitamin D
Hepatic metabolism of vitamin D
Renal metabolism of vitamin D
End-organ responsiveness

recently reported cases of congenital rickets. Sann et al. (52), and Moncrieff and Fadahunsi (53) both reported mothers with low serum 25(OH)D concentrations who gave birth to infants with congenital rickets. In each case, the mother was, by retrospective history, determined to have a low intake of vitamin D during the pregnancy. In addition, exposure to sunlight also was restricted in the case reported by Sann et al.; the mother had been on home bedrest for the last 9 weeks of her pregnancy (52).

Maternal malabsorption also has been reported in association with congenital rickets. In the report by Begum et al. (54), two mothers were described who delivered infants with congenital rickets; the mothers had unsuspected intestinal malabsorptive disease during pregnancy. One woman was found to have celiac disease while the other had a carcinoma of the head of the pancreas causing bile duct obstruction, cholestasis, and fat malabsorption. Although extensive studies are not available in the literature, it would seem that significant maternal intestinal malabsorption, especially producing steatorrhea and poor absorption of fat-soluble vitamins, can place the infant at risk for rickets.

Pre-eclampsia also has been observed in mothers whose infants subsequently develop rickets. Bosley et al. (55), reported six preterm infants who subsequently developed rickets. Four of these infants' mothers had severe pre-eclampsia. Another report by Zeidan and Bamford (56) described a preterm infant born to a mother with severe pre-eclampsia; the infant had radiological evidence of rickets at delivery. The presumed mechanism for the development

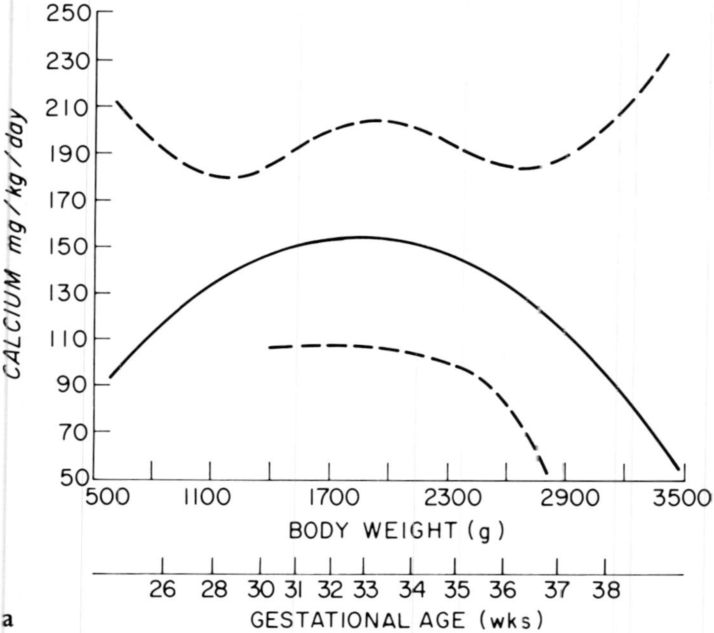

a

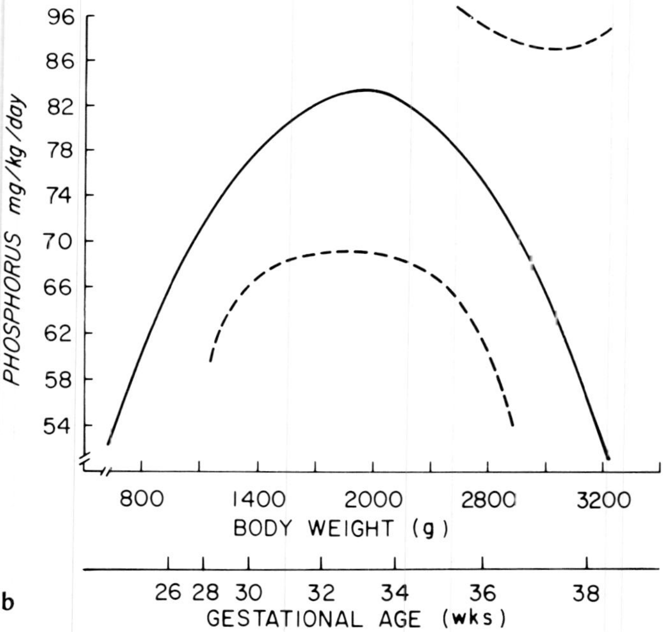

b

Figure 3 In utero (a) Ca and (b) P retention, as calculated by Thomas A. Picone, Senior Clinical Research Associate at Ross Laboratories (from ref. 257). Interrupted line represents 95% confidence limits.

of rickets in offspring of pre-eclamptic mothers is decreased transport of Ca and P to the fetus due to the "placental insufficiency" observed in this condition. In a study by Khattab and Forfar (57), it was observed that the cord blood Ca concentration was lower in infants of pre-eclamptic mothers than in normal pregnancies of similar gestation. No such difference in serum P was noted. From this study it has been suggested that placental transfer of Ca may be impaired in pre-eclampsia (57). Actual Ca transfer rates have not been measured, so a definite conclusion can not be drawn. Furthermore, many reported instances of rickets in infants of pre-eclamptic mothers have occurred in very early preterm infants, a group known to be at high risk for rickets for multiple reasons. As such, pre-eclampsia, may serve as an exacerbating factor, but appears rarely to be a principal cause of rickets of prematurity.

Formula and Human Milk Feedings. Deficiency of Ca and P is one of the main contributing factors to the development of rickets of prematurity. During the last trimester of pregnancy, the fetal skeleton accumulates about 80% of its total body Ca and P (58). Daily accretion rates during this period have been estimated at 120–140 mg Ca/kg and 60–75 mg P/kg (59,60) (Fig. 3). These accretion rates are the highest that an individual will have throughout life. With conventional feeding practices, it is difficult to supply the amounts of Ca and P required to meet intrauterine accretion rates (Table 2). Feedings of mature human milk, or commercial formula at 120 kcal/kg/day, would be expected to supply less than 60 mg Ca/kg/day or less than 90 mg Ca/kg/day, respectively (61,62). For P, the corresponding values would be less than 25 mg/kg/day or less than 70 mg/kg/day (61,62). Since absorption of these minerals is not 100%, even under ideal conditions, it becomes very clear that the preterm infant will not be able to meet the requirements for Ca and P necessary to maintain the intrauterine accretion rate.

With the resurgence of interest in human milk feeding, increasing numbers of preterm infants are being fed human milk. This practice has significant nutritional and immunological merits but, as mentioned, human milk alone is inadequate to meet the mineral needs of the growing preterm infant. Mature human milk contains about 340 mg Ca and 140 mg P/L (61). Many case reports are available describing preterm infants fed human milk who have developed rickets (63–67).

A phosphorus-depletion syndrome also has been described in preterm infants fed human milk (64–66,68). Characterized by hypophosphatemia, hypercalciuria, and hypophosphaturia, this condition appears to be due to P deficiency, which would secondarily impair Ca utilization and bone mineralization. Supplementation of the diet with Ca and P has resulted in resolution of the serum and urine abnormalities and has produced healing of rickets (64,65,68). This syndrome further emphasizes the importance of mineral deficiency in the development of rickets in the preterm infant.

Table 2 Comparison of Intrauterine Accretion Rates of Ca and P with Content of Various Formulas and Human Milk Feed at 120 Kcal/kg/day

	Ca (mg/kg/day)	P (mg/kg/day)
In utero accretion rate	120–140	60–75
Recommended daily intake[a]	up to 200	up to 113
Mature human milk[b]	61	25
Formula:		
PM 60/40 (Ross)	72	36
Similac (Ross)	92	70
Enfamil (Mead Johnson)	85	58
SMA (Wyeth)	79	59
Special Care (24 cal/oz) (Ross)	216	108
Enfamil Premature (24 cal/oz) (Mead Johnson)	143	72
SMA "Preemie" (24 cal/oz) (Wyeth)	113	60

[a]From Tsang, R. C. *Vitamin and Mineral Requirements in Preterm Infants*. New York, 1985, p. vii. Recommendation based on 2-week-old, stable, growing, 29-week gestation fetus.
[b]From ref. 61.

Soy formulas also have been associated with rickets of prematurity (49,69–71). Low retention of Ca and P has been observed with the use of soy-based formulas. Phytates are present in these preparations, which presumably form unabsorbable complexes with dietary phosphorus that thus restrict the bioavailability of P (70).

Prolonged Hyperalimentation. Several practices put the preterm infant at special risk of developing mineral deficiency and, subsequently, rickets. Many preterm infants have medical problems that can hinder the introduction of enteral feedings. As a result, these infants might receive parenteral alimentation for prolonged periods. There are many reports in the literature of preterm infants who develop rickets while receiving parenteral hyperalimentation (72–77). Because of solubility problems, it has been difficult to give adequate amounts of Ca and P in a single hyperalimentation solution without causing the precipitation of calcium phosphate crystals (72). Work by Poole et al. (78), Venkataraman et al. (79), and Eggert et al. (80) has shown that by careful manipulation of the dextrose concentration, choice of amino acid preparation, and adjustment of pH, the solubility of Ca and P can be improved (Fig. 4). The order of addition of minerals can also have a profound impact on solubility (79). Using the recommendations of Poole et al. (78) and Eggert et al. (80),

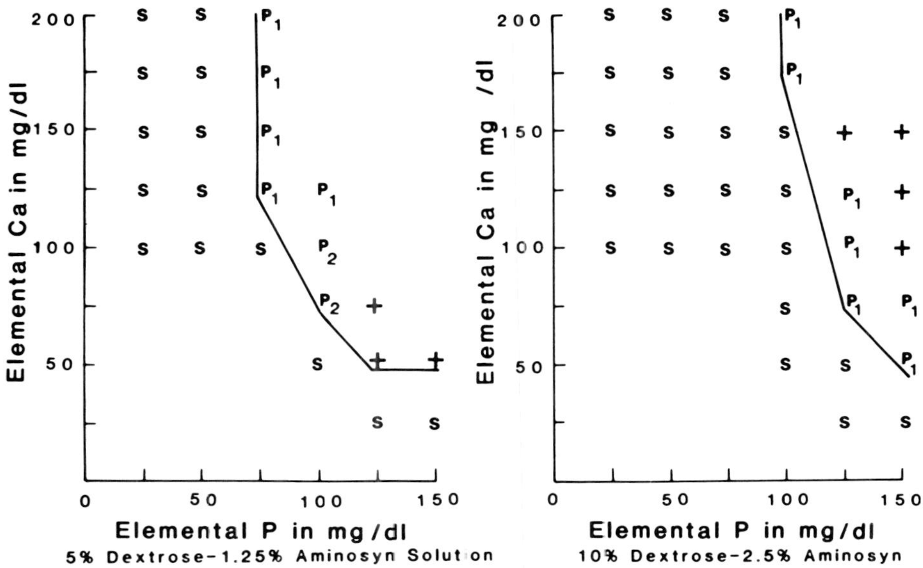

Figure 4 Solubility and stability of calcium (Ca) and phosphorus (P) in amino acid–dextrose solutions. Visual documentation of stability was confirmed by spectrophotometric absorbance studies. Precipitation observed in mixtures of Ca and P solutions at 4°C. +, immediate precipitate observed; P_1, precipitate in 24 hr; P_2, precipitate in 48 hr; S, no visible precipitate in 48 hr at 4°C. (From Venkataraman, P. S., Brissie, E. O., and Tsang, R. C. Stability of calcium and phosphate in neonatal parenteral nutrition solutions. *J. Pediatr. Gastroenterol. Nutr. 2*:641, 1983, with permission.)

hyperalimentation fluids can be prepared to administer Ca and P at rates comparable to the intrauterine accretion rates of these minerals.

Fat Malabsorption. Fat malabsorption also may contribute to mineral deficiency by reducing the bioavailability of Ca in the diet. The preterm infant appears to have an insufficient intraluminal bile salt concentration for establishment of a micelle phase and this appears to correlate with the steatorrhea observed (81,82). The unabsorbed fats are then available to interact with ionic Ca in the intestinal lumen and to form insoluble Ca soaps, which then are not available for absorption. With significant degrees of steatorrhea, Ca absorption can be greatly impaired, further reducing the supply of Ca to the developing skeleton. Although steatorrhea can be greatly reduced by administering a larger proportion of dietary fat as medium-chain triglycerides, this practice does not apparently enhance Ca absorption (83-85).

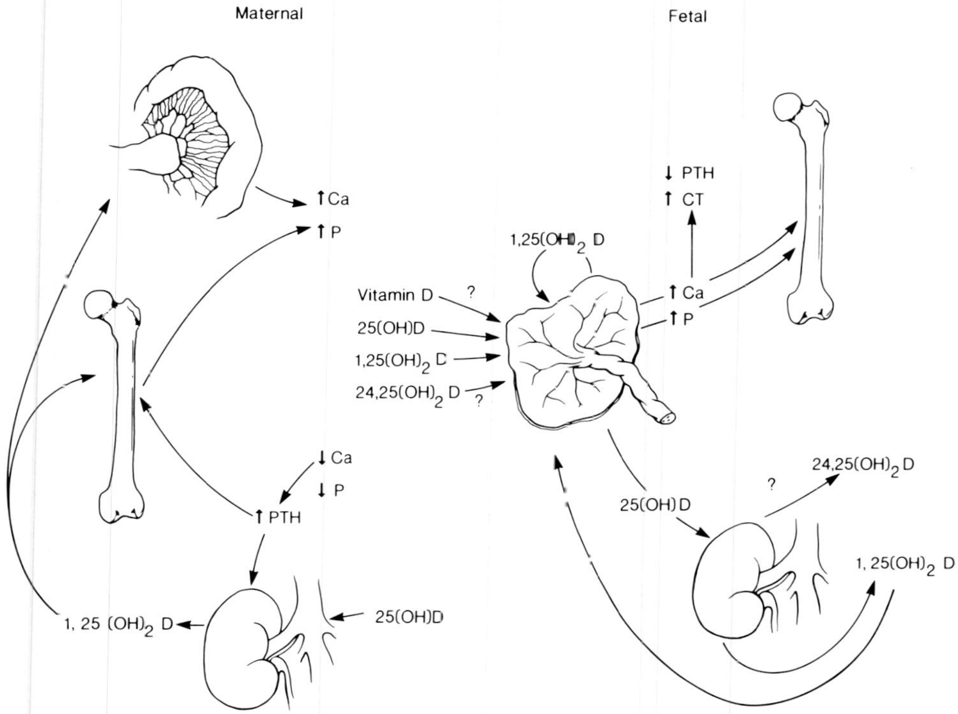

Figure 5 Maternal–fetal vitamin D metabolism. 25-Hydroxyvitamin D and 1,25-dihydroxyvitamin D cross the placenta from the maternal to the fetal circulation. The degree of placental transfer of vitamin D and its other metabolites is unclear. The placenta and the fetal kidney are capable of further metabolism of 25-hydroxyvitamin D, but the physiological significance of this with regard to placental calcium transport and fetal mineral homeostasis is unclear.

Diuretics. Furosemide, a potent loop diuretic, is well known to enhance urinary excretion of Ca (86,87). Preterm infants have been observed to develop urolithiasis and increased urinary Ca excretion while being treated with chronic furosemide therapy for a variety of medical conditions (88–91). Rickets of prematurity also has been noted in preterm infants receiving chronic diuretic therapy with furosemide (92). Other infants maintained on prolonged furosemide therapy have been shown to develop secondary hyperparathyroidism (93). In neonatal rats, Koo et al. demonstrated that chronic administration of furosemide resulted in growth failure and reduced bone mineral content proportional to the growth failure (94). In the case reports of preterm infants receiving chronic diuretics who have developed rickets of prematurity, their hospital courses usually have been complicated, with resultant poor nutritional intake. Ca, P, and vitamin

D intakes often have not been optimal and may have played roles in the evolution of rickets of prematurity. The use of diuretics possibly acts as an aggravating factor in the infants' inadequate Ca balance. Development of secondary hyperparathyroidism theoretically may compromise mineralization of bone through resorption. However, it is doubtful that diuretics are a primary cause of rickets of prematurity.

2. *Vitamin-D-Related Disorders*

The exact role of vitamin D in the development of rickets of prematurity is not clear (Fig. 5). Impaired fat-soluble vitamin absorption, decreased tissue stores of vitamin D, and organ immaturity with possible decreased responsiveness or actual end-organ resistance to the active metabolite of $1,25(OH)_2D$ theoretically may contribute to inappropriate mineral balance in the preterm infant, and the development of rickets.

Placental Transport of Vitamin D and D Metabolites. During pregnancy, the fetus presumably is dependent upon the mother, via placental transfer, for its supply of vitamin D or its metabolites. Placental transfer of vitamin D, 25(OH)D, and $1,25(OH)_2D$ has been demonstrated (82,95–98). Fetal serum concentrations of vitamin D_3 and D_2 have been found to be undetectable to very low, and it appears that 25(OH)D is the primary metabolite transferred across the placenta (99–101). The maternal and fetal concentrations of 25(OH)D are highly correlated at birth, with the former concentration being higher than the latter (102–105). The concentration of 25(OH)D at birth varies directly with the seasons, being highest in summer and lowest in winter, just as has been observed in maternal serum (106,107).

The source of $1,25(OH)_2D$ in the fetal circulation is not clear. As stated earlier, $1,25(OH)_2D$ has been observed to cross the placenta but other studies have suggested that the placenta is somewhat impermeable to this metabolite (108,109). There generally is no correlation between maternal and cord concentrations of $1,25(OH)_2D$ (100–102,105). In addition, the fetal kidney and the placenta have been shown to be capable of $1,25(OH)_2D$ production from 25(OH)D (111–116). Recent experiments in the sheep have demonstrated a fetal production rate (expressed as a function of body weight) for $1,25(OH)_2D$ almost three times that of the mother (117). From available evidence, it appears that the fetal/placental unit may be its own primary source of $1,25(OH)_2D$.

Less is known about placental transfer and metabolism of $24,25(OH)_2D$. Studies are conflicting as to the correlation between maternal and fetal concentrations at birth of this metabolite (99,100,103,118,119). Concentrations of $24,25(OH)_2D$ in maternal serum are slightly higher than or the same as those of the fetus (99,102,103,118). The contributions of placental transfer and fetal/placental unit production to the fetal blood concentration of $24,25(OH)_2D$ are not known.

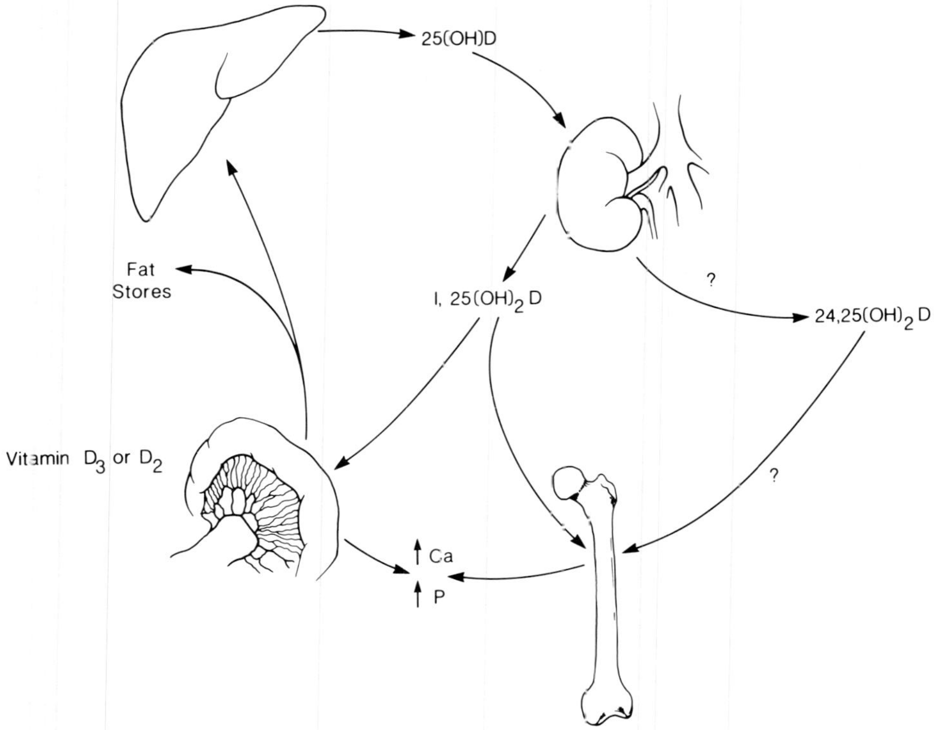

Figure 6 Preterm vitamin D metabolism. Once born, the preterm infant is dependent upon exogenous sources of vitamin D. Upon entering the circulation, vitamin D may be deposited in fat stores or hydroxylated in liver to 25(OH)D. Further hydroxylation in the kidney produces 1,25(OH)D, which then acts on the intestine to enhance Ca and phosphorus absorption, and on bone where it mediates mineral resorption. 24,25-Dihydroxyvitamin D may also be produced by the kidney, but its physiological significance is uncertain.

Experiments in weanling rats have demonstrated that adipose tissue serves as a storage site for vitamin D (120). About half of the vitamin D recovered from this site was unaltered vitamin D_3 and the other half represented other metabolites and esters of vitamin D. Preterm infants have decreased fat stores compared to full-term infants (60). Furthermore, unaltered vitamin D appears to cross the placenta to the fetus only in small quantities (99-101). As such, it would appear that adipose tissue will serve only as a minimal depot site for vitamin D in the preterm infant.

Ultraviolet Irradiation. Once born, the preterm infant essentially becomes dependent on dietary or parenteral vitamin D (Fig. 6), since ultraviolet light exposure generally will be minimal. The ability of the preterm infant to produce vitamin D in the skin through ultraviolet photoconversion of 7-dehydrocholesterol is unstudied; it is therefore not clear how effective a method this would be for maintaining vitamin D sufficiency.

Race. There is some evidence that an individual's race may have some influence on his or her vitamin D status. In the United Kingdom, vitamin-D-deficient rickets is a much more common disorder among the Asian immigrant population (121,122), mainly those from the Indian subcontinent. Specker et al., in a study of breast-feeding mothers in Cincinnati, have found that 25(OH)D serum concentrations were higher in white mothers and infants compared to their black counterparts (123). Hollis and Pittard (99) examined maternal and cord blood concentrations of vitamin D metabolites and found that white mothers had higher serum concentrations of vitamin D_3, $25(OH)D_3$, and $24,25(OH)_2D_3$ compared to blacks. The infants of both races had undetectable amounts of vitamin D in their cord blood, but white infants had higher concentrations of $25(OH)D_3$ and $24,25(OH)_2D_3$. Black mothers and infants had higher concentrations of $1,25(OH)_2D$ ($1,25(OH)_2D_3$ and $1,25(OH)_2D_2$ concentrations combined) than their white counterparts. No significant racial differences were noted with regard to vitamin D_2 metabolites.

The significance of race and its influence on an individual's vitamin D status are not clear. From the studies cited, there is some suggestion that race may have some influence, but the results probably also reflect different cultural and dietary influences. Since the neonates' mineral and vitamin D status probably are very dependent upon that of the mother and since, from available evidence, American blacks appear to be at higher risk of having a marginal vitamin D status (123,99), we believe that black infants probably should be considered at increased risk for rickets.

Dietary Vitamin D. Theoretically, absorption of vitamin D may be suboptimal in preterm infants. Absorption of vitamin D is linearly related to the dose administered, consistent with simple diffusion being the predominant mechanism by which vitamin D is absorbed (124). Vitamin D is absorbed to a greater extent in an acidic intraluminal environment than in an alkaline one (124). The presence of polyunsaturated fatty acids (linoleic and linolenic acid) has been observed to decrease the absorption of vitamin D (124). Moreover, micelle formation is essential for adequate absorption of fat soluble vitamins. The preterm infant is known to have a decreased intraluminal concentration of bile salts, which can impede micelle formation and result in reduced fat absorption (81,82). Reduced fat absorption, in turn, would increase the intraluminal concentration of polyunsaturated fats, which could further hinder vitamin D absorption. Furthermore, the neonate has reduced gastric acid production (125), which might influence intestinal intraluminal pH and reduce vitamin D absorption. Although vitamin D absorption in the preterm infants has been only minimally studied, it is clear that many factors can adversely influence its absorption.

Hepatic Metabolism of Vitamin D. Once absorbed, vitamin D must undergo C-25 hydroxylation in the liver before it can be further metabolized to its most active form. It is not known at what point in human fetal development 25-hydroxylation becomes functional. 25-Hydroxylase is a microsomal enzyme (46). In neonatal rats, the endoplasmic reticulum and its membrane-bound enzymes in hepatocytes do not appear to reach adult levels of activity until after the first week of life (126). In a study by Mendelsohn and Haddad (127), 25-hydroxylation activity was demonstrated in neonatal rats as early as 1 day after birth, but a documented increase in serum 25(OH)D concentration was not observed until 18 days after birth.

In work by Hillman and Haddad (128), an increase in serum 25(OH)D concentration was not observed until a gestational age of 36–38 weeks in preterm infants supplemented with vitamin D. This led to the speculation that 25-hydroxylation is not adequately functional until this time. In contrast, studies by other authors indicated that 25-hydroxylation reaches adequate activity at an earlier time. Markestad et al. (129,130), Glorieux et al. (131), Wolf et al. (132), Salle et al. (133), Robinson et al. (134), and Salle et al. (135), have demonstrated that preterm infants as young as 28 weeks of gestational age receiving supplements of vitamin D ranging from 500 to 2100 IU per day could maintain adequate serum concentrations of 25(OH)D (Fig. 7). Whether impairment of hepatic 25-hydroxylation is of clinical significance has not been determined. It is important to note that serum concentrations of 25(OH)D have not been consistently shown to correlate with the presence of rickets of prematurity (56, 136–142). Furthermore, elevated serum concentrations of $1,25(OH)_2D$ (the most active vitamin D metabolite) have been reported in preterm infants with rickets even with relatively low serum concentrations of 25(OH)D (143). Considering these observations, it would appear that any potential reduction in 25-hydroxylase activity in preterm infants is of minimal clinical significance.

Hepatic Disease. Liver disease has been associated with the development of rickets in both preterm and term infants. Neonatal hepatitis is strongly associated with the development of rickets (144,145). In one series, as many as 50% of infants with this disease subsequently developed rickets (145). The development of rickets does not seem to correlate with the severity of hepatic disease or the degree of steatorrhea experienced by these patients (145). Rickets is thought to be related to impaired hepatic conversion of vitamin D to 25(OH)D, producing a functional vitamin D deficiency. However, in adults 25-hydroxylation appears to be little affected in liver disease unless the disease is severe (146).

Infants receiving prolonged parenteral alimentation who have developed cholestasis have been reported with rickets (147). In these cases, it is not clear

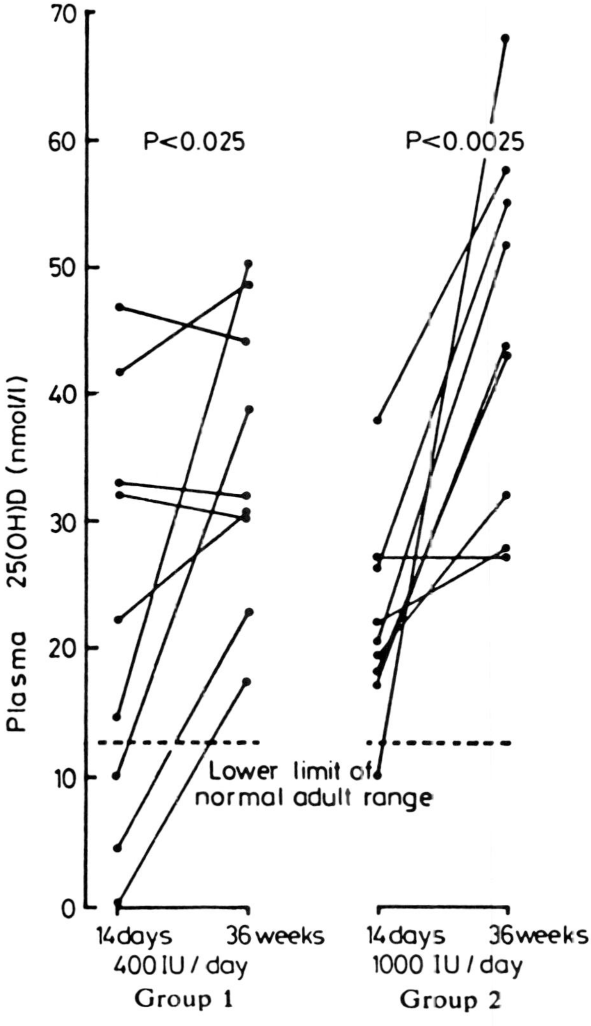

Figure 7 Plasma 25-OHD response to two daily dose regimens of vitamin D_3. Plasma concentrations measured at 14 days of life and 36 weeks postconceptual age. Group 1 had birthweights and gestational ages of 1420 ± 67 g and 31.3 ± 0.5 weeks, respectively. Group 2 had birthweights and gestational ages of 1562 ± 98 g and 30.1 ± 0.5, weeks, respectively (mean ± SEM). 1nmol of 25(OH)D/L = 40 ng of 25(OH)D/100 ml (from Robinson, M. J., Merrett, A. L., Tetlow, V. A., and Compston, J. E. Plasma 25-hydroxyvitamin D concentrations in preterm infants receiving oral vitamin D supplements. *Arch. Dis. Child.* 56:144, 1981, with permission).

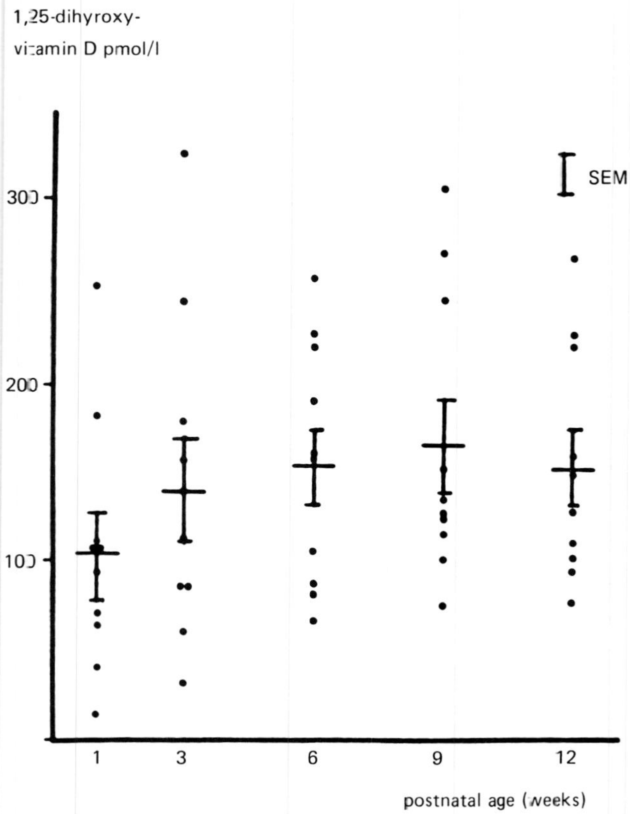

Figure 8 Individual concentrations and mean values (± SEM) of 1,25(OH)D in 10 low-birthweight infants without rickets (from Fetter, W. P. F., Mettau, J. W., Degenhart, H. J., Hoogenboezem, T., Molenaar, A., and Visser, H. K. A. Plasma 1,25-dihydroxyvitamin D concentration in preterm infants. *Acta Paediatr. Scand.* *74*:552, 1985, with permission).

that the cholestasis was a major factor in the development of bone disease, since many of these patients may have had Ca, P, or trace mineral deficiencies, which can cause metabolic bone disease. At present, cholestatic jaundice from prolonged hyperalimentation probably is not a major contributing factor to the development of rickets of prematurity.

Renal Metabolism of Vitamin D. There are no precise measurements of the preterm infants' ability to 1 alpha-hydroxylate 25(OH)D. From studies in fetal animals, the fetal kidney appears capable of producing 1,25$(OH)_2$D from 25(OH)D (111,112,148,149). After fetal nephrectomy in sheep during the latter part of pregnancy, a marked decrease in fetal serum 1,25$(OH)_2$D concentration was observed, consistent with the thesis that this organ is a primary site of production prior to term (150). In full-term infants, serum concentrations of 1,25$(OH)_2$D have been reported to increase to adult levels by 24 hr of age (110). Work by Markestad et al. (130), and Fetter et al. (151), in preterm infants with gestational ages of 28-36 weeks, demonstrated a significant increase in the concentration of 1,25$(OH)_2$D by the end of the first week of life (Fig. 8). Moreover, Glorieux et al. (131), in preterm infants ranging from 32-37 weeks of gestation, noted a threefold increase in 1,25$(OH)_2$D serum concentration by 5 days of age, but only in those infants that had received an oral supplement of 2100 IU vitamin D_3 per day. Furthermore, there are several reports of preterm infants with rickets who have markedly elevated serum concentrations of 1,25$(OH)_2$D at the time of diagnosis (137,143,149). From the studies presented, it can be concluded that renal 1 alpha-hydroxylase appears present during the latter portion of gestation and that within a week of birth it is sufficiently functional to meet the 1,25$(OH)_2$D requirements of the preterm infant.

As mentioned earlier, the exact role of the 24,25$(OH)_2$D metabolite is not known, but it has been speculated to have a role in bone mineralization (38,37). The ability of the preterm infant to perform 24-hydroxylation is unstudied. Fetal sheep and embryonic chick have been demonstrated to have functional 24-hydroxylase activity (148,149). In a study by Danan et al., the fetal rat was observed to have higher serum concentrations of 24,25$(OH)_2$D than its mother, but fetal concentrations were comparable to those of nonpregnant control rats (119). At the time of delivery, fetal concentrations of 24,25$(OH)_2$D have been found to be less than or nearly equal to maternal concentrations in humans, pigs, and cattle (101,103,118). In humans, both fetal cord and maternal serum concentrations tend to be below those of the general adult population (118). During the first year of life, concentrations of 24,25$(OH)_2$D tend to remain relatively constant and stay below those found in adults (152). When measured by Markestad et al., plasma concentrations of 24,25$(OH)_2$D were found to be consistently lower in preterm infants of 28-36 weeks gestational age than in adults (130). The values reported, however, are similar to those reported in normal infants who were born at term during the first year of life (130).

The activity of renal 24-hydroxylase appears to be regulated by 1,25$(OH)_2$D, and PTH (26-28,153-156). The administration of 1,25$(OH)_2$D to vitamin-D-deficient chicks and rats, or 1,25$(OH)_2$D administration in the culture media of rhesus monkey kidney cells, results in a marked increase in 24-hydroxylation of 25(OH)D (26-28,153). Using rhesus monkey kidney and vitamin-D-deficient chick kidney cells, it was observed that 24-hydroxylation was suppressed (26, 27) by the addition of PTH to the culture media. As noted earlier, preterm infants with rickets of prematurity can have elevated concentrations of 1,25$(OH)_2$D. Other affected infants also have been noted to have secondary hyperparathyroidism with elevated PTH concentrations (93). These two factors might act to suppress 24-hydroxylase activity in the preterm infant.

It would appear from the available information that the preterm infant probably can produce $24,25(OH)_2D$ from 25(OH)D, but some conditions may prevent optimal production of this metabolite. Whether the 24-hydroxylation step, and $24,25(OH)_2D$ are of physiological significance for the preterm infant has yet to be determined.

End-Organ Responsiveness. An important issue involving the role of vitamin D in rickets of prematurity is the responsiveness of target organs to $1,25(OH)_2D$. In the intestine, $1,25(OH)_2D$ interacts with a specific receptor on the enterocyte, which results in the production of calcium-binding protein (157) and stimulates the active absorption of Ca and P from the intestinal lumen (158). In rat pups born to vitamin-D-replete or vitamin-D-deficient mothers, no difference in active Ca transport, as measured in everted duodenal gut sacs, was observed until about the time of weaning (about 3 weeks of age) (159). At this time, active Ca transport was three times greater in pups born to vitamin-D-replete mothers than in their vitamin-D-deficient counterparts.

Neonatal rat pups have very low concentrations of calcium-binding protein in the intestine until about the time of weaning (17–22 days after birth) at which time a marked increase is noted (160). Halloran and DeLuca (161) have shown also in neonatal rats that at 14 days of age intestinal receptor for $1,25(OH)_2D$ is present at concentrations of about 10% of those found in the adult. This increases to 50% by 21 days of age and becomes comparable to adult concentrations by 28 days (161). From these studies it is clear that in the neonatal rat, intestinal responsiveness to $1,25(OH)_2D$ matures after delivery and is timed with the appearance of calcium-binding protein and receptors for this metabolite.

The timing of these events in humans is unknown. In a study by Senterre and Salle (162), Ca absorption was measured in preterm infants (mean gestational age, 32 weeks at birth) receiving breast milk with or without vitamin D supplementation and two other groups receiving a formula with or without vitamin D supplementation. Within both feeding groups, the vitamin-D-supplemented groups had significantly higher percentage absorption of Ca (human milk Ca was 49% with no supplemental D vs. 70% in the supplemented group; for the formula-fed group, 20% in the unsupplemented group vs. 32% in the supplemented group). It appears either that the vitamin-D-dependent active transport mechanism in the human intestine is present prior to the term date, or that intestinal maturation is accelerated by preterm delivery and occurs within 2–4 weeks of birth. Since the absorption of Ca was 49% and 20% in the non-D-supplemented groups, one additional implication is that non-D-dependent transport mechanisms for Ca are operative at this time as well.

Table 3 Diagnosis of Rickets of Prematurity

Serum:	
Ca	↓, NL, ↑
P	↓, NL
25(OH)D	↓, NL, ↑
1,25(OH)D	↑
PTH	NL, ↑
Alkaline phosphatase[a]	NL, ↑
Urine:	
Ca	NL, ↑[b]
P (tubular reabsorption)	↓, NL, ↑
Amino acids	NL, ↑

Summary of reported biochemical abnormalities associated with rickets of prematurity.
↑ = increased, NL = normal, ↓ = decreased
[a]Depressed activities observed in malnutrition and zinc deficiency.
[b]Increase in urinary Ca tends to be seen only with P depletion, as seen with breast milk feedings.

In a study by Shenai et al. (163), an experimental formula with high concentrations of Ca and P was used and preterm infants demonstrated mineral accretion rates similar to those reported during intrauterine life. Again, from this study it appears that mineral absorption mechanisms (whether D-dependent or D-independent) are not impaired in the preterm infant. In summary, intestinal end-organ responsiveness to $1,25(OH)_2D$ may be intact in preterm infants and may not be specifically relevant to the development of rickets of prematurity.

C. Presentation and Diagnosis

In classic vitamin-D-deficient rickets, infants will present with craniotabes, palpable or visible enlargement of the costochondral junction of the ribs (the "rachitic rosary"), and thickening of the wrists and ankles. Deformities of the spine, pelvis, and extremities along with ligamentous laxity and hypotonia also may be present (164). The classic signs of rickets are not always present when the diagnosis of rickets of prematurity is made (50,52,66,69,76,137,139). Preterm infants with rickets may have an enlarged anterior fontanel or a rachitic rosary (63–65,69,74,143). It is not uncommon for the diagnosis to be made as an incidental finding on a radiograph (56,69,75,77,138,139,165,166). Fractures of ribs or an extremity will often lead to the detection of rickets (67,69,76,77,137, 139,143,165,166). A rachitic respiratory distress syndrome also has been described, characterized by gradual progressive respiratory decompensation, occasionally associated with an expiratory wheeze (55,56,76,167,168). In such

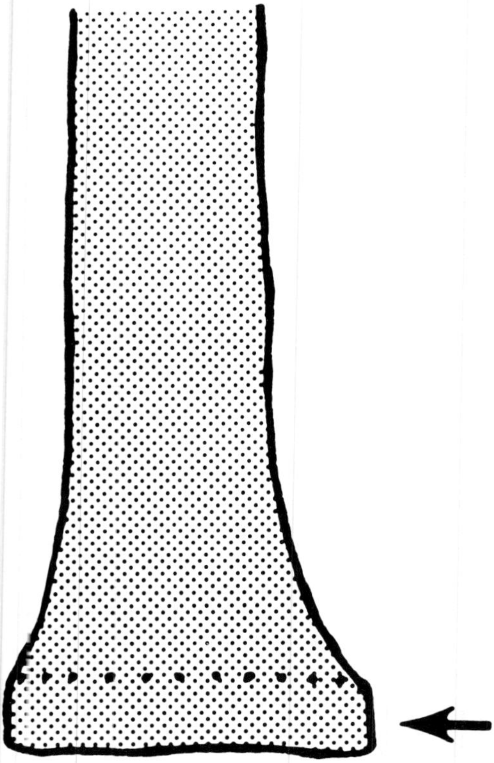

Figure 9 The Laval-Jeantet (L-J) ring (indicated by arrow) is the short straight segment of the distal metaphysis of the radius and/or ulna. This represents the surrounding perichondral ring and groove. The L-J ring is seen in normal infants. Loss of this structure is an early finding in infants with rickets and hypothyroidism (from Oestreich, A. E., and Crawford, A. H. *Atlas of Pediatric Orthopedic Radiology*. Thieme, Stuttgart, 1985, p. 159, with permission).

patients the chest x-ray often reveals the first evidence of rickets: demineralization of the ribs and splaying of the anterior rib ends. Resolution of respiratory symptoms is not observed until healing of rickets is noted.

Preterm infants usually will present with rickets from about a month of postnatal age to about 5 months of age, with 2–4 months being the most common time of diagnosis (49,50,63–65,67–70,74,76,92,137–140,143,147,167). In addition to physical findings, biochemical abnormalities often will be present at the time of diagnosis (Table 3). Unfortunately biochemical abnormalities can vary greatly in their pattern and usually are not diagnostic for rickets (Table 3). Serum Ca concentration is often normal, but occasionally will be low, or even elevated, especially if serum P concentrations are low (49,63,64,66,67,74,76, 77,92, 133,137-140,143,169,170). Serum P concentration may also be normal, but commonly will be depressed (49,63,64,66,67,70,74,76,92,137,138,140,143, 147,170). Measurements of serum 25(OH)D concentration may be low, normal, or high (49,56,63,66,136-142,169). In contrast, elevated concentrations of 1,25$(OH)_2$D have been reported in rickets of prematurity (49,63,64,66,75,137, 138,143). Serum concentrations of PTH have been variously reported as normal to elevated in rickets of prematurity (50,63-66,75,137,138,143).

Serum alkaline phosphatase activity can not be relied upon to make a biochemical diagnosis of rickets of prematurity. In most cases the activity of this enzyme will be increased (49,63,64,66,67,70,77,92,137-139,143,169,171-175) but, the presence of isoenzymes from non-bone sources, variations in the technique of measurement, and the wide normal range in growing infants undermine the reliability of alkaline phosphatase as a marker for rickets of prematurity. It also has been observed that malnourished children with rickets will have normal serum alkaline phosphatase activity (176). With institution of a high-protein diet, a significant elevation of alkaline phosphatase was observed. Zinc deficiency also will reduce serum alkaline phosphatase activity (177). Urinary findings may be significant. Hypercalciuria and very high tubular reabsorption of P may be observed when P deficiency is a major factor (64,65). These findings have also been observed in adults and experimental animals made P deficient (178-180). Supplementation with P results in a decrease in urinary Ca and the tubular reabsorption of P returns to normal. A generalized renal aminoaciduria, as is reported in classic vitamin-D-deficient rickets, also has been observed in rickets of prematurity (75,76,137,181,182).

Currently, radiographic studies remain the best means of diagnosing rickets of prematurity. A few points must be borne in mind when examining radiographs for evidence of rickets of prematurity. First, histologic changes are apparent in bone before rickets is detectable by x-rays. Second, during the first half-year of life, normally the distal surface of the ulnar metaphysis (the zone of provisional calcification) shows a slight degree of concavity. Finally, during the first year of life in normal hand radiographs, at the medial and lateral margins of the distal radial and ulnar metaphyses there is usually a longitudinal straight segment, the so called Laval-Jeantet ring (183) (Fig. 9).

The earliest radiographic findings in rickets of prematurity may be rarefaction of bone and loss of the straight edge of the Laval-Jeantet ring. The latter finding may also be present in hypothyroidism. Rarefaction of bone may be observed as early as the second week of postnatal life (184). Delayed ossification of the hamate and capitate growth centers beyond that expected by the individual's degree of prematurity (normal ossification has begun by 3 months in term infants) should suggest the diagnosis of rickets. If other secondary growth centers are present, their margins will be less sharp than normal. Metaphyseal cupping at

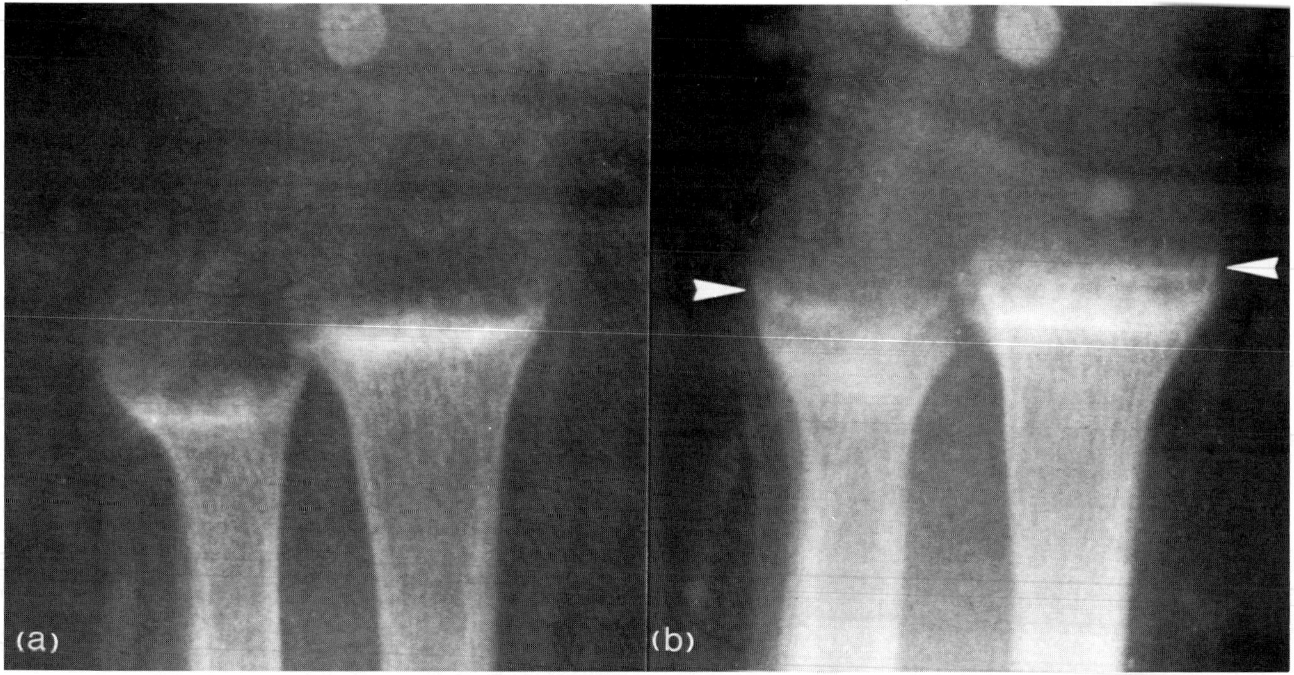

Figure 10 Radiograph of distal radius and ulna showing florid rickets. a. Absence of Laval-Jeantet ring. b. Radiograph taken 17 days later demonstrates healing calcification with reappearance of L-J ring (from Oestreich, A. E., and Crawford, A.H. *Atlas of Pediatric Radiology*. Thieme, Stuttgart, 1985, p. 159, with permission).

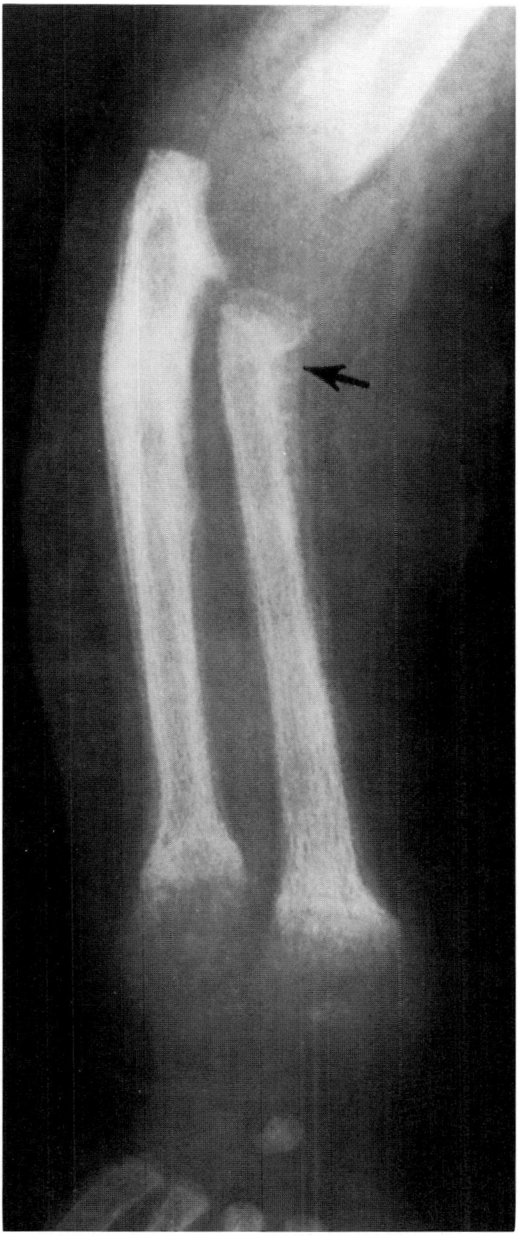

Figure 11 Marked rickets in an infant. The pertinent findings are the presence of cupped, frayed metaphysics; increased distance between the distal radius metaphysis and its indistinct growth center; and severe secondary hyperparathyroidism with washed-out, unsharp cortices. Dark arrow indicates fracture in proximal radius (from Oestreich, E., and Crawford, A. H. *Atlas of Pediatric Orthopedic Radiology*, Thieme, Stuttgart, 1985, p. 97, with permission).

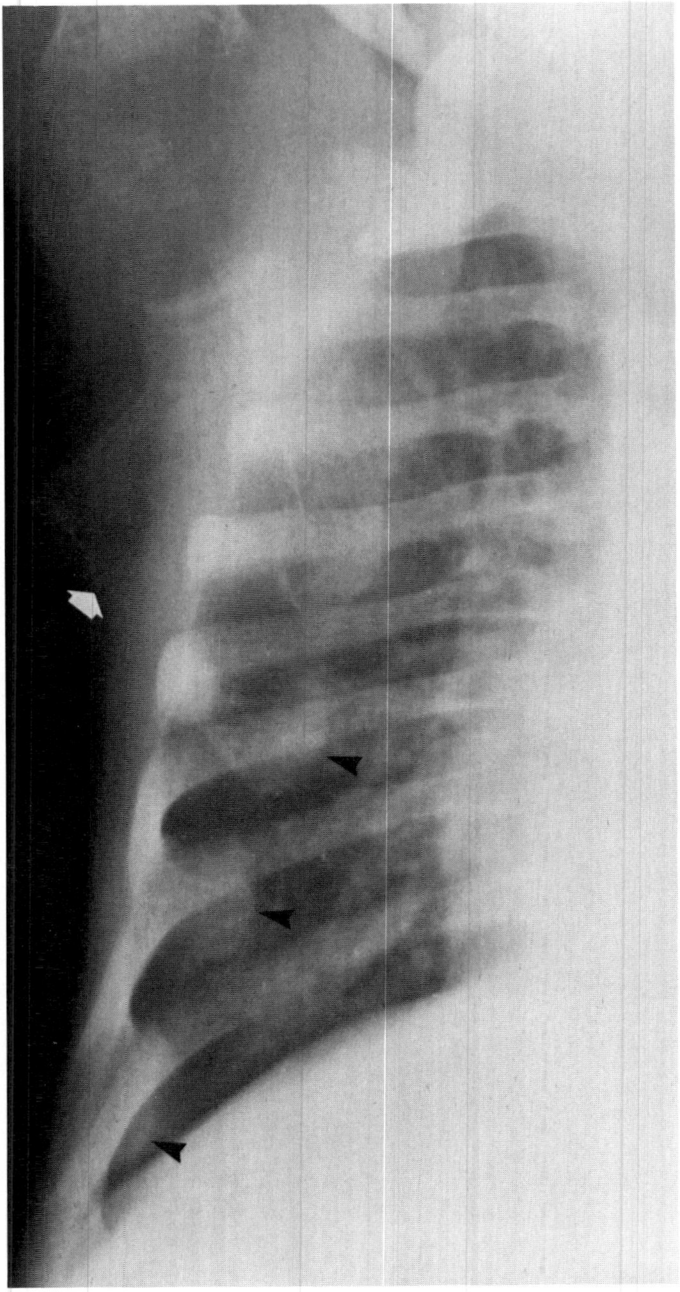

Figure 12 Radiological rachitic rosary (dark arrows). This radiograph demonstrates the splayed anterior rib ends of the rachitic rosary (from Oestreich, A. E., and Crawford, A. H. *Atlas of Pediatric Orthopedic Radiology*. Thieme, Stuttgart, 1985, p. 97, with permission).

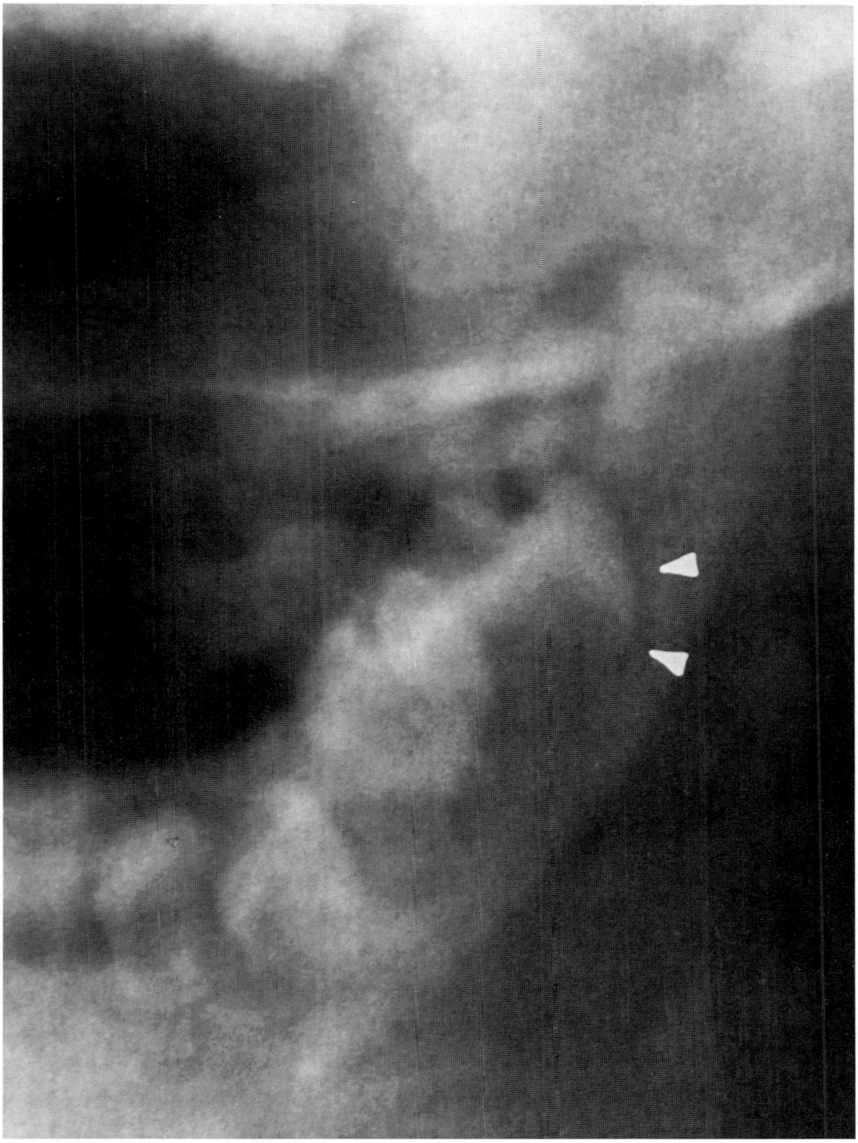

Figure 13 Absence of lamina dura surrounding teeth in the mandible, a manifestation of secondary hyperparathyroidism (arrowheads) (from Oestreich, A. E., and Crawford, A. H. *Atlas of Pediatric Orthopedic Radiology*. Thieme, Stuttgart, 1985, p. 98, with permission).

the ends of long bones (especially the distal ulna and radius) in excess of the normal concavity, along with fraying and transverse indexing of the metaphyseal margin, are radiological signs of rickets as might be observed in older children (Figs. 10, 11). Demineralization of the ribs with splaying of the anterior rib ends also can be observed on the chest radiograph in preterm infants with rickets (Fig. 12). Periosteal new bone formation may be noted along the inferior border of the mandible and the shafts of long bones. The former finding has been referred to as the "mandibular mantle" sign (168). Furthermore, signs of hyperparathyroidism (unless due to primary hyperparathyroidism) should suggest the diagnosis of rickets. Such signs are "washed-out" poorly defined cortices, multiple small fractures, loss of the lamina dura dense line around tooth roots, and loss of the well-defined line around the crypts of unerupted teeth (185) (Figure 12 and 13).

Besides the current radiological and biochemical tests, other experimental modalities may become available in the future and may prove of value in the diagnosis of rickets of prematurity. Photon absorptiometry is presently being utilized as a research tool to measure the mineral content of bone (186). In this method, a well-collimated photon beam from a ^{125}I or ^{241}Am source is moved across the bone to be scanned. The transmittance of the beam is measured with a scintillation photon detector that moves simultaneously with the source. Logarithmic transformations of the transmitted counts are plotted as an absorption curve, with the area under the resulting curve being proportional to the bone mineral mass in the cross-section of the scanned bone.

Work by Minton et al. (187), Greer et al. (188,189), Chan et al. (190,191), Roberts et al. (192), and Steichen et al. (193) have shown that this method can be successfully adapted to measurement of bone mineral content in infants (Figs. 14, 15). With the establishment of accurate norms for bone mineral content in preterm and term infants, this method should prove to be sensitive enough to detect significant bone demineralization before radiological evidence of rickets is apparent. At the current state of our knowledge, photon absorptiometry is useful only as a research tool.

Osteocalcin, the major noncollagenous bone protein, also may prove of value in the diagnosis of rickets of prematurity. In humans the protein contains two residues of the vitamin-K-dependent amino acid gamma-carboxyglutamic acid (194). With increased serum concentrations of $1,25(OH)_2D$, serum concentrations of this protein have been noted to increase (195). Increased serum concentrations of osteocalcin have been observed in disorders associated with increased bone resorption, such as hyperparathyroidism, Paget's disease, and recent fracture (196,197). Studies by Delmas et al. (198) have demonstrated increased serum concentrations of osteocalcin in conditions associated with increased bone turnover. At birth, cord serum values were consistently higher than maternal values (199). In a study by Pettifor et al., a group of very-low-birth-

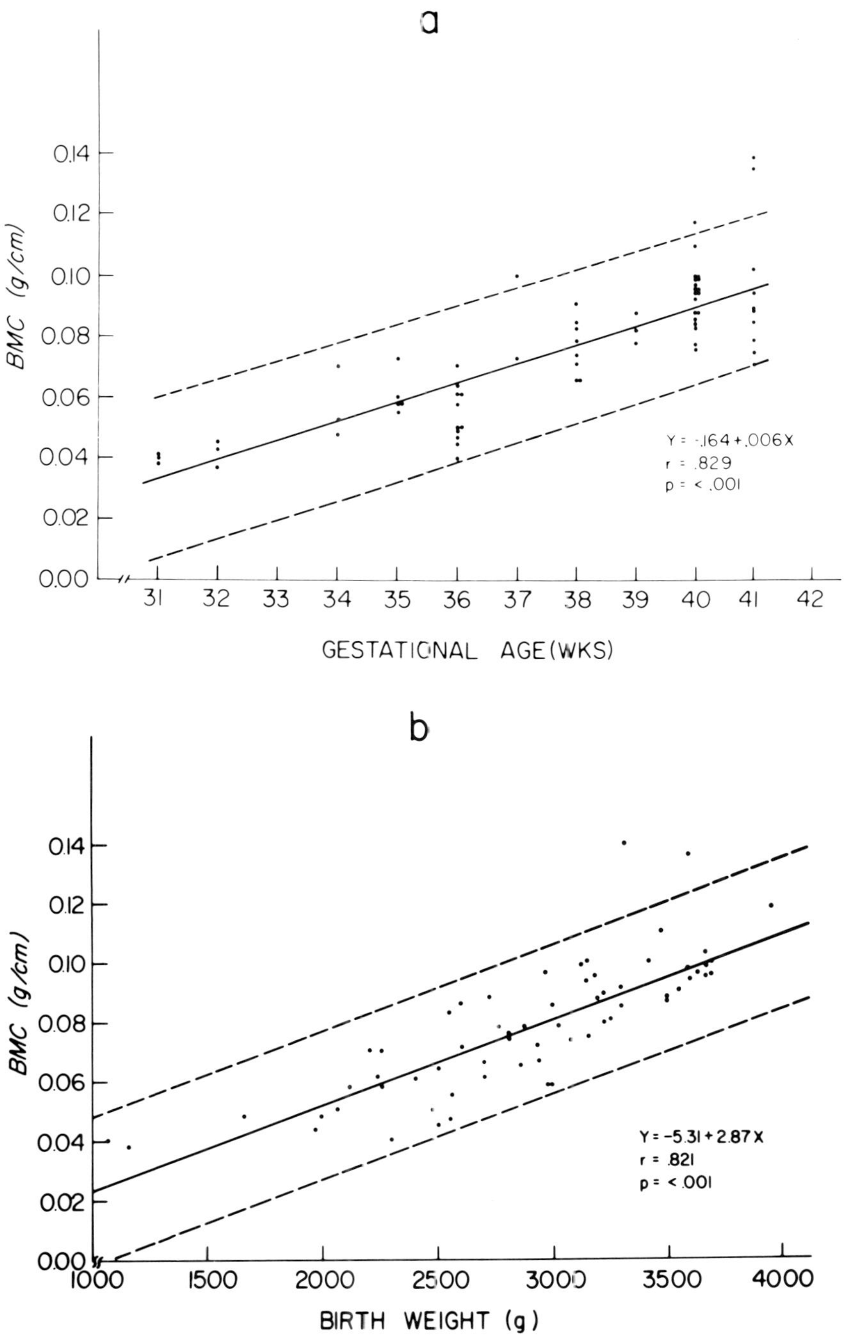

Figure 14 Bone mineral content (BMC) in preterm and term infants in relation to (a) gestational age and (b) birthweight. Lines indicate the regression line for BMC with the 95% confidence limits for the sample (from Minton, S. D., Steichen, J. J., and Tsang, R. C. Bone mineral content in term and preterm appropriate-for-gestational-age infants. *J. Pediatr. 95*:1039, 1979, with permission).

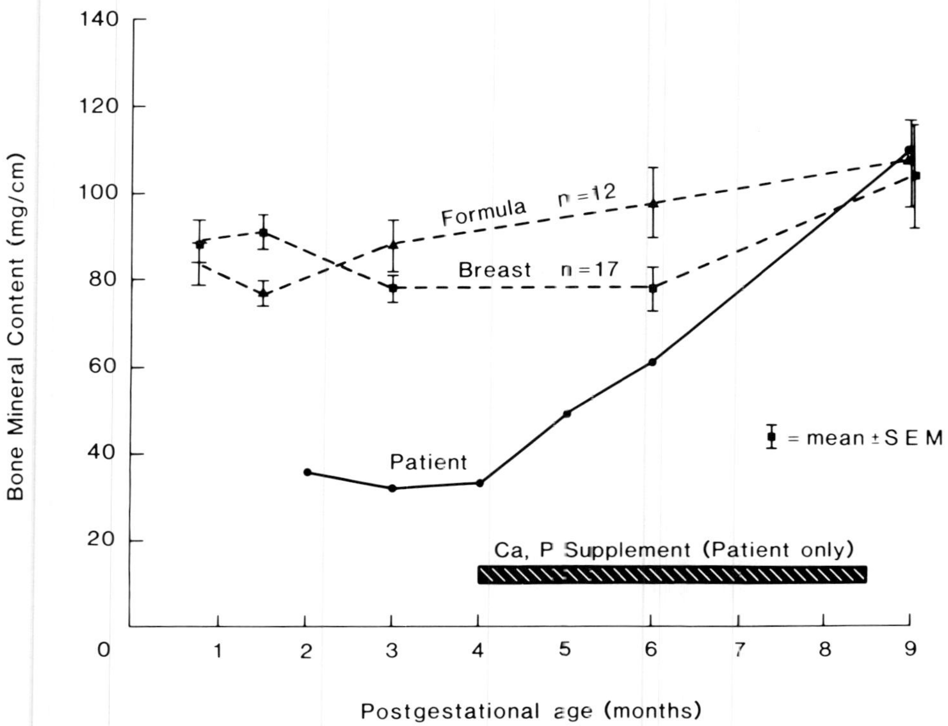

Figure 15 Bone mineral content of left radius shows response to Ca and P supplementation. Patient compared to 12 full-term formula-fed infants (Similac, 20 cal/oz) and 17 full-term breastfed infants (from Greer, F. R., Steichen, J. J., and Tsang, R. C. Calcium and phosphate supplements in breast milk-related rickets: Results in a very-low-birth-weight infant. *Am. J. Dis. Child. 136*:582, 1982, with permission).

weight infants demonstrated a significant rise in serum osteocalcin concentration after birth that was positively correlated with serum alkaline phosphatase activity (136). Since osteocalcin is a protein specific to bone and its production does not appear to be dependent on adequate body stores of zinc, it may not be subject to as many of the factors that make alkaline phosphatase an unreliable marker of bone disease in the preterm infant.

Gamma-carboxyglutamic acid (Gla), a breakdown product of osteocalcin and other vitamin-K-dependent proteins, can be measured in urine (200). If nonbone sources of Gla remain stable, changes in urinary excretion of this amino acid should reflect bone turnover or loss. In adult patients with osteoporosis, urinary Gla excretion has been found to be elevated, which is thought to be related to bone resorption in excess of formation. In Paget's disease of bone, urinary Gla excretion was found to be normal (201) and thought to represent a balance between bone formation and bone resorption. Measurement of urinary Gla excretion may be of potential value in rickets of prematurity, where bone resorption could be excessive due to secondary hyperparathyroidism and/or elevated serum $1,25(OH)_2D$ concentrations.

One additional bone protein that also may have some potential value in the diagnosis of rickets of prematurity is bone morphogenetic protein. This protein circulates in blood at detectable levels and is increased in growing children and in patients with Paget's disease (202). Like osteocalcin and Gla, bone morphogenetic protein may be a specific marker of bone turnover and might prove of value in detecting rickets of prematurity.

In summary, no one biochemical measurement is a reliable indicator of rickets of prematurity. For "screening purposes," it would seem reasonable to obtain measurements of serum Ca, P, and alkaline phosphatase. With the combination of a low serum P concentration (less than 4 mg/dl) and increased alkaline phosphatase activity (greater than 500 IU/L), a radiograph of the wrist is required to determine whether rickets is present. Even with normal results from screening tests, a radiograph of the wrist would still be of value at 3–4 months postnatal age, to ensure that rickets of prematurity is not missed. Urine "screening" for hypercalciuria (a urinary Ca level $>$ 100 mg/24 hr per 1.73 m^2) (203) and hypophosphaturia (a tubular reabsorption of P, expressed as a function of creatinine clearance, greater than 95%) also may be of value in early detection of rickets of prematurity.

D. Differential Diagnosis

Several conditions can present with bone disease in infancy and can be confused with rickets of prematurity or congenital rickets. With the use of a few historical facts and simple laboratory tests, these disorders usually can be readily differentiated.

Trace mineral deficiency can produce bone disease in preterm infants. Neonates with complicated clinical courses and who have required prolonged intravenous alimentation, or who have received suboptimal nutrition, are the most likely to present with this problem. Copper deficiency is the best characterized with regard to observed skeletal changes. Often, affected individuals will demonstrate osteoporosis with blurring and cupping of the metaphyses on radiographs of long bones (204–209). Subperiosteal new bone formation is a prominent feature (208,209). Copper deficiency also will be associated with failure to thrive, apathy, hypotonia, and seborrheic dermatitis. On laboratory examination, anemia with neutropenia will be observed along with decreased serum concentrations of copper and ceruloplasmin. Usually serum Ca and P concentrations will be normal, although hypocalcemia has been observed in one case report (207).

Zinc is another trace mineral associated with a well-recognized deficiency syndrome. In humans, affected individuals tend to present with skin manifestations characterized by a periorificial, exfoliative, erythematous dermatitis that may be associated with diarrhea (210–214). Depressed serum concentrations of zinc and zinc-dependent enzymes, such as alkaline phosphatase, also will be observed. In postnatal rats, pigs, and rhesus monkeys maintained on zinc-deficient diets, hypomineralization and maturational delay of the skeleton have been observed (215–217). A corresponding skeletal condition in the human has not been identified, but it remains a possibility.

Vitamin C deficiency has the potential of being confused with rickets of prematurity. Infants with scurvy may present with fractures and swelling of the costochondral junction. Radiographic osteopenia, subperiosteal hematomas with calcification, and a ground-glass appearance of the shafts of long bones are prominent features (218,219). Review of the dietary history should point to an inadequate intact of vitamin C, and a low plasma concentration of this vitamin (less than 0.2 mg/dl) (220) should confirm the diagnosis of scurvy.

Hypervitaminosis A is another condition that can present similarly to rickets. Clinical presentation is characterized by tender swellings (most commonly in the forearms), limitation of motion, hyperirritability, craniotabes, and, occasionally, fractures (219,221). Radiological features include thickening of the cortex and metaphyseal irregularity (219,221,222). As with scurvy, review of the dietary history usually reveals the cause of the infant's difficulties. Vitamin A intake is usually excessive and prolonged, 80,000–500,000 IU/day for more than 6 months. Persson et al. (222) have reported vitamin A intoxication in infants less than a year of age with relatively low daily dosage (18,000–60,000 IU per day) and for a briefer duration than usually expected (only 1–2 months). Confirmation of the diagnosis can be made by finding an elevated serum concentration of vitamin A (normal plasma concentration as measured in 3,500 preschool children: 33.7 μg/dl ± 7.6 μg/dl; mean ± S.D.) (223).

Hypophosphatasia is an inherited skeletal disorder that can present in the neonatal period. The spectrum of disease is variable, ranging from the severe congenital form, which can be confused with short-limbed dwarfism of osteogenesis imperfecta congenita, to a mild form that may not become evident until late in childhood (224). On radiographs, hypophosphatasia can resemble rickets with poor skeletal ossification and marked metaphyseal irregularities (184,224). Serum studies will reveal normal to elevated Ca levels, normal P levels, and markedly decreased alkaline phosphatase concentrations. Phosphoethanolamine excretion in the urine is increased (224). Hypophosphatasia is inherited as an autosomal recessive trait (224). Parental consanguinity, previously affected children, and a radiological picture similar to rickets, accompanied by normal serum mineral concentrations (or, occasionally, a high serum Ca concentration) and low alkaline phosphatase activity should make one entertain the possibility of this disorder.

The final group of disorders to be briefly considered are vitamin-D-dependent and vitamin-D-resistant rickets. It is unlikely that this group of inherited disorders of vitamin D metabolism would be confused with rickets of prematurity or congenital rickets. At birth, infants so affected appear perfectly normal and usually do not present with problems until a year of age, when they have difficulty walking and develop bowing of the extremities. Usually, by this time affected individuals have hypophosphatemia and elevated serum alkaline phosphatase activity. Serum concentrations of 25(OH)D are normal. Radiological and biochemical abnormalities usually are present before a year of age, but unless there is a positive family history of these conditions to prompt early investigation, the diagnosis usually is not made until later when clinical signs are more apparent (225-230).

E. Complications

The most common complication encountered in rickets of prematurity is fractures. The exact incidence of fractures in patients with this condition is not known, but from reported cases, a significant percentage of preterm infants present with fractures of ribs or long bones (67,69,76,77,137,139,143,165,166). Often retrospective review of x-rays will reveal previously unrecognized fractures (76,77,138,147,167). Brittle rachitic bones are more prone to fracture with little trauma. Routine handling by nursery personnel and chest physiotherapy apparently can provide sufficient force to result in broken bones. With resolution of rickets, healing of fractures is observed, and no long-term deformities have been reported.

In addition to fractures, a phosphate-depletion syndrome has been observed and may account for some of the problems encountered in rickets of prematurity. In adults, phosphate depletion has been associated with hypophosphatemia, hypophosphaturia, hypercalciuria, and increased resorption of skeletal Ca and P (178). Some reported constitutional symptoms have been anorexia, weakness, malaise, and bone pain (178,179,231). Acute respiratory failure (231) and impaired cardiac function (232,233) responsive to phosphate replacement also have been reported. Travis et al. have observed decreased erythrocyte 2,3-diphosphoglycerate and adenosine triphosphate, with a marked increase in red cell oxygen affinity in individuals who became hypophosphatemic while receiving parenteral nutrition (234).

The development of respiratory difficulty in the face of mild lung disease has been observed by Glasgow and Thomas, and others, in infants with rickets of prematurity (65,76,167,168). The respiratory difficulties were not observed to improve until healing of rickets was noted. The exact cause of this "rachitic respiratory distress" is not clear and has been presumed to be secondary to impaired structural support of the lungs by a demineralized rib cage that often has multiple fractures and/or muscular dysfunction. From what has been observed in adults, it would seem possible that phosphorus depletion, in addition to contributing to the development of rickets in the preterm infant, might, at least in part, explain some of the respiratory and cardiovascular problems these infants encountered.

F. Prevention and Therapy

The ideal preventive strategy or treatment for rickets of prematurity has not been defined. Resolution of bone lesions has been reported with administration of Ca alone (235), P alone (64,66), a combination of Ca and P (63,65,143), and extra vitamin D or one of its metabolites (67,76,77,92,137,138,140,147,236, 237). To confuse the issue further, spontaneous resolution of rickets in preterm infants also has been observed (49,140).

The "gold standard" that has been applied to term infants with regard to Ca and P requirements is the intrauterine accretion rate. As mentioned earlier, during the last trimester of pregnancy, the daily net accretion rates of Ca and P average between 120-140 mg/kg and 60-75 mg/kg, respectively. From review of the literature, Zeigler et al. (58) have estimated that the intestinal absorption rates for Ca and P in the preterm infant are 65% and 80%, respectively. A minimum daily intake of elemental Ca and P of 215 mg/kg and 90 mg/kg, respectively, might be expected to supply sufficient minerals to maintain the intrauterine accretion rates in the preterm infant. Whether normal bone development can be maintained on this or some other intake is not specifically known. With the use of human milk or conventional commercial formula, supplementation with Ca and P will be required to meet the intake of these minerals necessary to equal intrauterine accretion rates (Table 2). Formulas designed specifically for the preterm infant, with high Ca and P contents, may prove successful in meeting the special mineral requirements of these infants (163).

When supplementation is instituted, care must be taken in choosing the preparations of Ca and P. Liquid preparations tend to be easier to use, in that they are more readily mixed with the infant's feedings. Calcium lactate in its tablet form is poorly soluble in milk, so that the calcium in solution will be less than the intended amount (238). Ca glubionate, Ca gluceptate, and Ca gluconate all come in liquid preparations and are readily available. Ca glubionate, however, in its proprietary liquid forms, contains 20% sucrose and has a high osmolarity. It has been observed to produce increased frequency of stooling in preterm infants (239) and diarrhea in young infants (238). Thus, Ca gluconate and Ca gluceptate would appear to be the most appropriate Ca salts to use in supplementing preterm infant feedings.

The administration of phosphate as a supplement also presents its problems. In the form of its monobasic salt, P can present a significant acid load to the preterm infant's kidney, and lead to the development of metabolic acidosis. By administering a mixture of mono and dibasic P salts, this problem can be avoided (240). Both sodium and potassium P salts are available; sodium and potassium overload therefore must be guarded against. As such, the P supplement should be manipulated to meet the special electrolyte requirements of each infant.

A further problem that can be encountered is the precipitation of Ca and P when the two supplements are mixed together. To avoid this problem, the P should be added to the milk first and thoroughly mixed before the Ca is added. This allows the P to complex with other constituents in the feeding so that it is not available to precipitate with Ca. Another alternative might be to administer the Ca and P supplements at separate times, for example, before and after a feeding. However, this mode of administration might result in alternating swings in the concentrations of Ca and P. Since this approach has never been studied, it cannot be recommended.

When instituting mineral supplementation, the initial dosage could be started at about half the final desired concentration and increased by 25% every 3–4 days. During supplementation, serum Ca and P concentrations and urinary fractional excretion of Ca and P should be monitored at least once or twice a week. Hypercalcemia and hyperphosphatemia should be avoided and the dosage of supplements adjusted if these occur. With phosphorus depletion, the urinary fractional excretion of Ca is elevated and the excretion of P is very near zero (64). In this situation the aim of supplementation should be to maintain the fractional excretion of P in the 3-5% range; a marked decrease in the urinary fractional excretion of Ca also should be observed (65,240).

An alternative to the use of Ca and P supplements is the use of complementary formulas with high Ca and P contents. Commercial introduction of special preterm infant formulas allows a choice of formula with varying strengths of Ca and P fortification. Use of these preparations alone or in combination with standard formulas or human milk allows a wide range of possible nutrient Ca and P concentrations. Unfortunately there is little direct evidence that mixtures of formulas are effective in preventing bone demineralization.

The administration of P without Ca as a supplement probably should be avoided. Although this approach has been used successfully to treat rickets of prematurity in the past, it is not without its hazards. Carey et al. (241) have reported a group of four preterm infants fed human milk who had markedly increased urinary losses of P once the supplement was begun. In this group, 45–100% of the supplemental P was lost in the urine (241). Sann et al. (242) also have observed in P-supplemented preterm infants fed human milk an increase in serum immunoreactive PTH compared to unsupplemented infants. Although this was not commented on by the authors, we would suggest that the P load would result in transient hypocalcemia and secondary hyperparathyroidism. In addition, the supplemented infants had serum $1,25(OH)_2D$ concentrations that were markedly elevated and not statistically different from those of the unsupplemented control. We would infer, therefore, that there was still a Ca deficiency in these infants, which served to stimulate increased production of $1,25(OH)_2D$ in spite of P supplementation.

The bone effects of P supplementation alone may be complex. First, P supplementation without Ca, as mentioned, may produce sufficient hypocalcemia to stimulate parathyroid activity. Increased serum PTH concentrations result in increased urinary P excretion. Secondary hyperparathyroidism results in bone resorption and ultimately osteitis fibrosa. Second, in the face of Ca depletion, the supplemental P possibly cannot be properly utilized; the increased P brought into the circulation through $1,25(OH)_2D$ stimulated intestinal absorption of P or the P released through bone resorption may be eliminated in the urine. Thus P supplementation alone theoretically might aggravate the bone demineralization observed in preterm infants.

The role of vitamin D in the management and prevention of rickets of prematurity is controversial. Preterm infants have been managed with a wide range of vitamin D and its metabolites. From current evidence, as stated earlier, it appears that the preterm infant is capable of maintaining a normal to elevated serum concentration of $1,25(OH)_2D$, the most active vitamin D metabolite (137,139,143). Although treatment with 1 alpha (OH)D, a synthetic analog of $1,25(OH)_2D$, has been successfully used in the treatment of rickets of prematurity (140,237), its high potency and potential for toxicity probably prevent its routine use. Moreover, the theoretical small increase in Ca absorption in the presence of the metabolite, in comparison to the much greater absorption achievable by increased Ca content in formula, make the clinical use of the metabolite impractical.

Finally, 1-alpha(OH)D and $1,25(OH)_2D$ may be toxic to renal function. These concerns have been raised in renal failure patients who showed deterioration of renal function while receiving these vitamin D metabolites (243,244). The loss of renal function was probably related to hypercalcemia produced by excessive dosages of 1-alpha(OH)D or $1,25(OH)_2D$ (245–248). Renal calcifications have been observed in neonatal rats treated with 1-alpha(OH)D (249) and increased sensitivity to the effects of $1,25(OH)_2D$ on serum Ca have been observed in suckling rats (250). Without further study, these concerns, and the finding that $1,25(OH)_2D$ does not appear to be deficient in rickets of prematurity, question the justification for using this metabolite or its analog in rickets of prematurity.

It has been suggested that 25(OH)D, $24,25(OH)_2D$, or some as yet unidentified vitamin D metabolite might be necessary for normal bone development. In vitamin-D-deficient adults with osteomalacia, Bordier et al. (38) found that treatment with 1,25$(OH)_2D_3$ or 24,25$(OH)_2D_3$ alone produced only partial healing of bone lesions as measured by bone biopsy. In contrast, individuals who received D_3, 25$(OH)D_3$, or a combination of 1,25$(OH)_2D_3$ and 24,25$(OH)_2D_3$ showed complete healing. In rats, experimental work also points to the possible importance of other vitamin D metabolites. In a group of rats made rachitic by means of a low-phosphorus, vitamin-D-deficient diet, Atkin et al. (251), treated them with 1-alpha$(OH)D_3$, 1,25$(OH)_2D_3$, or 24,25$(OH)_2D_3$ alone, or vitamin D_3 in combination with a diet of normal phosphorus content. As in the study by Bordier et al. (38), the rats treated with 1-alpha$(OH)D_3$ or 1,25$(OH)_2D_3$ demonstrated only partial healing of their rickets; 24,25$(OH)_2D_3$ given alone while the animals were still on the low-P diet and vitamin D_3 with normal P intake resulted in healing of rickets. Additional studies utilizing rats have demonstrated inhibition of bone collagen production by 1,25$(OH)_2D$ (252) while 24,25$(OH)_2D$ has been found to inhibit the bone resorption mediated by 1,25$(OH)_2D$ (253). In contrast to the studies cited above, Miller et al. (254) found normal bone modeling and mineralization on histological studies of weanling rats treated with a 24,24-difluoro-25(OH)D, in which the fluorines block the 24-hydroxylation of 25(OH)D. Since bone was normal in spite of the blockage of 24-hydroxylation, the authors concluded that the 24-hydroxylation step per se, and therefore 24,25$(OH)_2D$, was not essential for normal bone mineralization.

Although other metabolites of vitamin D besides 1,25$(OH)_2D$ may be of importance in bone mineralization and development, current information is not sufficient to support the use of these metabolites in the management or prevention of rickets of prematurity. Further studies are required to define the toxicities as well as the physiological actions of these metabolites before they can be safely used in preterm infants. In keeping with these concerns, the traditional dosage of 400 IU of vitamin D per day would seem sufficient and reasonable for the prevention and treatment of rickets of prematurity, when used in association with Ca and P supplementation.

As a final point, it should be emphasized again that the ideal means of preventing or treating rickets of prematurity is not known. Even with extreme attention to intakes of Ca, P, and vitamin D, rickets of prematurity may still be observed. This was demonstrated in a recent report by Koo et al. (255) of a very-low-birthweight infant who developed rickets of prematurity while receiving amounts of Ca and P that should have been sufficient to sustain the intrauterine accretion rates of these minerals, as well as a normal intake of vitamin D.

IV. SUMMARY

Rickets of prematurity is a common disorder of low-birthweight infants, which often presents as an incidental finding at 2-4 months of age. Deficiency of Ca and P appears to be the primary causative factor in the development of this condition, although further work is required to elucidate better the role of vitamin D and its metabolites in this disease. Meticulous attention to Ca and P intakes with attempts to approximate intrauterine accretion rates may prevent rickets of prematurity. Furthermore, supplemental Ca and P can be used to treat this condition once it develops. Standard dosages of vitamin D (i.e., 400 IU/day) appear to be sufficient to meet the needs of the preterm infant; higher dosages do not seem to give additional benefit in the prevention or treatment of rickets of prematurity.

REFERENCES

1. Blum, J. W., Fischer, J. A., Schwoerer, D., Hunziker, W., and Binswanger, U. Acute parathyroid hormone response: Sensitivity, relationship to hypocalcemia, and rapidity. *Endocrinology 95*:753–759 (1974).
2. Chang, H. Y. Grafts of parathyroid and other tissues to bone. *Anat. Rec. 111*:23–47 (1951).
3. Barnicot, N. A. The local action of the parathyroid and other tissues on bone in intracerebral grafts. *J. Anat. 82*:233–248 (1948).
4. Talmage, R. V., and Kraintz, F. W. Progressive changes in renal phosphate and calcium excretion in rats following parathyroidectomy or parathyroid administration. *Proc. Soc. Exp. Biol. Med. 87*:263–267 (1954).
5. Jahan, I., and Pitts, R. F. Effect of parathyroid on renal tubular reabsorption of phosphate and calcium. *Am. J. Physiol. 155*:42–49 (1948).
6. Rasmussen, H., Wong, M., Bikle, D., and Goodman, D. B. P. Hormonal control of the renal conversion of 25-hydroxycholecalciferol to 1,25-dihydroxycholecalciferol. *J. Clin. Invest. 51*:2502–2504 (1972).
7. Armbrecht, H. J., Wongsurawat, N., Zenser, T. V., and Davis, B. B. Effect of PTH and 1,25$(OH)_2D_3$ on renal 25$(OH)D_3$ metabolism, adenylate cyclase, and protein kinase. *Am. J. Physiol. 246*:E102–E107 (1984).
8. Kenny, A. D. *Intestinal Calcium Absorption and its Regulation*. CRC Press, Boca Raton, FL, 1981, pp. 91–102.
9. Chase, L. R., and Slatopolsky, E. Secretion and metabolic efficacy of parathyroid hormone in patients with severe hypomagnesemia. *J. Clin. Endocrinol. Metab. 38*:363–371 (1974).
10. Suh, S. M., Tashjian, A. H., Matsuo, N., Parkinson, D. K., and Fraser, D. Pathogenesis of hypocalcemia in primary hypomagnesemia: Normal end-organ responsiveness to parathyroid hormone, impaired parathyroid gland function. *J. Clin. Invest. 52*:153–160 (1973).
11. McMillan, P. J., Hooker, W. H., and Deftos, L. J. Distribution of calcitonin-containing cells in the human thyroid. *Am. J. Anat. 140*:73–80 (1974).
12. Wolfe, H. J., Voelkel, E. F., and Tashjian, A. H. Distribution of human calcitonin-containing cells in the normal adult human thyroid gland: A correlation of morphology with peptide content. *J. Clin. Endocrinol. Metab. 38*: 688–694 (1974).

13. Parthemore, J. G., and Deftos, L. J. Calcitonin secretion in normal human subjects. *J. Clin. Endocrinol. Metab. 47*:184–188 (1978).
14. Heath, H., and Sizemore, G. W. Plasma calcitonin in normal man: Differences between men and women. *J. Clin. Invest. 60*:1135–1140 (1977).
15. Care, A. D., Bruce, J. B., Boelkins, J., Kenny, A. D., Conaway, H., and Anast C. S. Role of pancreozymin–cholecystokinin and structurally related compounds as calcitonin secretogogues. *Endocrinology 89*:262–271 (1971).
16. Sizemore, G. W., and Go, V. L. W. Stimulation tests for diagnosis of medullary thyroid carcinoma. *Mayo Clin. Proc. 50*:53–66 (1975).
17. Holtrop, M. E., Raisz, L. G., and Simmons, H. A. The effects of parathyroid hormone, colchicine, and calcitonin on the ultrastructure and the activity of osteoclasts in organ culture. *J. Cell Biol. 60*:346–355 (1974).
18. Ardaillou, R. Kidney and calcitonin. *Nephron 15*:250–260 (1975).
19. Bijvoet, O. L. M., van der Sluys Veer, J., de Vries, H. R., and van Koppen, A. T. J. Natriuretic effect of calcitonin in man. *N. Engl. J. Med. 284*:681–688 (1971).
20. Holick, M. F. The cutaneous photosynthesis of previtamin D_3: A unique photoendocrine system. *J. Invest. Dermatol. 76*:51–58 (1981).
21. Ponchon, G., and DeLuca, H. F. The role of the liver in the metabolism of vitamin D. *J. Clin. Invest. 48*:1273–1279 (1969).
22. Olson, E. B., Knutson, J. C., Bhattacharyya, M. H., and DeLuca, H. F. The effect of hepatoctomy on the synthesis of 25-hydroxyvitamin D. *J. Clin. Invest. 57*:1213–1220 (1976).
23. Langman, C. B., Favus, M. J., Bushinsky, D. A., and Coe, F. L. Effects of dietary calcium restriction on 1,25-dihydroxyvitamin D_3 net synthesis by rat proximal tubules. *J. Lab. Clin. Med. 106*:286–292 (1985).
24. Shain, S. A. The *in vitro* metabolism of 25-hydroxycholecalciferol to 1,25-dihydroxycholecalciferol by chick renal tubules. *J. Biol. Chem. 247*:4404–4413 (1972).
25. Spanos, E., Freake, H., MacAuley, S. J., and MacIntyre, I. Regulation of vitamin D metabolism by calcium and phosphate ions in isolated renal tubules. *Biochem. J. 196*:187–193 (1981).
26. Tanaka, Y., Lorenc, R. S., and DeLuca, H. F. The role of 1,25-dihydroxyvitamin D_3 and parathyroid hormone in the regulation of chick renal 25-hydroxyvitamin D_3-24-hydroxylase. *Arch. Biochem. Biophys. 171*:521–526 (1975).
27. Juan, D., and DeLuca, H. F. The regulation of 24,25-dihydroxyvitamin D_3 production in cultures of monkey kidney cells. *Endocrinology 101*:1184–1193 (1977).
28. Tanaka, Y., and DeLuca, H. F. Stimulation of 24,25-dihydroxyvitamin D_3 production by 1,25-dihydroxyvitamin D_3. Science 183:1198–1200 (1974).
29. Harrison, H. E., and Harrison, H. C. Vitamin D and permeability of intestinal mucosa to calcium. *Am. J. Physiol. 208*:370–374 (1965).
30. Holick, M. F., Schnoes, H. K., and DeLuca, H. F. Identification of 1,25-dihydroxycholecalciferol, a form of vitamin D_3 metabolically active in the intestine. *Proc. Natl. Acad. Sci. USA 68*:803–804 (1971).

31. Karsenty, G., Lacour, B., Ulmann, A., Piérandréi, E., Drüeke, T. Phosphate fluxes in isolated enterocytes from vitamin D replete and vitamin D deficient rats—early effects of calcitrol. *Pflügers Arch. 403*:151–155 (1985).
32. Raisz, L. G., Trummel, C. L., Holick, M. F., and DeLuca, H. F. 1,25-Dihydroxycholecalciferol: A potent stimulator of bone resorption in tissue culture. *Science 175*:768–769 (1972).
33. Brommage, R., and Neuman, W. F. Mechanism of mobilization of bone mineral by 1,25-dihydroxyvitamin D_3. *Am. J. Physiol. 237*:E113–E120 (1979).
34. Raisz, L. G. Physiologic and pharmacologic regulation of bone resorption. *N. Engl. J. Med. 282*:909–916 (1970).
35. Rasmussen, H., and Bordier, P. J. *The Physiological and Cellular Basis of Metabolic Bone Disease*. Baltimore, Williams & Wilkins, 1974.
36. Galus, K., Szymendera, J., Zaleski, A., and Schreyer, K. Effect of 1 alpha-hydroxyvitamin D_3 and 24R,25-dihydroxyvitamin D_3 on bone remodeling. *Calcif. Tissue Int. 31*:209–213 (1980).
37. Kanis, J. A., Cundy, T., Bartlett, M., Smith, R., Heynen, G., Warner, G. T., and Russell, R. G. G. Is 24,25-dihydroxycholecalciferol a calcium-regulating hormone in man? *Br. Med. J. 1*:1382–1386 (1978).
38. Bordier, P., Rasmussen, H., Marie, P., Miravet, L., Gueris, J., and Ryckwaert, A. Vitamin D metabolites and bone mineralization in man. *J. Clin. Endocrinol. Metab. 46*:284–294 (1978).
39. Tanaka, Y., and DeLuca, H. F. The control of 25-hydroxyvitamin D metabolism by inorganic phosphorus. *Arch. Biochem. Biophys. 154*:566–574 (1973).
40. Boyle, I. T., Gray, R. W., and DeLuca, H. F. Regulation by calcium of in vivo synthesis of 1,25-dihydroxycholecalciferol and 21,25-dihydroxycholecalciferol. *Proc. Natl. Acad. Sci. USA 68*:2131–2134 (1971).
41. Garabedian, M., Holick, M. F., DeLuca, H. F., and Boyle, I. T. Control of 25-hydroxycholecalciferol metabolism by parathyroid glands. *Proc. Natl. Acad. Sci. USA 69*:1673–1676 (1972).
42. Sommerville, B. A., Fox, J., and Care, A. D. The *in vitro* metabolism of 25-hydroxycholecalciferol by pig kidney: Effect of low dietary levels of calcium and phosphorus. *Br. J. Nutr. 40*:159–162 (1978).
43. Swaminathan, R., Sommerville, B. A., and Care, A. D. Metabolism *in vitro* of 25-hydroxycholecalciferol in chicks fed on phosphorus-deficient diets. *Clin. Sci. Mol. Med. 54*:197–200 (1978).
44. Bikle, D. D., and Rasmussen, H. The ionic control of 1,25-dihydroxyvitamin D_3 production in isolated chick renal tubules. *J. Clin. Invest. 55*:292–298 (1975).
45. Hughes, M. R., Brumbaugh, P. F., and Haussler, M. R. Regulation of serum 1 alpha, 25-dihydroxyvitamin D_3 by calcium and phosphate in the rat. *Science 190*:578–579 (1975).
46. Fraser, D. R. Regulation of the metabolism of vitamin D. *Physiol. Rev. 60*: 551-613 (1980).
47. Suda, T., Horiuchi, N., and Sasaki, S. Direct control by calcium of 25-hydroxycholecalciferol-1-hydroxylase activity in chick kidney mitochrondria. *Biochem. Biophys. Res. Commun. 54*:512–518 (1973).

48. Armbrecht, H. J., Wongsurawat, N., Zenser, T. V., and Davis, B. B. *In vitro* modulation of renal 25-hydroxyvitamin D_3 metabolism by vitamin D_3 metabolites and calcium. *Arch. Biochem. Biophys. 220*:52–59 (1983).
49. Callenbach, J. C., Sheehan, M. B., Abramson, S. J., and Hall, R. T. Etiologic factors in rickets of very low-birth-weight infants. *J. Pediatr. 98*:800–805 (1981).
50. Koo, W. W. K., Gupta, J. M., Nayanar, V. V., Wilkinson, M., and Posen, S. Skeletal changes in preterm infants. *Arch. Dis. Child. 57*:447–452 (1982).
51. Maxwell, J. P. Further studies in adult rickets (osteomalacia) and foetal rickets. *Proc. R. Soc. Med. 28*:265–300 (1934).
52. Sann, L., David, L., Frederich, A., Bovier-Lapierre, M., Bourgeois, J., Romand-Monier, M., and Bethenod, M. Congenital rickets: Study of the evolution of secondary hyperparathyroidism. *Acta Paediatr. Scand. 66*: 323–327 (1977).
53. Moncrieff, M., and Fadahunsi, T. O. Congenital rickets due to maternal vitamin D deficiency. *Arch. Dis. Child. 49*:810–811 (1974).
54. Begum, R., Coutinho, M. de L., Dormandy, T. L., and Yudkin, S. Maternal malabsorption presenting as congenital rickets. *Lancet 1*:1048–1052 (1986).
55. Bosley, A. R. J., Verrier-Jones, E. R., and Campbell, M. J. Aetiological factors in rickets of prematurity. *Arch. Dis. Child. 55*:683–686 (1980).
56. Zeidan, S., and Bamford, M. Congenital rickets with maternal pre-eclampsia. *J. R. Soc. Med. 77*:426–427 (1984).
57. Khattab, A. K., and Forfar, J. O. The interrelationship between calcium, phosphorus and glucose levels in mother and infant in conditions commonly associated with "placental insufficiency." *Biol. Neonate 18*:1–16 (1971).
58. Ziegler, E. E., Biga, R. L., and Fomon, S. J. Nutritional requirements of the premature infant. In: *Textbook of Pediatric Nutrition* (R. M. Suskind, ed.). Raven Press, New York, 1981, pp. 29–39.
59. Shaw, J. C. L. Evidence for defective skeletal mineralization in low-birth-weight infants: The absorption of calcium and fat. *Pediatrics 57*:16–25 (1976).
60. Ziegler, E. E., O'Donnell, A. M., Nelson, S. E., and Fomon, S. J. Body composition of the reference fetus. *Growth 40*:329–341 (1976).
61. Fomon, S. J., and Filer, L. J. Milks and formulas. In: *Infant Nutrition*, 2nd ed. (S. J. Fomon, ed.). Philadelphia, W. B. Saunders, 1974, pp. 359–407.
62. Gross, S. J., David, R. J., Bauman, L., and Tomarelli, R. M. Nutritional composition of milk produced by mothers delivering preterm. *J. Pediatr. 96*:641–644 (1980).
63. Greer, F. R., Steichen, J. J., and Tsang, R. C. Calcium and phosphate supplements in breast milk-related rickets: Results in a very-low-birth-weight infant. *Am. J. Dis. Child. 136*:581–583 (1982).
64. Sagy, M., Birenbaum, E., Balin, A., Orda, S., Barzilay, Z., and Brish, M. Phosphate-depletion syndrome in a premature infant fed human milk. *J. Pediatr. 96*:683–685 (1980).

65. Rowe, J. C., Wood, D. H., Rowe, D. W., and Raisz, L. G. Nutritional hypophosphatemic rickets in a premature infant fed breast milk. *N. Engl. J. Med. 300*:293–296 (1979).
66. Koo, W. W. K., Antony, G., and Stevens, L. H. S. Continuous nasogastric phosphorus infusion in hypophosphatemic rickets of prematurity. *Am. J. Dis. Child. 138*:172–175 (1984).
67. Keipert, J. A. Rickets with multiple fractured ribs in a premature infant. *Med. J. Aust. 1*:672–675 (1970).
68. Rowe, J., Rowe, D., Horak, E., Spackman, T., Saltzman, R., Robinson, S., Philipps, A., and Raye, J. Hypophosphatemia and hypercalciuria in small premature infants fed human milk: Evidence for inadequate dietary phosphorus. *J. Pediatr. 104*:112–117 (1984).
69. Kulkarni, P. B., Hall, R. T., Rhodes, P. G., Sheehan, M. B., Callenbach, J. C., Germann, D. R., and Abramson, S. J. Rickets in very low-birth-weight infants. *J. Pediatr. 96*:249–252 (1980).
70. Kulkarni, P. B., Dorand, R. D., Bridger, W. M., Payne, J. H., Montiel, D. C., and Hill, J. G. Rickets in premature infants fed different formulas. *South Med. J. 77*:13–16 (1984).
71. Shenai, J. P., Jhaveri, B. M., Reynolds, J. W., Huston, R. K., and Babson, S. G. Nutritional balance studies in very low-birth-weight infants: Role of soy formula. *Pediatrics 67*:631–637 (1981).
72. Knight, P. J., Buchanan, S., and Clatworthy, H. W. Calcium and phosphate requirements of preterm infants who require prolonged hyperalimentation. *J.A.M.A. 243*:1244–1246 (1980).
73. Kien, C. L., Browning, C., Jona, J., and Starshak, R. J. Rickets in premature infants receiving parenteral nutrition: A case report and review of the literature. *J.P.E.N. 6*:152–156 (1982).
74. Leape, L. L., and Valaes, T. Rickets in low birth weight infants receiving total parenteral nutrition. *J. Pediatr. Surg. 11*:665–674 (1976).
75. The, T. S., Kollee, L. A. A., Boon, J. M., and Monnens, L. A. H. Rickets in a preterm infant during intravenous alimentation. *Acta Paediatr. Scand. 72*:769–771 (1983).
76. Geggel, R. L., Pereira, G. R., and Spackman, T. J. Fractured ribs: Unusual presentation of rickets in premature infants. *J. Pediatr. 93*:680–682 (1978).
77. Gefter, W. B., Epstein, D. M., Anday, E. K., and Dalinka, M. K. Rickets presenting as multiple fractures in premature infants on hyperalimentation. *Radiology 142*:371–374 (1982).
78. Poole, R. L., Rupp, C. A., and Kerner, J. A. Calcium and phosphorus in neonatal parenteral nutrition solutions. *J.P.E.N. 7*:358–360 (1983).
79. Venkataraman, P. S., Brissie, E. O., and Tsang, R. C. Stability of calcium and phosphorus in neonatal parenteral nutrition solutions. *J. Pediatr. Gastroenterol. Nutr. 2*:640–643 (1983).
80. Eggert, L. D., Rusho, W. J., MacKay, M. W., and Chan, G. M. Calcium and phosphorus compatibility in parenteral nutrition solutions for neonates. *Am. J. Hosp. Pharm. 39*:49–53 (1982).

81. Watkins, J. B., Ingall, D., Szczepanik, P., Klein, P. D., and Lester, R. Bile-salt metabolism in the newborn: Measurement of poor size and synthesis by stable isotope technic. *N. Engl. J. Med. 288*:431–434 (1973).
82. Lavy, U., Silverberg, M., and Davidson, M. Role of bile acids in fat absorption in low birth weight infants. *Pediatr. Res. 5*:387 (1971).
83. Barltrop, D., and Oppe, T. E. Absorption of fat and calcium by low birth-weight infants from milks containing butterfat and olive oil. *Arch. Dis. Child 48*:496–501 (1973).
84. Tantibhedhyangkul, P., and Hashim, S. A. Medium-chain triglyceride feeding in premature infants: Effects on calcium and magnesium absorption. *Pediatrics 61*:537–545 (1978).
85. Huston, R. K., Reynolds, J. W., Jensen, C., and Buist, N. R. M. Nutrient and mineral retention and vitamin D absorption in low-birth-weight infants: Effect of medium-chain triglycerides. *Pediatrics 72*:44–48 (1983).
86. Edwards, B. R., Baer, P. G., Sutton, R. A. L., and Dirks, J.H. Micropuncture study of diuretic effects on sodium and calcium reabsorption in the dog nephron. *J. Clin. Invest. 52*:2418–2427 (1973).
87. Toft, H., and Roin, J. Effect of frusemide administration on calcium excretion. *Br. Med. J. 1*:437–438 (1971).
88. Noe, H. N., Bryant, J. F., Roy, S., and Stapleton, F. B. Urolithiasis in preterm neonates associated with furosemide therapy. *J. Urol. 132*:93–94 (1984).
89. Hufnagle, K. G., Khan, S. N., Penn, D., Cacciarelli, A., and Williams, P. Renal calcifications: A complication of long-term furosemide therapy in preterm infants. *Pediatrics 70*:360-363 (1982).
90. Savage, M. O., Wilkinson, A. R., Baum, J. D., and Roberton, N. R. C. Frusemide in respiratory distress syndrome. *Arch. Dis. Child. 50*:709–713 (1975).
91. Goldsmith, M. A., Bhatia, S. S., Kanto, W. P., Kutner, M. H., and Rudman, D. Gluconate calcium therapy and neonatal hypercalciuria. *Am. J. Dis. Child. 135*:538–543 (1981).
92. Chudley, A. E., Brown, D. R., Holzman, I. R., and Oh, K. S. Nutritional rickets in 2 very low birthweight infants with chronic lung disease. *Arch. Dis. Child. 55*:687–690 (1980).
93. Venkataraman, P. S., Han, B. K., Tsang, R., and Daugherty, C. C. Secondary hyperparathyroidism and bone disease in infants receiving long-term furosemide therapy. *Am. J. Dis. Child. 137*:157–1161 (1983).
94. Koo, W. W. K., Guan, Z. P., Tsang, R. C., Laskarzewski, P., and Neuman, V. Growth failure and decreased bone mineral of newborn rats with chronic furosemide therapy. *Pediatr. Res. 20*:74–78 (1986).
95. Devaskar, U. P., Ho, M., Devaskar, S. U., and Tsang, R. C. 25-Hydroxy- and 1 alpha, 25-dihydroxyvitamin D: Maternal–fetal relationship and the transfer of 1,25-dihydroxyvitamin D_3 across the placenta in an ovine model. *Dev. Pharmacol. Ther. 7*:213–220 (1984).
96. Care, A. D., Ross, R., Pickard, D. W., Weatherley, A. J., Garel, J. M., Manning, R. M., Allgrove, J., Papapoulos, S., and O'Riordan, J. L. H. Calcium homeostasis in the fetal pig. *J. Dev. Physiol. 4*:85–106 (1982).

97. Haddad, J. G., Boisseau, V., and Avioli, L. V. Placental transfer of vitamin D_3 and 25-hydroxycholecalciferol in the rat. *J. Lab. Clin. Med. 77*: 908–915 (1971).
98. Hidiroglou, M., and Williams, C. J. Transfer of tritium-labeled vitamin D_3 and 25-hydroxyvitamin D_3 in ovine placenta. *Am. J. Vet. Res. 42*:140–141 (1981).
99. Hollis, B. W., and Pittard, W. B. Evaluation of the total fetomaternal vitamin D relationships at term: Evidence for racial differences. *J. Clin. Endocrinol. Metab. 59*:652–657 (1984).
100. Goff, J. P., Horst, R. L., and Littledike, E. T. Effect of the maternal vitamin D status at parturition on the vitamin D status of the neonatal calf. *J. Nutr. 112*:1387–1393 (1982).
101. Goff, J. P., Horst, R. L., and Littledike, E. T. Effect of low vitamin D status at parturition on the vitamin D status of neonatal piglets. *J. Nutr. 114*:163–169 (1984).
102. Seino, Y., Ishida, M., Yamaoka, K., Ishii, T., Hiejima, T., Ikehara, C., Tanaka, Y., Matsuda, S., Shomotsuji, T., Yabuuchi, H., Morimoto, S., and Onishi, T. Serum calcium regulating hormones in the perinatal period. *Calcif. Tissue Int. 34*:131–135 (1982).
103. Weisman, Y., Occhipinti, M., Knox, G., Reiter, E., and Root, A. Concentrations of 24,25-dihydroxyvitamin D and 25-hydroxyvitamin D in paired maternal-cord sera. *Am. J. Obstet. Gynecol. 130*:704–707 (1978).
104. Hillman, L. S., and Haddad, J. G. Human perinatal vitamin D metabolism I: 25-hydroxyvitamin D in maternal and cord blood. *J. Pediatr. 84*:742–749 (1974).
105. Delvin, E. E., Glorieux, F. H., Salle, B. L., David, L., and Varenne, J. P. Control of vitamin D metabolism in preterm infants: Feto-maternal relationships. *Arch. Dis. Child. 57*:754–757 (1982).
106. Kuroda, E., Okano, T., Mizuno, N., Kobayashi, T., Kodama, S., Ninomiya, M., Morishita, Y., and Matsuo, T. Plasma levels of 25-hydroxyvitamin D_2 and 25-hydroxyvitamin D_3 in maternal, cord and neonatal blood. *J. Nutr. Sci. Vitaminol. (Tokyo) 27*:55–65 (1981).
107. Bouillon, R., Van Assche, F. A., and Van Baelen, H. Influence of the vitamin D-binding protein on the serum concentration of 1,25-dihydroxyvitamin D_3. Significance of the free 1,25-dihydroxyvitamin. *J. Clin. Invest. 67*:589–596 (1981).
108. Ross, R., Care, A. D., Taylor, C. M., Pelc, B., and Sommerville, B. The transplacental movement of metabolites of vitamin D in the sheep. In: *Vitamin D: Basic Research and Clinical Application* (A. W. Norman, K. Schafer, D. Von Herrath, H. G. Grigoleit, J. W. Coburn, H. F. DeLuca, E. B. Marver, and T. Suda, eds.). Walter de Gruyter, Berlin/New York, 1979, pp. 341–344.
109. Lester, G. E., Gray, T. K., and Lorenc, R. S. 25-Hydroxyvitamin D_3 metabolism in the pregnant rat: Maternal–fetal relationships. *Biol. Neonate 39*:232–238 (1981).

110. Steichen, J. J., Tsang, R. C., Gratton, T. L., Hamstra, A., and DeLuca, H. F. Vitamin D homeostasis in the perinatal period: 1,25-Dihydroxyvitamin D in maternal, cord, and neonatal blood. *N. Engl. J. Med. 302*:315–319 (1980).
111. Sunaga, S., Horiuchi, N., Takahashi, N., Okuyama, K., and Suda, T. The site of 1 alpha, 25-dihydroxyvitamin D_3 production in pregnancy. *Biochem. Biophys. Res. Commun. 90*:948–955 (1979).
112. Fenton, E., and Britton, H. G. 25-Hydroxycholecalciferol 1 alpha-hydroxylase activity in the kidney of the fetal, neonatal and adult guinea pig. *Biol. Neonate 37*:254–256 (1980).
113. Whitsett, J. A., Ho, M., Tsang, R. C., Norman, E. J., and Adams, K. G. Synthesis of 1,25-dihydroxyvitamin D_3 by human placenta *in vitro. J. Clin. Endocrinol. Metab. 53*:484–488 (1981).
114. Weisman, Y., Harell, A., Edelstein, S., David, M., Spirer, Z., and Golander, A. 1 alpha, 25-Dihydroxyvitamin D_3 and 24,25-dihydroxyvitamin D_3 *in vitro* synthesis by human decidua and placenta. *Nature 281*:317–319 (1979).
115. Tanaka, Y., Halloran, B., Schnoes, H. K., and DeLuca, H. F. *In vitro* production of 1,25-dihydroxyvitamin D_3 by rat placental tissue. *Proc. Natl. Acad. Sci. USA 76*:5033–5035 (1979).
116. Delvin, E. E., Arabian, A., Glorieux, F. H., and Mamer, O. A. *In vitro* metabolism of 25-hydroxycholecalciferol by isolated cells from human decidua. *J. Clin. Endocrinol. Metab. 60*:880–885 (1985).
117. Ross, R., Chen, M. H., Halbert, K., and Tsang, R. C. High *in vivo* fetal production rates of 1,25-dihydroxyvitamin D_3 in sheep. *Pediatr. Res. 20*: 334A (1986).
118. Hillman, L. S., Slatopolsky, E., and Haddad, J. G. Perinatal vitamin D metabolism. IV. Maternal and cord serum 24,25-dihydroxyvitamin D concentrations. *J. Clin. Endocrinol. Metab. 47*:1073–1077 (1978).
119. Danan, J. L., Delorme, A. C., Benassayag, C., Vallette, G., and Cuisinier-Gleizes, P. 25-Hydroxyvitamin D and 24,25-dihydroxyvitamin D in maternal plasma, fetal plasma and amniotic fluid in the rat. *Biochem. Biophys. Res. Commun. 95*:453–460 (1980).
120. Rosenstreich, S. J., Rich, C., and Volwiler, W. Deposition in and release of vitamin D_3 from body fat: Evidence for a storage site in the rat. *J. Clin. Invest. 50*:679–687 (1971).
121. Goel, K. M., Sweet, E. M., Logan, R. W., Warren, J. M., Arneil, G. C., and Shanks, R. A. Florid and subclinical rickets among immigrant children in Glasgow. *Lancet 1*:1141–1145 (1976).
122. Preece, M. A., Ford, J. A., McIntosh, W. B., Dunnigan, M. G., Tomlinson, S., and O'Riordan, J. L. H. Vitamin-D deficiency among Asian immigrants to Britain. *Lancet 1*:907–910 (1973).
123. Specker, B. L., Tsang, R. C., and Hollis, B. W. Effect of race and diet on human-milk vitamin D and 25-hydroxyvitamin D. *Am. J. Dis. Child. 139*: 1134–1137 (1985).

124. Hollander, D. Intestinal absorption of vitamins A, E, D., and K. *J. Lab. Clin. Med. 97*:449–462 (1981).
125. Agunod, M., Yamaguchi, N., Lopez, R., Luhby, A. L., and Glass, G. B. J. Correlative study of hydrochloric acid, pepsin, and intrinsic factor secretion in newborns and infants. *Am. J. Dis. 14*:400–414 (1969).
126. Dallner, G., Siekevitz, P., and Palade, G. E. Synthesis of microsomal membranes and their enzymatic constituents in developing rat liver. *Biochem. Biophys. Res. Commun. 20*:135–141 (1965).
127. Mendelsohn, M., and Haddad, J. G. Postnatal fall and rise of circulating 25-hydroxyvitamin D in the rat. *J. Lab. Clin. Med. 86*:32–37 (1975).
128. Hillman, L. S., and Haddad, J. G. Perinatal vitamin D metabolism: II. Serial 25-hydroxyvitamin D concentrations in sera of term and premature infants. *J. Pediatr. 86*:928–935 (1975).
129. Markestad, T., Aksnes, L., Finne, P. H., and Aarskog, D. Vitamin D nutritional status of premature infants supplemented with 500 IU vitamin D_2 per day. *Acta Paediatr. Scand. 72*:517–520 (1983).
130. Markestad, T., Aksnes, L., Finne, P. H., and Aarskog, D. Plasma concentrations of vitamin D metabolites in premature infants. *Pediatr. Res. 18*: 269–272 (1984).
131. Glorieux, F. H., Salle, B. L., Delvin, E. E., and David, L. Vitamin D metabolism in preterm infants: Serum calcitriol values during the first five days of life. *J. Pediatr. 99*:640–643 (1981).
132. Wolf, H., Gräff, V., and Offerman, G. The vitamin D_3 requirement for premature infants. In: *Vitamin D, Basic Research and Its Clinical Application* (A. W. Norman, K. Schaefer, D. Von Herrath, H. Grigoleit, J. W. Coburn, H. F. DeLuca, E. B. Marver, and T. Suda, eds.). Walter de Gruyter, Berlin, 1979, pp. 349–352.
133. Salle, B. L., David, L., Glorieux, F. H., Delvin, E., Senterre, J., and Renaud, H. Early oral administration of vitamin D and its metabolites in premature neonates. Effect on mineral homeostasis. *Pediatr. Res. 16*:75–78 (1982).
134. Robinson, M. J., Merrett, A. L., Tetlow, V. A., and Compston, J. E. Plasma 25-hydroxyvitamin D concentrations in preterm infants receiving oral vitamin D supplements. *Arch. Dis. Child. 56*:144–145 (1981).
135. Salle, B. L., Glorieux, F. H., Delvin, E. E., David, L. S., and Meunier, G. Vitamin D metabolism in preterm infants: Serial serum calcitriol values during the first four days of life. *Acta Paediatr. Scand. 72*:203–206 (1983).
136. Pettifor, J. M., Stein, H., Herman, A., Ross, F. P., Blumenfeld, T., and Moodley, G. P. Mineral homeostasis in very low birth weight infants fed either on mother's milk or pooled pasteurized preterm milk. *J. Pediatr. Gastroenterol. Nutr. 5*:248–253 (1986).
137. Chesney, R. W., Hamstra, A. J., and DeLuca, H. F. Rickets of prematurity: Supranormal levels of serum 1,25-dihydroxyvitamin D. *Am. J. Dis. Child. 135*:34–37 (1981).

138. Hoff, N., Haddad, J., Teitelbaum, S., McAlister, W., and Hillman, L. S. Serum concentrations of 25-hydroxyvitamin D in rickets of extremely premature infants. *J. Pediatr. 94*:460–466 (1979).
139. Markestad, T., Aksnes, L., Finne, P. H., and Aarskog, D. Plasma concentrations of vitamin D metabolites in a case of rickets of prematurity. *Acta Paediatr. Scand. 72*:759–761 (1983).
140. McIntosh, N., Livesey, A., and Brooke, O. G. Plasma 25-hydroxyvitamin D and rickets in infants of extremely low birthweight. *Arch. Dis. Child. 57*:848–850 (1982).
141. Seino, Y., Ishii, T., Shimotsuji, T.,Ishida, M., andYabuuchi, H. Plasma active vitamin D concentration in low birthweight infants with rickets and its response to vitamin D treatment. *Arch. Dis. Child. 56*:628–632 (1981).
142. Seino, Y., Shimotsuji, T., Ishida, M., Ishii, T., and Yabuuchi. H. Rickets in infancy and childhood. *Endocrinol. Jpn. 1*:95–100 (1979).
143. Steichen, J. J., Tsang, R. C., Greer, F. R., Ho, M., and Hug. G. Elevated serum 1,25 dihydroxyvitamin D concentrations in rickets of very low-birth-weight infants. *J. Pediatr. 99*:293–298 (1981).
144. Kobayashi, A., Kawai, S., Utsunomiya, T., and Ohbe, Y. Bone disease in infants and children with hepatobiliary disease. *Arch. Dis. Child. 19*:641–646 (1974).
145. Yu, J. S., Walker-Smith, J. A., and Burnard, E. D. Rickets: A common complication of neonatal hepatitis. *Med. J. Aust. 1*:790–792 (1971).
146. Krawitt, E. L., Grundman, M. J., and Mawer, E. B. Absorption, hydroxylation, and excretion of vitamin D_3 in primary biliary cirrhosis. *Lancet 2*: 1246–1249 (1977).
147. Toomey, F., Hoag, R., Batton, D., and Vain, N. Rickets associated with cholestasis and parenteral nutrition in premature infants. *Radiology 142*: 85–88 (1982).
148. Kooh, S. W., and Vieth, R. 25-Hydroxyvitamin D metabolism in the sheep fetus and lamb. *Pediatr. Res. 14*:360–363 (1980).
149. Moriuchi, S., and DeLuca, H. F. Metabolism of vitamin D_3 in the chick embryo. *Arch. Biochem. Biophys. 164*:165–171 (1974).
150. Ross, R., Care, A. D., Robinson, J. S., Pickard, D. W., and Weatherly, A. J. Perinatal $1,25(OH)_2D_3$ in the sheep: Involvement of foetal $1,25(OH)_2D_3$ in the maintenance of the transplacental calcium gradient. In: *Hormonal Control of Calcium Metabolism: Proceedings of the Seventh International Conference on Calcium Regulating Hormones.* (D. V. Cohen, R. V. Talamage, and J. L. Mathews, eds.). Excerpta Medica, Amsterdam, 1981, p. 382
151. Fetter, W. P. F., Mettau, J. W., Degenhart, H. J., Hoogenboezem, T., Molenaar, A., and Visser, H. K. A. Plasma 1,25-dihydroxyvitamin D concentrations in preterm infants. *Acta Paediatr. Scand. 74*:549–554 (1985).
152. Markestad, T. Plasma concentrations of 1,25-dihydroxyvitamin D, 24,25-dihydroxyvitamin D, and 25,26-dihydroxyvitamin D in the first year of life. *J. Clin. Endocrinol. Metab. 57*:755–759 (1983).

153. Turner, R. T., Bell, N. H., and Baylink, D. J. The renal metabolism of 25-hydroxyvitamin D_3 in the rat: Regulation by 1,25-dihydroxyvitamin D_3. *Calcif. Tissue Int. 35*:438–442 (1983).
154. MacIntyre, I., Colston, K. W., Evans, I. M. A., Lopez, E., MacAuley, S. J., Piegnoux-Deville, J., Spanos, E., and Szelke, M. Regulation of vitamin D: An evolutionary view. *Clin. Endocrinol. 5*(suppl):85 S–95 S (1976).
155. DeLuca, H. F., and Schnoes, H. K. Metabolism and mechanism of action of vitamin D. *Annu. Rev. Biochem. 45*:631–666 (1976).
156. Larkins, R. G., MacAuley, S. J., and MacIntyre, I. Feedback control of vitamin D metabolism by a nuclear action of 1,25-dihydroxycholecalciferol on the kidney. *Nature 252*:412–414 (1974).
157. Charles, M. A., Martial, J., Zolock, D., Morrissey, R., and Baxter, J. D. Regulation of calcium-binding protein messenger RNA by 1,25-dihydroxycholecalciferol. *Calcif. Tissue Int. 33*:15–18 (1981).
158. Schachter, D., and Rosen, S. M. Active transport of Ca^{45} by the small intestine and its dependence on vitamin D. *Am. J. Physiol. 196*:357–362 (1959).
159. Halloran, B. P., and DeLuca, H. F. Calcium transport in small intestine during early development: Role of vitamin D. *Am. J. Physiol. 239*:G473–G479 (1980).
160. Bruns, M. E. H., Bruns, D. E., and Avioli, L. V. Vitamin D-dependent calcium-binding protein of rat intestine: Changes during postnatal development and sensitivity to 1,25-dihydroxycholecalciferol. *Endocrinology 105*:934–938 (1979).
161. Halloran, B. P., and DeLuca, H. F. Appearance of the intestinal cytosolic receptor for 1,25-dihydroxyvitamin D_3 during neonatal development in the rat. *J. Biol. Chem. 256*:7338–7342 (1981).
162. Senterre, J., and Salle, B. Calcium and phosphorus economy of the preterm infant and its interaction with vitamin D and its metabolites. *Acta Paediatr. Scand. 296* (Suppl):85–92 (1982).
163. Shenai, J. P., Reynolds, J. W., and Babson, S. G. Nutritional balance studies in very-low-birth-weight infants: Enhanced nutrient retention rates by an experimental formula. *Pediatrics 66*:233–238 (1980).
164. Barness, L. A. Nutrition and nutritional disorders. In: *Nelson Textbook of Pediatrics*, 12th ed. (R. E. Behrman, V. C. Nelson, W. E. Nelson, eds.). W. B. Saunders, Philadelphia, 1983, pp. 179–183.
165. Koo, W. W. K., Oestreich, A. E., Sherman, R., Tsang, R. C., Steichen, J. J., and Young, L. W. Radiological case of the month: Osteopenia, rickets, and fractures in preterm infants. *Am. J. Dis. Child. 139*:1045–1046 (1985).
166. Lewin, P. K., Reid, M., Reilly, B. J., Swyer, P. R., and Fraser, D. Iatrogenic rickets in low-birth-weight infants. *J. Pediatr. 78*:207–210 (1971).
167. Glasgow, J. F. T., and Thomas, P. S. Rachitic respiratory distress in small preterm infants. *Arch. Dis. Child. 52*:268–273 (1977).
168. Thomas, P. S., and Glasgow, J. F. T. The "mandibular mantle"—a sign of rickets in very low birth weight infants. *Br. J. Radiol. 51*:93–98 (1978).

169. Davies, D. P., Hughes, C. A., and Moore, J. R. Rickets in preterm infants. *Arch. Dis. Child. 53*:88–89 (1978).
170. Lyon, A. J., McIntosh, N., Wheeler, K., and Brooke, O. G. Hypercalcemia in extremely low birthweight infants. *Arch. Dis. Child. 59*:1141–1144 (1984).
171. Pettifor, J. M., Isdale, J. M., Sahakian, J., and Hansen, J. D. L. Diagnosis of subclinical rickets. *Arch. Dis. Child. 55*:155–157 (1980).
172. Glass, E. J., Hume, R., Hendry, G. M. A., Strange, R. C., and Forfar, J. O. Plasma alkaline phosphatase activity in rickets of prematurity. *Arch. Dis. Child. 57*:373–376 (1982).
173. McIntosh, N., Williams, J. E., Lyon, A. J., and Wheeler, K. A. Diagnosis of rickets of prematurity. *Lancet 2*:869 (1984).
174. Kovar, I., Mayne, P., and Barltrop, D. Plasma alkaline phosphatase activity: A screening test for rickets in preterm neonates.
175. Kovar, I., and Mayne, P. Plasma alkaline phosphatase activity in the preterm neonate. *Acta Paediatr. Scand. 70*:501–506 (1981).
176. Reddy, V., and Srikantia, S. G. Serum alkaline phosphatase in malnourished children with rickets. *J. Pediatr. 71*:595–597 (1967).
177. Adeniyi, F. A., and Heaton, F. W. The effect of zinc deficiency on alkaline phosphatase and its isoenzymes. *Br. J. Nutr. 43*:561–569 (1980).
178. Lotz, M., Zisman, E., and Bartter, F. C. Evidence for a phosphorus-depletion syndrome in man. *N. Engl. J. Med. 278*:409–415 (1968).
179. Lotz, M., Ney, R., Bartter, F. C., and Smith, H. Osteomalacia and debility resulbint from phosphorus depletion. *Trans. Assoc. Am. Physicians 77*: 281–295 (1964).
180. Goldfarb, S., Westby, G. R., Goldberg, M., and Agus, Z. S. Renal tubular effects of chronic phosphate depletion. *J. Clin. Invest. 59*:770–779 (1977).
181. Chisolm, J. J., and Harrison, H. E. Aminoaciduria in vitamin D deficiency state in premature infants and older infants with rickets. *J. Pediatr. 60*: 206–219 (1962).
182. Cifuentes, R. F., Kooh, S. W., and Radde, I. C. Vitamin D deficiency in a calcium-supplemented very low-birth-weight infant. *J. Pediatr. 96*:252–255 (1980).
183. Oestreich, A. E. Rontgendiagnostic metabolischer knochenkrankheiten im kindesalter. *Rontgenpraxis 32*:114–120 (1979).
184. Caffey, J. *Pediatric X-Ray Diagnosis*. Year Book Medical Publishers, Chicago, 1972, pp. 1222–1231.
185. Oestreich, A. E., and Crawford, A. H. *Atlas of Pediatric Orthopedic Radiology*. Thieme, Stuttgart, 1985.
186. Cameron, J. R., and Sorenson, J. Measurement of bone mineral in vivo: An improved method. *Science 142*:230–232 (1963).
187. Minton, S. D., Steichen, J. J., and Tsang, R. C. Bone mineral content in term and preterm appropriate-for-gestational-age infants. *J. Pediatr. 95*: 1037–1042 (1979).

188. Greer, F. R., Searcy, J. E., Levin, R. S., Steichen, J. J., Steichen-Asche, P. S., and Tsang, R. C. Bone mineral and serum 25-hydroxyvitamin D concentrations in breast-fed infants with and without supplemental vitamin D: One-year follow up. *J. Pediatr. 100*:919–922 (1982).
189. Greer, F. R., Searcy, J. E., Levin, R. S., Steichen, J. J., Steichen-Asch, P., and Tsang, R. C. Bone mineral content and serum 25-hydroxyvitamin D concentration in breast-fed infants with and without supplemental vitamin D. *J. Pediatr. 98*:696–701 (1981).
190. Chan, G. M., Roberts, C. C., Folland, D., and Jackson, R. Growth and bone mineralization of normal breast-fed infants and the effects of lactation on maternal bone mineral status. *Am. J. Clin. Nutr. 36*:438–443 (1982).
191. Chan, G. M., and Mileur, L. J. Posthospitalization growth and bone mineral status of normal preterm infants: Feeding with mother's milk or standard formula. *Am. J. Dis. Child. 139*:896–898 (1985).
192. Roberts, C. C., Chan, G. M., Folland, D., Rayburn, C., and Jackson, R. Adequate bone mineralization in breast-fed infants. *J. Pediatr. 99*:192–196 (1981).
193. Steichen, J. J., Gratton, T. L., and Tsang, R. C. Osteopenia of prematurity: The cause and possible treatment. *J. Pediatr. 96*:528–534 (1980).
194. Poser, J. W., Esch, F. S., Ling, N. C., and Price, P. A. Isolation and sequence of the vitamin K-dependent protein from human bone: Undercarboxylation of the first glutamic acid residue. *J. Biol. Chem. 255*:8685–8691 (1980).
195. Price, P. A., and Baukol, S. A. 1,25-Dihydroxyvitamin D_3 increases serum levels of the vitamin K-dependent bone protein. *Biochem. Biophys. Res. Commun. 99*:928–935 (1981).
196. Price, P. A., Parthemore, J. G., and Defto, L. J. New biochemical marker for bone metabolism: Measurement by radioimmunoassay of bone Gla protein in the plasma of normal subjects and patients with bone disease. *J. Clin. Invest. 66*:878–883 (1980).
197. Slovik, D. M., Gundberg, C. M., Neer, R. M., and Lian, J. B. Clinical evaluation of bone turnover by serum osteocalcin measurements in a hospital setting. *J. Clin. Endocrinol. Metab. 59*:228–230 (1984).
198. Delmas, P. D., Wahner, H. W., Mann, K. G., and Riggs, B. L. Assessment of bone turnover in postmenopausal osteoporosis by measurement of serum bone Gla-protein. *J. Lab. Clin. Med. 102*:470–476 (1983).
199. Shima, M., Seino, Y., Tanaka, Y., Yabuuchi, H., Tsutsumi, C., and Moriuchi, S. Bone gamma-carboxyglutamic acid containing protein in the perinatal period. *Acta Paediatr. Scand. 74*:674–677 (1985).
200. Kuwada, M., and Katayama, K. A high-performance liquid chromatographic method for the simultaneous determination of gamma-carboxyglutamic acid and glutamic acid in proteins, bone, and urine. *Anal. Biochem. 117*:259–265 (1981).
201. Gundberg, C. M., Lian, J. B., Gallop, P. M., and Steinberg, J. J. Urinary gamma-carboxyglutamic acid and serum osteocalcin as bone markers: Studies in osteoporosis and Paget's disease. *J. Clin. Endocrinol. Metab. 57*:1221–1225 (1983).

202. Urist, M. R., and Hudak, R. T. Radioimmunoassay of bone morphogenetic protein in serum: A tissue-specific parameter of bone metabolism. *Proc. Soc. Exp. Biol. Med. 176*:472–475 (1984).
203. Karlén, J., Aperia, A., and Zetterström, R. Renal excretion of calcium and phosphate in preterm and term infants. *J. Pediatr. 106*:814–819 (1985).
204. Heller, R. M., Kirchner, S. G., O'Neil, J. A., Hough, A. J., Howard, L., Kramer, S. S., and Green, H. L. Skeletal changes of copper deficiency in infants receiving prolonged total parenteral nutrition. *J. Pediatr. 92*:947–949 (1978).
205. Al-Rashid, R. A., and Spangler, J. Neonatal copper deficiency. *N. Engl. J. Med. 285*:841–843 (1971).
206. Ashkenazi, A., Levin, S., Djaldetti, M., Fishel, E., and Benvenisti. D. The syndrome of neonatal copper deficiency. *Pediatrics 52*:525–533 (1973).
207. Sann, L., David, L., Galy, G., and Romand-Monier, M. Copper deficiency and hypocalcemic rickets in a small-for-date infant. *Acta Paediatr. Scand. 67*:303–307 (1978).
208. Griscom, N. T., Craig, J. N., and Neuhauser, E. B. D. Systemic bone disease developing in small premature infants. *Pediatrics 48*:883–895 (1971).
209. Yuen, P., Lin, H. J., and Hutchison, J. H. Copper deficiency in a low birthweight infant. *Arch. Dis. Child. 54*:553–555 (1979).
210. Blom, I., Jameson, S., Krook, F., Larsson-Stymne, B., and Wranne, L. Zinc deficiency with transitory acrodermatitis enteropathica in a boy of low birth weight. *Br. J. Dermatol. 104*:459–464 (1980).
211. Aggett, P. J., Atherton, D. J., More, J., Davey, J., Delves, H. T., and Harries, J. T. Symptomatic deficiency in breast-fed preterm infant. *Arch. Dis. Child. 55*:547–550 (1980).
212. Hambridge, K. M. Zinc deficiency in man: Its origins and effects. *Phil. Trans. R. Soc. Lond. B294*:129–144 (1981).
213. Bonifazi, E., Rigillo, N., DeSimone, B., and Meneghini, C. L. Acquired dermatitis due to zinc deficiency in a premature infant. *Acta Derm. Venereol. (Stock.) 60*:449–451 (1980).
214. Shaw, J. C. L. Trace metal requirements of preterm infants. *Acta Paediatr. Scand. 296 (suppl)*:93–100 (1982).
215. Odutuga, A. A. Effects of low-zinc status and essential fatty acid deficiency on bone development and mineralization. *Comp. Biochem. Physiol. 71A*:383–388 (1982).
216. Leek, J. C., Vogler, J. B., Gershwin, M. E., Golub, M. S., Hurley, L. S., and Hendrickx, A. G. Studies of marginal zinc deprivation on rhesus monkeys. V. Fetal and infant skeletal effects. *Am. J. Clin. Nutr. 40*:1203–1212 (1984).
217. Miller, E. R., Luecke, R. W., Ullrey, D. E., Baltzer, B. V., Bradley, B. L., and Hoefer, J. A. Biochemical, skeletal and allometric changes due to zinc deficiency in the baby pig. *J. Nutr. 95*:278–286 (1968).
218. Harrison, H. E., and Harrison, H. C. *Disorders of Calcium and Phosphate Metabolism in Childhood and Adolescence*. W. B. Saunders, Philadelphia, 1979.

219. Maroteaux, P. *Bone Diseases of Childhood*, J. B. Lippincott, Philadelphia, 1979.
220. Schanler, R. J., and Nichols, B. L. The water-soluble vitamins C, B_1, B_2, B_6, and niacin. In: *Vitamin and Mineral Requirements in Preterm Infants* (R. C. Tsang, ed.). Marcel Dekker, New York, 1985, p. 41.
221. Caffey, J. Chronic poisoning due to excess of vitamin A. *Am. J. Roentgenol. 65*:12–26 (1951).
222. Persson, B., Tunell, R., and Ekengren, K. Chronic vitamin A intoxication during the first half year of life. *Acta Paediatr. Scand. 54*:49–60 (1965).
223. Owen, G. M., Garry, P. J., Lubin, A. H., and Kram, K. M. Nutritional status of preschool children: Plasma vitamin A. *J. Pediatr. 78*:1042–1044 (1971).
224. Beighton, P. *Inherited Disorders of the Skeleton*. Churchill Livingstone, New York, 1978.
225. Marx, S. J., Spiegel, A. M., Brown, E. M., Gardner, D. G., Downs, R. W., Attie, M., Hamstra, A. J., and DeLuca, H. F. A familial syndrome of decrease in sensitivity to 1,25-dihydroxyvitamin D. *J. Clin. Endocrinol. Metab. 47*:1303–1310 (1978).
226. Fraser, D., Scriver, C. R. Familial forms of vitamin D-resistant rickets revisited. X-linked hypophosphatemia and autosomal recessive vitamin D dependency. *Am. J. Clin. Nutr. 29*:1315–1329 (1976).
227. Parfitt, A. M. Hypophosphatemic vitamin D refractory rickets and osteomalacia. *Orthop. Clin. North Am. 3*:653–680 (1972).
228. Griffin, J. E., and Zerwekh, J. E. Impaired stimulation of 25-hydroxyvitamin D-24-hydroxylase in fibroblasts from a patient with vitamin D-dependent rickets, type II. A form of receptor-positive resistance to 1,25-dihydroxyvitamin D_3. *J. Clin. Invest. 72*:1190–1199 (1983).
229. Silver, J., Landau, H., Bab, I., Shvil, Y., Friedlaender, M. M., Rubinger, D., and Popovtzer, M. M. Vitamin D-dependent rickets type I and II. Diagnosis and response to therapy. *Isr. J. Med. Sci. 21*:53–56 (1985).
230. Arnaud, C., Maijer, R., Reade, T., Scriver, C. R., and Whelan, D. T. Vitamin D dependency: An inherited postnatal syndrome with secondary hyperparathyroidism. *Pediatrics 46*:871–880 (1970).
231. Newman, J. H., Neff, T. A., and Ziporin, P. Acute respiratory failure associated with hypophosphatemia. *N. Engl. J. Med. 296*:1101–1103 (1977).
232. O'Connor, L. R., Wheeler, W. S., and Bethune, J. E. Effect of hypophosphatemia on myocardial performance in man. *N. Engl. J. Med. 297*:901–903 (1977).
233. Darsee, J. R., and Nutter, D. O. Reversible severe congestive cardiomyopathy in three cases of hypophosphatemia. *Ann. Intern. Med. 89*:867–870 (1978).
234. Travis, S. F., Sugerman, H. J., Ruberg, R. L., Dudrick, S. J., Delivoria-Papadopoulos, M., Miller, L. D., and Oski, F. A. Alterations of red-cell glycolytic intermediates and oxygen transport as a consequence of hypophosphatemia in patients receiving intravenous hyperalimentation. *N. Engl. J. Med. 285*:763–768 (1971).

235. Kooh, S. W., Fraser, D., Reilly, B. J., Hamilton, J. R., Gall, D. G., and Bell, L. Rickets due to calcium deficiency. *N. Engl. J. Med. 297*:1264–1266 (1977).
236. Tullock, A. L. Rickets in the premature. *Med. J. Aust. 1*:137–140 (1974).
237. Kovar, I. Z., Mayne, P., and Wallis, J. Neonatal rickets in one of identical twins. *Arch. Dis. Child. 57*:792–794 (1982).
238. Harrison, H. E., and Harrison, H. C. *Disorders of Calcium and Phosphate Metabolism in Childhood and Adolescence*. W. B. Saunders, Philadelphia, 1979.
239. Brown, D. R., Tsang, R. C., and Chen, I-W. Oral calcium supplementation in premature and asphyxiated neonates. *J. Pediatr. 89*:973–977 (1976).
240. Koo, W. K., and Tsang, R. C. Rickets in infants. In: *Current Therapy in Neonatal-Perinatal Medicine 1985–1986*. (N. M. Nelson, ed.). B. C. Decker, Philadelphia, 1985, pp. 299–304.
241. Carey, D. E., Goetz, C. A., Horak, E., and Rowe, J. C. Phosphorus wasting during phosphorus supplementation of human milk feedings in preterm infants. *J. Pediatr. 107*:790–794 (1985).
242. Sann, L., Loras, B., David, L., Durr, F., Simonnet, C., Baltassat P., and Bethenod, M. Effect of phosphate supplementation to breast fed very low birthweight infants on urinary calcium excretion, serum immunoreactive parathyroid hormone and plasma 1,25-dihydroxy-vitamin D concentration. *Acta Paediatr. Scand. 74*:664–668 (1985).
243. Christiansen, C. Rødbro, P., Christensen, M. S., Hartnack, B., and Transbøl, I. Deterioration of renal function during treatment of chronic renal failure with 1,25-dihydroxycholecalciferol. *Lancet 2*:700–703 (1978).
244. Christiansen, C., Rødbro, P., Christensen, M. S., and Hartnack, B. Is 1,25-dihydroxy-cholecalciferol harmful to renal function in patients with chronic renal failure? *Clin. Endocrinol. 15*:229–236 (1981).
245. Massry, S. G., and Goldstein, D. A. Is calcitriol [$1,25(OH)_2D_3$] harmful to renal function? *J.A.M.A. 242*:1875–1876 (1979).
246. Paterson, C. R. Hypercalcemia in alphacalcidol therapy. *Postgrad. Med. J. 57*:431–432 (1981).
247. Compston, J. E., Horton, L. W. L., and Laker, M. F. Vitamin-D analogues and renal function. *Lancet 1*:386 (1979).
248. Nordin, B. E. C. Vitamin-D analogues and renal function. *Lancet 2*:1259 (1978).
249. Dostal, L. A., Toverud, S. U., and Peach, R. Renal calcification in suckling rats after high doses of calcitriol (1,25-dihydroxycholecalciferol). *Arch. Pathol. Lab. Med. 108*:410–415 (1984).
250. Dostal, L. A., and Toverud, S. U. Enhanced sensitivity of young suckling rats to the toxic effects of 1,25-dihydroxyvitamin D_3. *Calcif. Tissue Int. 35*:432–437 (1983).
251. Atkin, I., Pita, J. C., Ornoy, A., Agundez, A., Castiglione, G., and Howell, D. S. Effects of vitamin D metabolites on healing of low phosphate vitamin D-deficient induced rickets in rats. *Bone 6*:113–123 (1985).

252. Raisz, L. G., Maina, D. M., Gworek, S. C., Dietrich, J. W., and Canalis, E. M. Hormonal control of bone collagen synthesis *in vitro*: Inhibitory effect of 1-hydroxylated vitamin D metabolites. *Endocrinology 102*: 731–735 (1978).
253. Mahgoub, A. Interaction between 24R, 25-dihydroxycholecalciferol and 1,25-dihydroxycholecalciferon on ^{45}Ca release from bone *in vitro. Calcif. Tissue Int. 33*:663–666 (1981).
254. Miller, S. C., Halloran, B. P., DeLuca, H. F., Yamada, S., Takayama, H., and Jee, W. S. S. Studies on the role of 24-hydroxylation of vitamin D in the mineralization of cartilage and bone of vitamin D-deficient rats. *Calcif. Tissue Int. 33*:489–497 (1981).
255. Koo, W. W. K., Oestreich, A. E., Sherman, R., Buckley, D., Tsang, R. C., and Steichen, J. J. Failure of high calcium and phosphorus supplementation in the prevention of rickets of prematurity. *Am. J. Dis. Child. 140*: 857–858 (1986).
256. Schanler, R. J., and Nichols, B. L. The water-soluble vitamins C, B_1, B_2, B_6, and niacin. In: *Vitamin and Mineral Requirements in Preterm Infants*. (R. C. Tsang, ed.). Marcel Dekker, New York, 1985, p. 41.
257. Widdowson, E. M., and Spray, C. M. Chemical development in utero. *Arch. Dis. Child. 26*:205–214 (1951).

6

Familial Hypophosphatemia

Binita R. Shah, Irma Fiordalisi, and Laurence Finberg

SUNY Health Science Center at Brooklyn, Brooklyn, New York

I. INTRODUCTION

Familial hypophosphatemia (FH) is a genetically determined inability to reabsorb phosphate from the proximal renal tubule, the major site for phosphate reabsorption, with resultant phosphaturia and hypophosphatemia. When hypophosphatemia is significant, rickets or osteomalacia occurs. In regions where nutritional rickets is relatively uncommon, patients with familial hypophosphatemic rickets (FHR) far outnumber the former in metabolic clinics since these patients must return regularly over a lifetime. Albright et al. in 1937 reported a child with hypophosphatemic rickets responding to massive doses of vitamin D and introduced the term vitamin-D-resistant rickets (1). The same entity has been subsequently reported under a variety of names including renal hypophosphatemic rickets, familial hypophosphatemic rickets, X-linked hypophosphatemic rickets, and genetic primary hypophosphatemic rickets (2-5). Vitamin-D-resistant rickets is a misnomer; utilizing a pharmacological property of vitamin D in high dose that differs from its physiological actions does not overcome the resistance. Affected family members may have only mild rachitic deformities or short stature or hypophosphatemia as an isolated finding. Hence FH is the preferred term; the additional descriptor "familial" is important since most varieties of rickets are hypophosphatemic.

II. GENETICS

The most common mode of inheritance in FH is X-linked dominant with variable penetrance, with males being more severely affected than females. Autosomal dominant and recessive modes of inheritance have been described in rare kindreds (5,6) and a number of patients appear without a family history, presumably signifying appearance of a mutant gene.

III. PATHOPHYSIOLOGY

FH is classified as a primary defect in phosphate metabolism; it was relatively recently recognized, however, that vitamin D and calcium homeostasis is abnormal as well, but the traditional classification remains useful. The extracellular phosphorous concentration is the result of the interactions of the gastrointestinal absorption, urinary excretion, and bone metabolism. The kidney plays a major role in phosphorous homeostasis by regulating tubular reabsorption of phosphate (TRP). Maximal reabsorption of phosphate normalized to glomerular filtration rate (TmP/GFR) reflects the actual renal handling of phosphate. Normal TRP ranges from 80 to 95% and normal TmP/GFR is 3.3-8.2 mg/dl in children (ages 6-13.9 years) (2,7). The pathogenesis of FH includes a selective disorder of TRP leading to massive phosphate leak. The TRP is reduced to 42-72% and TmP/GFR is decreased to $<$2.0 mg/dl in these patients (8). Urinary phosphate wasting is thus massive, with values in excess of 20 mg/kg per day. Phosphaturia is selective; patients do not have glycosuria, increased aminoaciduria, or potassium or bicarbonate wasting.

There is also impaired conversion of 25-hydroxyvitamin D (25-OH-D) to 1,25-dihydroxyvitamin D (1,25$(OH)_2$D) (4,9-12). In untreated patients, the concentration of 25-OH-D is normal while concentration of 1,25 $(OH)_2$D is either low or normal. However, since hypophosphatemia is a strong stimulus for mitochondrial 1-α-hydroxylase activity higher than normal concentrations of 1,25$(OH)_2$D would be expected. Parathyroid hormone (PTH) stimulation in normal controls has been shown to increase serum 1,25$(OH)_2$D values 218% above the baseline, while in patients with FH this response is blunted and elevation is only about 68% (12). Also patients with FH who develop secondary hyperparathyroidism on treatment continue to have low levels of 1,25$(OH)_2$D (4). Inappropriately low 1,25$(OH)_2$D levels for the degree of hypophosphatemia suggest impaired 25-hydroxyvitamin D-1α-hydroxylase activity. Defective transport of phosphate across the intestinal mucosa as well as calcium malabsorption is described. Patients with FHR have high fecal excretion of calcium and phosphorus and their urinary calcium excretion is low (3,13,14). Hypophosphatemia prevents bone mineralization, thus flow of calcium from extracellular fluid is diminished and the eucalcemic state (with normal concentration of PTH) is maintained.

IV. CLINICAL MANIFESTATIONS

An affected infant with FHR appears normal at birth with normophosphatemia. Transplacental phosphate transfer to the fetus is adequately maintained, even from a hypophosphatemic mother, and the fetal skeleton is normally mineralized. The infant continues to grow normally over the first few months of life. Presumably the physiologically low GFR of a young infant prevents excessive phosphate leak, thus maintaining a normal serum phosphorus concentration (normal values, see Table 3, Chap. 4). However, if a mother with FH offers her low-phosphate breast milk to an affected infant, nutritional phosphate deficiency rickets may precede the expression of the genetic trait. The serum phosphorus values usually decrease in the second half of the first year coincident with diminished growth velocity. With a known family history, serial determinations of fasting serum phosphorous with elevated alkaline phosphatase levels will confirm the diagnosis before the appearance of rachitic deformities. When early biochemical events are unrecognized, patients usually present with deformities of the weight-bearing extremities in the second year of life. Genu varum, waddling gait secondary to coxa vara, and medial tibial torsion are common deformities. Somatic growth failure secondary to hypophosphatemia and rachitic deformities contribute to short stature. Genu valgum and craniosynostosis are occasionally seen. Dental eruption is usually not delayed and enamel hypoplasia is uncommon, though spontaneous tooth abscesses have been described. Typical features of vitamin D deficiency such as rachitic rosary, craniotabes, muscular hypotonia, and vertebral and pelvic deformities are seen uncommonly in children with FHR.

Table 1 Diagnostic Features of Familial Hypophosphatemic Rickets

Serum
Normocalcemia
Hypophosphatemia
Elevated alkaline phosphatase activity
Normal 25-OH-D concentration
"Normal" or low $1{,}25(OH)_2D$ concentration
Usually normal iPTH concentration
Urine
Isolated massive phosphate excretion
Normal amino acid excretion
Reduced calcium excretion

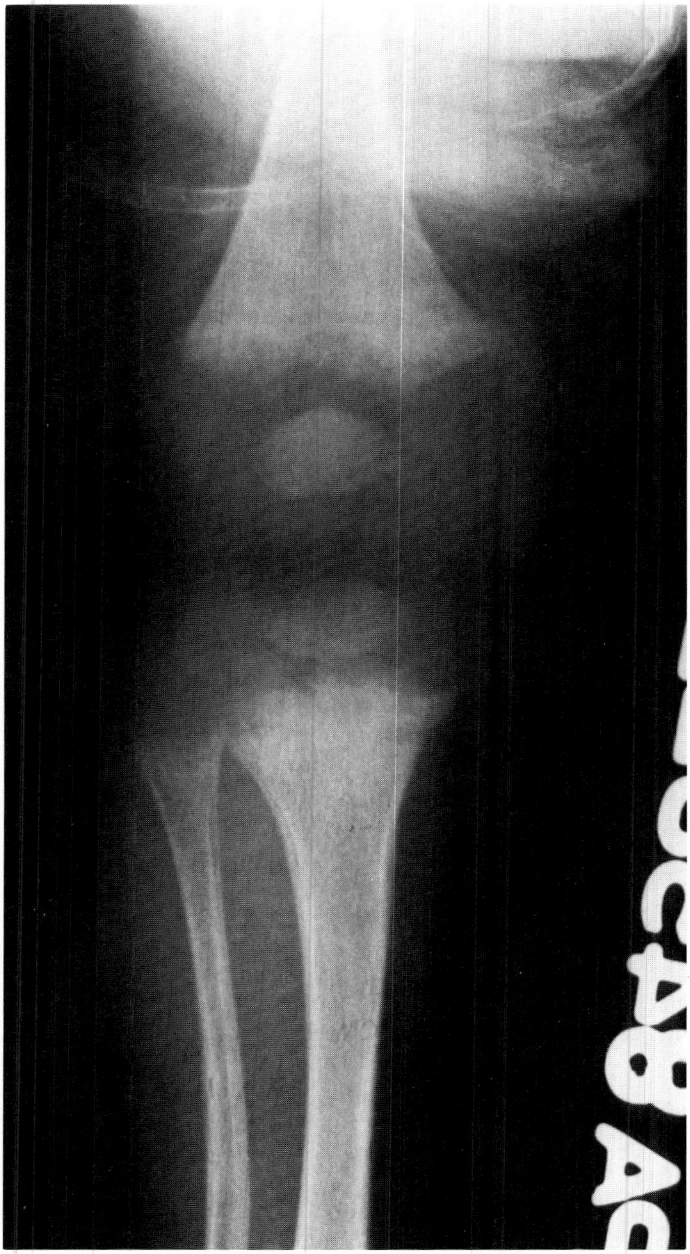

Figure 1 Familial hypophosphatemic rickets. Anteroposterior view of the knee. Note the radiolucent zone of unmineralized osteoid separating metaphysis from epiphysis. The shaggy appearance ("fraying") of the metaphyses represents bony projections protruding into the mass of unmineralized osteoid.

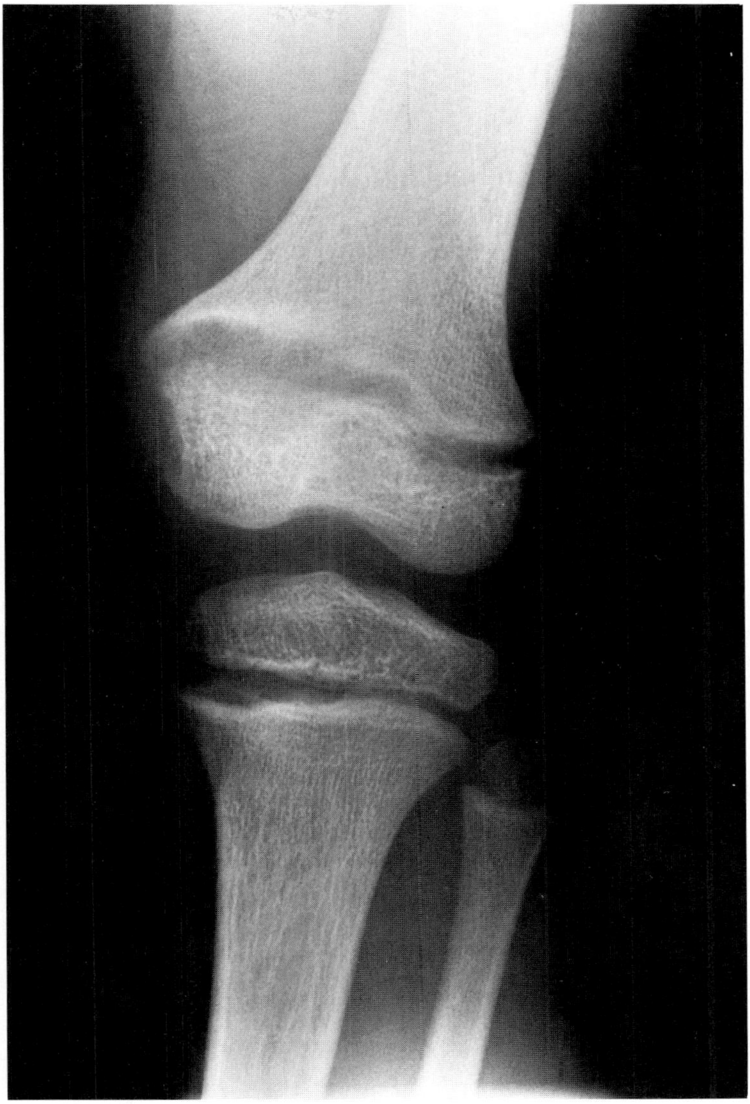

Figure 2 Familial hypophosphatemic rickets. Anteroposterior view of the knee. Note the wedge-shaped metaphyseal defect of the medial aspect of the distal femur and proximal tibia. Clinically, there was a genu varum deformity.

V. DIAGNOSIS

The diagnosis of FHR (Table 1) is made by presence of fasting hypophosphatemia, normocalcemia, elevated alkaline phosphatase levels and normal 25-OH-D concentrations. Parathyroid function as measured by system immunoreactive PTH (iPTH) is usually normal or only mildly elevated. Serum concentration of $1,25(OH)_2D$ is "normal" or low. Urinary phosphate wasting is prominent, while calcium excretion is reduced. Urinary amino acid excretion is normal. Roentgenographic findings show a hazy, indistinct metaphysis with a frayed appearance and an increased lucency (unmineralized osteoid) between epiphysis and metaphysis. The metaphysis may appear widened and its contour may be cupped or concave. These changes are best seen in children under the age of 4 at the distal end of the femur and proximal end of the tibia and fibula. At later ages, the radius and ulna are also useful sites to examine. The rapidly growing weight-bearing lower extremities make the knee joint the preferred site for confirmation and follow-up of rachitic changes (Fig. 1). The diaphysis may show a coarse trabecular pattern. In long-standing rickets of FH, a wedge-shaped defect of the weight-bearing side of the proximal tibial metaphysis, secondary to abnormal weight thrust, is a characteristic finding. Thus patients with genu varum have a metaphyseal defect medially while in genu valgum they have a lateral defect (Fig. 2).

VI. DIFFERENTIAL DIAGNOSIS

Conditions that mimic FHR include physiological bowing, Blount's disease, oncogenous rickets, nutritional phosphate deficiency, metaphyseal dysostosis, Fanconi's syndrome, distal renal tubular acidosis and vitamin D deficiency, and vitamin-D-dependent rickets (Table 2). Physiological bowing occurs in early childhood with normal serum biochemical and radiological findings. Blount's disease is characterized by normal serum biochemical values but diagnostic beak-like projection (aseptic necrosis) of the proximal tibial metaphysis medially.

Oncogenous rickets or osteomalacia is characterized by skeletal deformities, bone pain, and muscle weakness. As in children with FH, these patients have hypophosphatemia and hyperphosphaturia. Serum concentrations of calcium, iPTH, and 25-OH-D are normal, while the concentration of $1,25(OH)_2D$ is low. This form of rickets usually occurs in association with benign tumors of mesenchymal origin such as nonossifying fibromas, histiocytomas, fibroangiomas, or, rarely, with malignant tumors such as sarcomas. Various sites at which these tumors are seen include bone, nasal antrum, pharynx, skin, subcutaneous tissue, and muscle. These tumors secrete a substance (unidentified to date) that leads to phosphaturia and impaired vitamin D metabolism. Excision of the tumor corrects hypophosphatemia and $1,25(OH)_2D$ concentration also returns to normal

Table 2 Hypophosphatemic Disorders of Childhood

Disorders of renal tubular phosphate reabsorption with impaired production of $1,25(OH)_2D$
Familial hypophosphatemic rickets
Oncogenous rickets
Hypophosphatemic bone disease
Disorders of renal tubular phosphate reabsorption:
Fanconi's syndrome[a]
Congenital: cystinosis, tyrosinosis, Lowe's syndrome, Wilson's disease, hereditary fructose intolerance
Acquired: heavy metal poisoning, ingestion of outdated tetracycline
Idiopathic
Renal tubular acidosis[a]
Hereditary hypophosphatemic rickets with hypercalciuria
Nutritional phosphate deficiency
Total parenteral alimentation
Low-phosphate feedings in low-birthweight infants
Malabsorption (e.g., $Al(OH)_2$ intake)
Secondary to increased PTH secretion
Primary hyperparathyroidism
Vitamin-D-deficiency rickets
Vitamin-D-dependent rickets, type I
Vitamin-D-dependent rickets, type II

[a]Systemic acidosis may impair conversion of 25-OH-D to $1,25(OH)_2D$, resulting in low serum levels of calcitriol.

with resolution of symptoms. Glycinemia, glycinuria, glycosuria, and aminoaciduria have also been described in patients with this form of rickets. Patients with acquired hypophosphatemic rickets or osteomalacia should undergo complete roentgenographic examination and/or bone scan to search for tumors (15,16).

Hypophosphatemic rickets secondary to deficient phosphate intake is seen in very-low-birthweight premature infants given unsupplemented feedings such as human milk or standard formulas, or if they are receiving intravenous total parenteral nutrition for a prolonged period of time. Phosphorus and calcium available through these feedings are inadequate for optimal mineralization of the bones of these rapidly growing preterm infants. On the other hand, nutritional phosphate deficiency in children receiving a mixed diet is almost impossible because of the high content of phosphate in all foods derived from vegetable or animal sources. Phosphorus deficiency leading to rickets is characterized by hypophosphatemia, normal or increased serum calcium concentrations, and increased serum concentrations of $1,25(OH)_2D$ and alkaline phosphatase. Serum

Table 3 A Comparison of High-Dose Vitamin D Treatment in Nutritional Vitamin D Deficiency and Familial Hypophosphatemia

	A 6-Month-Old Patient With Nutritional Vitamin-D-Deficiency Rickets			A 2-Year-Old Patient with Familial Hypophosphatemic Rickets		
	Ca (mg/dl)	P (mg/dl)	Alkaline Phosphatase (U/L)	Ca (mg/dl)	P (mg/dl)	Alkaline Phosphatase (U/L)
Normal Values	8.5-10.5	4.0-6.2	109-265	8.5-10.5	4.0-6.2	95-218
Day						
0	7.1	3.4	1576	8.5	3.5	1342
			Ergocalciferol 600,000 U by mouth			
4	8.7	5.0	1554	8.9	3.8	1231
17	10.1	5.6	1072	9.4	3.7	1141
				Calcitriol and phosphate supplements		
42	10.1	5.8	291	10.2	3.2	581

concentration of iPTH is normal. Urinary phosphorus excretion is markedly reduced while hypercalciuria is prominent (17). Biochemical findings thus differentiate this form of rickets from FHR.

Metaphyseal dysostosis mimics this form of rickets radiographically but shows normal serum concentrations of calcium, phosphorus, and alkaline phosphatase. Fanconi's syndrome describes a variety of renal tubular defects resulting in at least two of the following: renal glycosuria, generalised aminoaciduria, renal hypophosphatemia, and bicarbonate wasting. Causes include certain inborn metabolic errors that result in accumulation of metabolites and damage to renal tubular cells, nephrotoxicity secondary to heavy metal, phenol, or cresol poisoning may also manifest as Fanconi's syndrome. Growth failure and rickets or osteomalacia due to hypophosphatemia with renal phosphate wasting are typical sequelae.

Vitamin-D-deficiency and vitamin-D-dependent rickets (types I and II) are associated with hypocalcemia, secondary hyperparathyroidism, and increased urinary aminoaciduria. Serum 25-OH-D concentration is decreased in vitamin-D-deficiency rickets while $1,25(OH)_2D$ concentration is decreased in vitamin-D-dependent rickets, type I, and markedly increased in type II. With an absent or doubtful positive family history for FH, one may administer a single large dose of vitamin D (e.g., 600,000 U vitamin D_3); in FHR, unlike vitamin-D-deficiency rickets, serum phosphorus levels do not rise and hypophosphatemia persists (Table 3).

Distal renal tubular acidosis is characterized by a failure of distal tubular cells to maintain a H^+ ion gradient and therefore to excrete an acid urine, systemic metabolic acidemia, polyuria, hypokalemia, renal hypophosphatemia, increased urinary calcium excretion, increased renal tubular reabsorption of citrate, and nephrocalcinosis. The disorder is inherited in either autosomal dominant or autosomal recessive fashion. Although renal tubular reabsorption of phosphate is almost entirely a proximal tubular function, this mechanism may be disrupted by the acidosis leading to hypophosphatemia and rickets. The bony lesions here heal with bicarbonate therapy and correction of acidosis.

VII. TREATMENT

The principles of therapy are promotion of linear growth without skeletal deformities, avoidance of drug toxicity, and genetic counseling. The most successful treatment strategies include phosphate supplements given around the clock sufficiently to raise extracellular phosphate concentration in conjunction with pharmacological dosages of a form of vitamin D. Vitamin D increases intestinal absorption of calcium and phosphorus. Supraphysiological dosages of vitamin D (cholecalciferol or ergocalciferol) administered alone have induced healing of rickets but have often led to vitamin D intoxication. Phosphate supplement alone often leads to secondary hyperparathyroidism by reducing calcium absorption from the intestinal tract. Increased levels of PTH can aggravate the bone disease both directly and indirectly by exaggerating the preexisting phosphate leak. Despite high dosages of vitamin D_2, vitamin D_3, or 25-hydroxyvitamin D (calcidiol), therapeutic levels of $1,25(OH)_2D$ may not be achieved since these patients are not adequately able to convert 25-OH-D to $1,25(OH)_2D$. Thus of available vitamin D preparations, 1,25-dihydroxyvitamin D_3 (calcitriol) is preferred. It is the most active vitamin D metabolite and offers a considerable margin of safety because of its shorter half-life; thus, if an excess dosage is given inadvertently, the hypercalcemia is transient. It is available commercially containing 0.25 or 0.50 μg of active metabolite per capsule. The initial dosage is between 0.25 and 0.50 μg given every 12 hr. The appropriate dosage of calcitriol is the amount necessary to normalize intestinal calcium absorption, which is determined indirectly by serum calcium concentration and urinary calcium excretion. Excessive calcitriol intake leads to hyperabsorption of calcium, hypercalciuria, and hypercalcemia, whereas with low calcitriol intake calcium malabsorption and decreased urinary calcium excretion characteristic of FH continue. By maintaining increased calcium absorption in the face of high phosphate intake, secondary hyperparathyroidism is prevented. The normal range of calcium in a 24 hr urine collection in children is 1-4 mg/kg, or a calcium/creatinine ratio (expressed as mg calcium/mg creatinine) between 0.05 and 0.25 in either a 12-24 hr collection or a single voided specimen (5,18). The earliest danger signal of vitamin D excess is hypercalciuria, which occurs before hypercalcemia. Close monitoring thus prevents hypercalcemia, nephrocalcinosis, and renal insufficiency. Renal ultrasonography is the diagnostic modality of choice for the detection of nephrocalcinosis; plain abdominal radiographs may show entirely normal findings (19).

Phosphate supplements are started with a small amount and gradually increased to a total of 1-1.5 g phosphate for infants and 1.5-2.5 g for older children. The total amount is divided into four or five doses to ensure a relatively constant concentration of phosphate in the extracellular fluid. Preparations currently available include Neutra-phos, Neutra-phos-K (both in powder and capsule form), and K-Phos (tablet form). The complications of therapy are diarrhea and noncompliance because of the formulation's unpleasant taste. Healing of rickets is confirmed biochemically and radiographically. Hypophosphatemia in the fasting state persists despite radiographic evidence of healing while alkaline phosphatase levels return to normal. Growth velocity and improvement in the deformities are important indicators to monitor. Parental education and patient compliance are important determinants of overall success in therapy. Medical therapy must be continued at least until skeletal maturation. Some patients may need therapy into adulthood to prevent osteomalacia.

Corrective osteotomies may be necessary for severe leg deformities. The preferred time, however, depends on severity (and disability) as well as response to medical treatment. If medical therapy is initiated early and is aggressive, most patients will not require surgery. Early surgical intervention without adequate medical therapy may result in reappearance of deformities. If surgery is warranted, calcitriol therapy should be discontinued several days prior to operation to avoid immobilization hypercalcemia and should not be resumed until after complete mobilization. However, phosphate supplements should be continued during the entire perioperative period.

All family members should be screened for short stature, rachitic deformities, and hypophosphatemia. Appropriate genetic counseling should be provided. To date, prenatal diagnosis is not possible.

Diuretics have recently been used along with calcitriol and phosphate supplements in a small group of children with FHR (20). Hydrochlorothiazide in combination with amiloride was shown to result in an elevation of the renal tubular threshold for phosphate, with an elevation of serum phosphate concentration. Both these diuretics, with their hypocalciuric properties, also help to maintain urinary calcium excretion in the normal range, thus allowing continued use of calcitriol. High calcitriol along with a low-phosphate regimen may be necessary in a rare patient to suppress secondary hyperparathyroidism. Long-term studies with a larger number of patients are desirable before such regimens can be considered beneficial or safe.

Development of parathyroid "autonomy" has been claimed to occur secondary to chronic hyperstimulation by oral phosphate supplements. A few patients with FH who developed hypercalcemic hyperparathyroidism have been reported; this probably represents coincidence of two separate diseases rather than a complication of therapy (21).

VIII. CLINICAL AND BIOCHEMICAL VARIANTS

Two clinical entities that share hereditary renal phosphate leak with FH but differ distinctly in some aspects have been described recently: hereditary hypophosphatemic rickets with hypercalciuria (HHRH) and hypophosphatemic bone disease (HBD).

A. Hereditary Hypophosphatemic Rickets with Hypercalciuria

This entity (22), described among closely related members of a single Bedouin tribe, manifests in early childhood with rickets, short stature, normocalcemia, and hypophosphatemia with isolated renal phosphate leak. Two important features differentiate HHRH from FH. Marked hypercalciuria and elevated serum $1,25(OH)_2D$ concentrations are characteristic findings in HHRH, while $1,25(OH)_2D$ concentrations are low or "normal" and urinary calcium excretion is low in FH. Also, serum iPTH concentration is low (suppressed by increased calcium absorption from the intestinal tract secondary to elevated $1,25(OH)_2D$ levels) in HHRH while it is normal or mildly elevated in FH. A significiant number of asymptomatic family members in this tribe also showed "idiopathic" hypercalciuria alone without associated bone disease (23). Hereditary renal phosphate leak results in hypophosphatemia, which in turn stimulates $1,25(OH)_2D$ production in the renal tubule. An appropriately elevated $1,25(OH)_2D$ concentration results in hyperabsorption of calcium and phosphorus from the intestine, leading to an increased renal filtered load of calcium and consequent hypercalciuria. The degree of hypophosphatemia appears to determine whether patients will have bone disease or not, since patients with hypercalciuria alone have relatively milder hypophosphatemia. Patients with HHRH have been treated effectively with phosphate supplements alone with good results. The mode of inheritance suggests an autosomal recessive pattern.

B. Hypophosphatemic Bone Disease

This is characterized by short stature and rachitic limb deformities in early childhood (24). The serum concentrations of calcium, iPTH, and 25-OH-D are normal, alkaline phosphatase levels are normal or elevated, and phosphorus concentration is low. The serum levels of $1,25(OH)_2D$ are normal; as compared with patients with FHR are significantly higher (9), although still inappropriate for the degree of hypophosphatemia. At low endogenous concentration of phosphate anion, net TRP is normal; however, TRP is below normal with an artificially raised concentration of phosphate. Even though TmP/GFR is reduced in both HBD and FH, fractional renal excretion of filtered phosphate is normal in the fasting hypophosphatemic state in HBD while it is markedly increased at the comparable serum phosphate level in FH. Phosphaturic response to bovine PTH also differs in both HBD and FH. Thus at comparable concentrations of serum phosphorus in HBD and FH, the bone disease and renal handling of phosphate are different. The bone disease is less severe in HBD. Typical findings are sclerosis, coarse trabeculae, and increased density with bowing of the long bones, but not rickets. HBD is inherited as an autosomal dominant trait, though sporadic occurrence is seen and some patients with HBD may have family members with FHR or isolated hypophosphatemia. Treatment with calcitriol alone has resulted not only in improvement in bone mineralization but also a rise of TRP leading to a rise in serum phosphorus concentration in some patients (24,25).

IX. CASE PRESENTATIONS

A. Patient P. F.

Patient P. F. was first seen at 4 months of age when his mother, who had FHR herself, brought him to visit one of the authors (L. F.). His perinatal history was normal, with birthweight and length at the 50th percentiles. He was receiving a soy-based infant formula. His physical examination was normal but his length and weight had shifted to below the 25th and 50th percentiles, respectively. Because of his family history (Fig. 3) serum analyses were performed (Table 4); rickets was confirmed radiographically. Vitamin D deficiency was not suspected based on the family history, adequate dietary vitamin D intake, and normal serum concentration of 25-OH-D. Serum concentration of $1,25(OH)_2D$ was numerically "normal" but distinctly low in the face of hypophosphatemia. He was given calcitriol 0.25 μg twice daily and phosphate supplement in small divided doses that were gradually increased to 1200 mg daily. After 1 year of treatment he continues to have fasting hypophosphatemia; alkaline phosphatase activity is normal for age and he has shown radiographic evidence of healing.

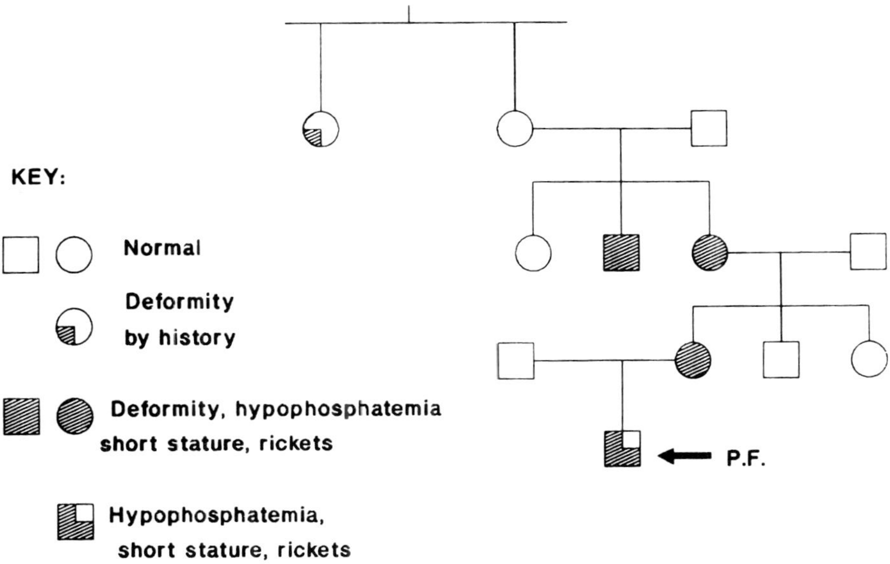

Figure 3 X-linked dominant inheritance of familial hypophosphatemia.

The family history is compatible with X-linked dominant inheritance. His great-grandmother did not have noticeable deformity and no serum levels are available. Incomplete expression of the gene is common among females, probably functioning according to the Lyon hypothesis. Noteworthy is that during treatment of his rickets, P. F.'s great-uncle developed renal failure from injudicious administration of vitamin D and subsequent toxicity.

This patient had hypophosphatemia at an early age and the relatively mild elevation of his serum iPTH concentration is incompletely understood. If dietary calcium and phosphate availability is diminished in the face of diminished production of $1{,}25(OH)_2D$ and suboptimal absorption of calcium from the intestinal tract, secondary hyperparathyroidism may occur and exacerbate the phosphate leak. It is possible that this patient' soy milk feeding with its low bioavailability of phosphate and calcium contributed to early development of hypophosphatemia and rickets. About 20% of the phosphorus in soy formula is present as phytic phosphorus; phosphate absorption across the intestine is inhibited by phytates, leading to greater fecal loss of phosphorus. Term infants fed soy formula have shown decreased bone mineral content and high $1{,}25(OH)_2D$ concentration due to decreased absorption and availability of calcium and phosphorus from soy milk feedings (26,27).

Table 4 Biochemical Data: Serum Concentrations in Patients with Familial Hypophosphatemic Rickets

	Calcium (mg/dl)	Phosphorus (mg/dl)	Alkaline Phosphatase (U/L)	25-OH-D (ng/ml)	$1,25(OH)_2D$ (pg/ml)	iPTH (pg/ml)
Normal range	8.5–10.5	4.0-6.2	1 mo–1 yr: 109-265 1-6 yrs: 95-218	10–58	15-60	50-330 (for Ca 8.8-10.4)
Patient P.F.	9.3	2.2	456	37	24	407/9.3
Patient A. R.	9.9	2.2	865	25	40	80/9.9

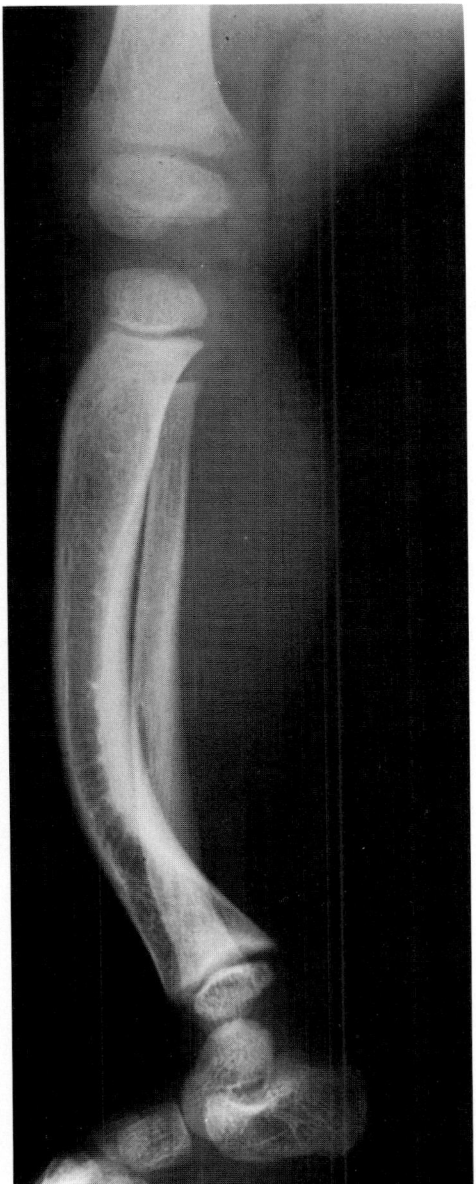

Figure 4 Same patient as in Figure 2, 12 months after treatment. Anteroposterior bowing of tibia is marked and there is thickening of the posterior cortex of tibia and fibula, an adaptive response to the marked bowing. Note that the rickets seen in Figure 2 is less conspicuous and there is marked sclerosis as a result of healing.

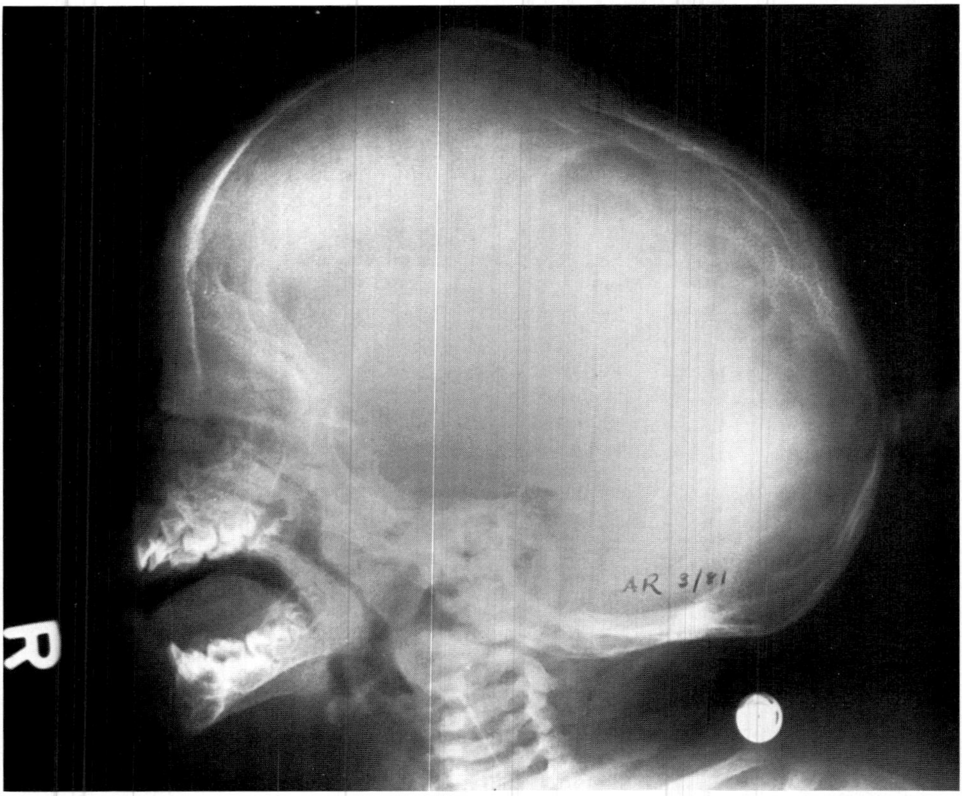

Figure 5 Same patient as in Figures 2 and 3: Lateral radiograph of skull. Note the elongated appearance with pansynostosis. Marked textural changes indicate increased intracranial pressure.

B. Patient A. R.

A 3-year-old boy was referred with severe genu varum deformity and short stature. His height was 83 cm (height-age, 20 months); his weight and head circumference were at the 10th and 5th percentile, respectively. He had scaphocephaly, lateral bowing of both femora, anterior bowing of both tibiae, and waddling gait (Figs. 2, 4) (chemical analyses of his serum are shown in Table 4). There was no evidence of hepatic or renal disease. He was diagnosed as having craniosynostosis (Fig. 5) with increased intracranial pressure at the age of 11 months. This was confirmed radiographically by computed tomographic scan and he had undergone craniectomy. Diagnosis of FHR was made and he was started on calcitriol and phosphate supplement.

Craniosynostosis is well-described in FHR, it occurs less frequently in other forms of rickets including vitamin D deficiency. One-third of 59 children under 9 years of age with rickets reportedly had craniosynostosis (28). Craniosynostosis and raised intracranial pressure is also seen in vitamin D intoxication (29), thus care must be taken to determine the cause. Unfortunately, FHR was not suspected in this patient when he was evaluated for craniosynostosis, resulting in a delay in diagnosis and severe bony deformities. With aggressive medical therapy, he has shown significant improvement in bowing and growth velocity. At the age of 7 years, he continues to take 1.75 μg calcitriol and 1500 mg phosphate supplement daily. He had occasional transient episodes of hypercalciuria but not hypercalcemia. Screening of the family members is negative for rachitic deformities, short stature, or hypophosphatemia, this patient represents a sporadic occurrence of FHR.

REFERENCES

1. Albright, F., Butler, A. M., and Bloomberg, E. Rickets resistant to vitamin D therapy. *Am. J. Dis. Child. 54*:529–547 (1937).
2. Chan, J. C. M., Alon, U., and Hirschman, G. M. Renal hypophosphatemic rickets. *J. Pediatr. 106*:533-544 (1985).
3. Short, E. M., Binder, H. J., and Rosenberg, L. E. Familial hypophosphatemic rickets: Defective transport of inorganic phosphate by intestinal mucosa. *Science 179*:700-702 (1973).
4. Chesney, R. W., Mazess. R. B., Rose, P., Hamstra, A. J., and DeLuca, H. F. Supranormal 25-hydroxyvitamin D and subnormal 1,25-dihydroxyvitamin D: Their role in X-linked hypophosphatemic rickets. *Am. J. Dis. Child. 134*:140-143 (1980).
5. Harrison, H. E., and Harrison, H. C Disorders of calcium and phosphate metabolism in childhood and adolescence. In: *Major Problems in Clinical Pediatrics*. (A. J. Schaffer and M. Markowitz, eds.). WB Saunders, Philadelphia, 1979.
6. Stamp, T. C. B., and Baker, L. R. I. Recessive hypophosphatemic rickets, and possible aetiology of the "vitamin D-resistant" syndrome. *Arch. Dis. Child 51*:360-365 (1976).
7. Kruse, K., Kracht, U., and Gopfert, G. Renal threshold phosphate concentration ($TmPo_4$/GFR). *Arch. Dis. Child. 57*:217-223 (1982).
8. Alon, U., and Chan, J. C. M. Effects of parathyroid hormone and 1,25-dihydroxyvitamin D_3 on tubular handling of phosphate in hypophosphatemic rickets. *J. Clin. Endocrinol. Metab. 58*:671-675 (1984).
9. Scriver, C. R., Reade, T. M., DeLuca, H. F., and Hamstra, A. J. Serum 1,25-dihydroxyvitamin D levels in normal subjects and in patients with hereditary rickets or bone disease. *N. Engl. J. Med. 299*:976-979 (1978).

10. Mason, R. S., Rohl, P. G., Lissner, D., and Posen, S. Vitamin D metabolism in hypophosphatemic rickets. *Am. J. Dis. Child. 136*:909-913 (1982).
11. Glorieux, F. H., Marie, P. J., Pettifor, J. M., and Delvin, E. E. Bone response to phosphate salts, ergocalciferol, and calcitriol in hypophosphatemic vitamin D-resistant rickets. *N. Engl. J. Med. 303*:1023–1031 (1980).
12. Lyles, K. W., and Drezner, M. K. Parathyroid hormone effects on serum 1,25-dihydroxyvitamin D levels in patients with X-linked hypophosphatemic rickets: Evidence for abnormal 25-hydroxyvitamin D-1-hydroxylase activity. *J. Clin. Endocrinol. Metab. 54*:638-644 (1982).
13. Condon, J. R., Nassim, J. R., and Rutter, A. Defective intestinal phosphate absorption in familial and non-familial hypophosphatemia. *Br. Med. J. 3*: 138–141 (1970).
14. Stickler, G. B., Beabout, J. W., and Riggs, B. L. Vitamin D-resistant rickets: Clinical experience with 41 typical familial hypophosphatemic patients and 2 atypical nonfamilial cases. *Mayo. Clin. Proc. 45*:197-218 (1970).
15. Parker, M. S., Klein, I., Haussler, M. R., and Mintz, D. H. Tumor induced osteomalacia: Evidence of a surgically correctable alteration in vitamin D metabolism. *J.A.M.A. 245*:492–493 (1981).
16 Kukumoto, Y., Tarui, S., Tsukiyama, K., Ichihara, K., Moriwaki, K., Nonaka, K., Mizushima, T., Kobyayashi, Y., Dokoh, S., Fukunaga, M., and Morita, R. Tumor-induced vitamin D-resistant hypophosphatemic osteomalacia associated with proximal renal tubular dysfunction and 1,25-dihydroxyvitamin D deficiency. *J. Clin. Endocrinol. Metab. 49*:873-878 (1979).
17. Rowe, J. C., and Carey, D. E. Phosphorus deficiency syndrome in very low birth weight infants. *Pediatr. Clin. North Am. 34*:997-1017 (1987).
18. Harrison, H. E. Primary hypophosphatemic rickets and growth retardation. *Growth, Genetics & Hormones 2*:1–4 (1986).
19. Goodyer, P. R., Kronick, J. B., Jequier, S., Reade, T. M., and Scriver, C. R. Nephrocalcinosis and its relationship to treatment of hereditary rickets. *J. Pediatr. 111*:700-704 (1987).
20. Alon, U., and Chan, J. C. M. Effects of hydrochlorothiazide and amiloride in renal hypophosphatemic rickets. *Pediatrics 75*:754-763 (1985).
21. Kleerekoper, M., Coffey, R., Greco, T., Nichols, S., Cooke, N., Murphy, W., and Avioli, L. V. Hypercalcemic hyperparathyroidism in hypophosphatemic rickets. *J. Clin. Endocrinol. Metab. 45* 86–94 (1977).
22. Tieder, M., Modai, D., Samuel, R., Arie, R., Halabe, A., Bab, I., Gabizon, D., and Liberman, U. A. Hereditary hypophosphatemic rickets with hypercalciuria. *N. Engl. J. Med. 312*:611-617 (1985).
23. Tieder, M., Modai, D., Shaked, U., Samuel, R., Arie, R., Halabe, A., Maor, J., Weissgarten, J., Averbukh, Z., Cohen, N., Edelstein, S., and Liberman, U. "Idiopathic" hypercalciuria and hereditary hypophosphatemic rickets. *N. Engl. J. Med. 316*:125-129 (1987).
24. Scriver, C. R., MacDonald, W., Reade, T., Glorieux, F. H., and Nogrady, B. Hypophosphatemic nonrachitic bone disease: An entity distinct from X-linked hypophosphatemia in the renal defect, bone involvement, and inheritance. *Am. J. Med. Genet. 1*:101-117 (1977).

25. Scriver, C. R., Reade, T., Halal, F., Costa, T., Cole, D E. C. Autosomal hypophosphatemic bone disease responds to 1,25-$(OH)_2D_3$. *Arch. Dis. Child.* *56*:203-207 (1981).
26. Shenai, J. P., Jhaveri, B. M., Reynolds, J. W., Huston, R. K., and Babson, S. G. Nutritional balance studies in very low-birthweight infants: Role of soy formula. *Pediatrics* *67*:631-637 (1981).
27. Steinchen, J. J., Schell, D., and Tsang, R. C. Decreased bone mineral content (BMC) and high 1,25-dihydroxyvitamin D (1,25$(OH)_2D$) in infants fed a soy protein based or a cow protein based formula. *Calcif Tissue Int.* *34*: S36 (1982).
28. Reilly, B. J., Leeming, J. M., and Fraser, D. Craniosynostosis in the rachitic spectrum. *J. Pediatr.* *64*:396-405 (1964).
29. Carlsen, N. L. T., Krasilnikoff, P. A., and Eiken, M. Premature cranial synostosis in X-linked hypophosphatemic rickets: Possible preceipitation by 1-alpha-OH-cholecalciferon intoxication. *Acta Paediatr Scand.* *73*:149-154 (1984).

7

Deficiencies in the Effector System for 1,25-Dihydroxyvitamin D

STEPHEN J. MARX

National Institute of Diabetes, Digestive, and Kidney Diseases, Bethesda, Maryland

CHAS EIL

Naval Hospital and Uniformed Services University of the Health Sciences, Bethesda, Maryland

URI A. LIBERMAN

National Institute of Diabetes, Digestive, and Kidney Diseases, Bethesda, Maryland, and Beilinson Medical Center, Petah-Tikva, Israel

M. MICHAEL BLIZIOTES, MARK S. NANES, JULIA BARSONY, and MARIA LUISA BRANDI

National Institute of Diabetes, Digestive, and Kidney Diseases, Bethesda, Maryland

I. NORMAL ACTIONS OF $1,25(OH)_2D$

1,25-Dihydroxyvitamin D ($1,25(OH)_2D$, calcitriol) is a hormonally active secosteroid with a mechanism of action analogous to that of the true steroids. Through its interaction with nuclei of target cells in many different organs, it controls a spectrum of responses (many proven so far only in vitro). These responses can be classified into four categories: (1) transepithelial transport of minerals: this "classic" response to calciferols results in increased calcium flux into serum across intestinal mucosa and, to a lesser degree, across bone surface and the renal tubule, (2) regulation of calciferol metabolism: $1,25(OH)_2D$ affects the concentrations (synthesis rate?) of 7-dehydrocholesterol in skin and the concentration of 25(OH)D, $1,25(OH)_2D$, and $24,25(OH)_2D$ in serum, not to mention concentrations in serum for a host of additional oxidation products in this pathway, (3) regulation of peptide synthesis and secretion: effects (either stimulatory or inhibitory) on a number of target peptides have been documented mostly in vitro (calcium-binding protein in intestine, collagen and osteocalcin in bone, parathyroid hormone and prolactin in their secretory cells, and interleukin-2 in T lymphocytes) and many others may be affected; (4) inhibition of proliferation and stimulation of cell differentiation: this seems to be important in conversion of macrophage-related stem cells to osteoclast or to other multinucleate giant cells and in maturation of skin and hair epithelium.

The dominant action of $1,25(OH)_2D$ in vivo is on intestinal transport of calcium, and it may be possible to replace all important actions of $1,25(OH)_2D$ by ensuring alternative methods to deliver calcium into blood.

II. RESISTANCE TO $1,25(OH)_2D$

A. Definition

We define resistance to $1,25(OH)_2D$ as a state in which abnormally high concentrations of $1,25(OH)_2D$ in blood are associated with a normal or deficient response. Although active transport of calcium by duodenum is the response of central importance in vivo, that parameter is difficult to measure directly. In clinical settings the relation between serum concentration of calcium and $1,25(OH)_2D$ is usually used as an index of this response. Resistance of serum calcium response to $1,25(OH)_2D$ can take several forms, typefied by defects in maximal response capacity, defects in response sensitivity, or mixed defects (this last includes lack of measurable response that cannot be assigned to the former two categories) (Fig. 1) (1).

B. States That Mimic Target Tissue Resistance to $1,25(OH)_2D$

Deficient function of calcitriol target cells can be mimicked by several states in which serum concentrations of $1,25(OH)_2D$ rise to compensate or to attempt to compensate for large imbalances in fluxes of calcium (or even phosphate) (1). Examples of this include growing adolescents (such as the Bantu) with diets severely deficient in calcium, neonates (with rapidly mineralizing skeleton) born prior to the third trimester of gestation, and patients with renal wastage of calcium. Another example is selective wasting of phosphate by the kidney (2); this causes hypophosphatemia, secondary elevation of $1,25(OH)_2D$, increased intenstinal absorption of calcium, PTH suppression, and hypercalciuria. The secondary rise of $1,25(OH)_2D$ is in part maladaptive (causing absorptive hypercalciuria), and patients with this syndrome benefit only from phosphate replacement; calciferols are not beneficial. All these groups are presumed to have normal target cell interaction in vivo with $1,25(OH)_2D$, and all but those with dietary calcium deficiency have normal response of net intestinal calcium flux to $1,25(OH)_2D$.

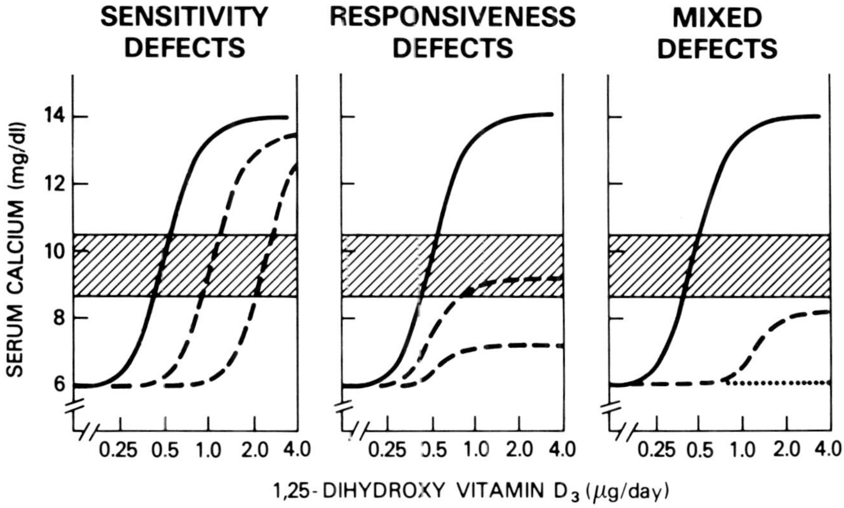

Figure 1 Variants in resistance of serum calcemic response to $1,25(OH)_2D_3$. Stippled zone indicates normal serum calcium; solid line is normal response (assuming a baseline of $1,25(OH)_2D$ deficiency and constant calcium intake) (from Ref. 1).

C. Regulation of Response to $1,25(OH)_2D$ in Target Cells

Cellular responsivity to $1,25(OH)_2D$ can be regulated in vivo. Tissue concentrations of $1,25(OH)_2D$ receptor in the gut are low in utero in the rat but rise dramatically at 2-3 weeks postpartum in association with development of $1,25(OH)_2D$-responsivivity for intestinal transport of calcium (3). Glucocorticoids can regulate concentrations of $1,25(OH)_2D$ receptors; in the rat, glucocorticoids increase receptor concentrations, while in the mouse, glucocorticoids decrease them. In general $1,25(OH)_2D$ receptor concentrations are higher in dividing than in quiescent cells. It is highly probable that a host of factors will be shown to regulate responsivity to $1,25(OH)_2D$ at the level of the receptor and beyond it.

D. Hereditary Resistance to $1,25(OH)_2D$ in Humans

1. Clinical Spectrum of Hereditary Resistance to $1,25(OH)_2D$

The general features of hereditary resistance to $1,25(OH)_2D$ (also called hereditary vitamin D dependency type II or hereditary pseudovitamin D deficiency type II) are rickets or osteomalacia, alopecia, hypocalcemia, secondary hyperparathyroidism, and high serum concentrations of $1,25(OH)_2D$ before or during treatment with calciferols. Each of these general features has shown a wide spectrum, but there are consistent correlations among all these features.

Transmission and Demographics. In about half the kindreds reported to date, parental consanguinity or similar disease in siblings has strongly suggested autosomal recessive inheritance. Parents have been reported as normal, but detailed studies have not been done. In several cases, subtle abnormalities have been suggested from analyses of receptor function of skin fibroblasts from parents (4).

There has been a striking clustering of cases close to the Mediterranean (5). This clustering is true for kindreds showing all types of cellular defect (see below); therefore, it is not simply a clustering of one mutation.

Serum Calcium and Calcemic Response to Calciferols. In the mildest forms of disease there is normocalcemia, mild secondary hyperparathyroidism, and mild elevation of $1,25(OH)_2D$ concentrations. Most reported patients, however, have had more severe dysfunction with hypocalcemia prior to treatment. Deficient intestinal calcium transport response to $1,25(OH)_2D$ has been documented only in a minority of these patients but is assumed to be severely depressed in all.

Approximately half of these patients have shown calcemic responses to high doses of calciferols (Fig. 2), in some patients, even hypercalcemia has been provoked by vigorous therapy (Fig. 2) (6). Some patients can respond satisfactorily to "natural" precursors of $1,25(OH)_2D$ (i.e., D_2 or $25(OH)D_3$), and a serum $1,25(OH)_2D$ concentration as high as 19,000 pg/ml has been documented in a patient receiving $25(OH)D_3$ (5). Other patients have remained hypocalcemic with high doses of calciferols (7); some of these cases have been judged to lack a calcemic response without having received sufficient therapeutic trials. An adequate trial must include (a) supplemental calcium by mouth, (b) a very high dosage of calciferol analog that ensures maintenance of high serum concentrations of $1,25(OH)_2D$ (this can be accomplished by treatment with $1,25(OH)_2D_3$ or $1a(OH)D_3$ at dosages in the range of 20-60 μg/day or by administering high dosages of $1,25(OH)_2D$ precursors and documenting that repeated measurements of $1,25(OH)_2D$ are above 2000 pg/ml), and (c) a duration of therapy (about 3 months) sufficient to mineralize depleted bones and thus allow recovery from the hypocalcemia of "hungry bones." In patients without clear calcemic response to calciferols, some therapies remain promising. In patients with no calcemic response to high dosages of calciferols, provision of calcium alone (by oral administration of high dosages: 2-4 g elemental calcium/day) could ameliorate many disturbances. Calcium can also be administered in extremely high dosages intravenously, particularly to overcome severe by reversible symptoms and signs resulting from chronic disease (8). A dramatic response to such treatment may be highly effective in promoting cooperation from the patients and family. Several patients have shown suppression of secondary

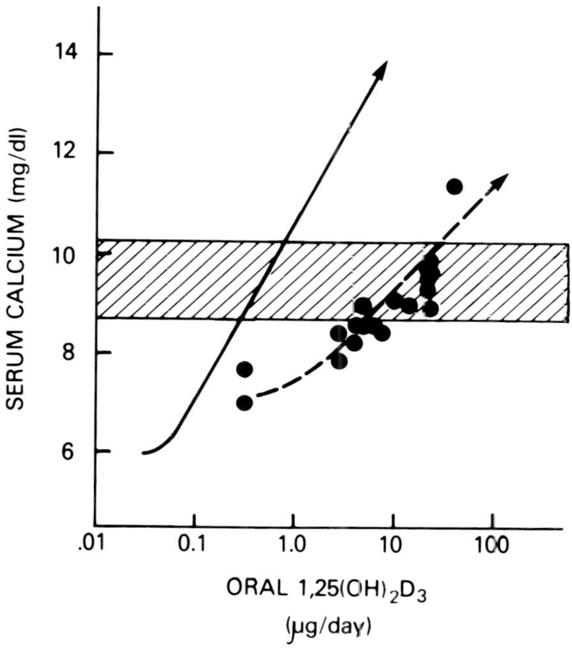

Figure 2 Serum calcemic response as function of 1,25(OH)$_2$D$_3$ dosage in patient with hereditary resistance to 1,25(OH)$_2$D. Stippled zone indicates normal serum calcium; solid line is normal response (assuming baseline of 1,25(OH)$_2$D deficiency and constant calcium intake) (modified from Ref. 1).

hyperparathyroidism and amelioration of hypophosphatemia despite continuation of hypocalcemia with high dosages of calciferols (9). This could represent a direct action of calciferols on the kidney or the parathyroid gland independent of actions mediated through serum ionized calcium.

Age at Presentation. The affected child appears normal at birth, because fetal mineral homeostasis is determined largely by maternal concentrations of calcium and phosphate. It seems likely, however, that abnormalitis in serum concentrations of 1,25(OH)$_2$D may be recognizable even in the first week of life. Most cases recognized to date have been in children who presented with rickets prior to age 3 years. When affected siblings have been evaluated prospectively, chemical disturbances have been evident prior to age 6 months. A small minority of patients have not shown rickets, but have presented with osteomalacia as late as age 45 (10). All patients with late presentation have been normocalcemic, and they represent the mildest manifestation of the disease.

Alopecia. Approximately half of reported patients have shown total alopecia or sparse hair (11). The alopecia can be present from birth, but typically hair is lost gradually between ages 3 and 6 months. Alopecia is a characteristic of the most severely affected patients, it is always associated with early age of presentation and it is always present in patients with no calcemic response to calciferols. Although some patients with alopecia have shown satisfactory calcemic responses to calciferols, none have shown improvement of hair growth. The clear association of alopecia with severe resistance to $1{,}25(OH)_2D$ indicates a role for this hormone in metabolism of the hair follicle.

Response of Calciferol Metabolizing Enzymes. Concentrations of 25(OH)D or vitamin D in serum or 7-dehydrocholesterol in skin have not been analyzed closely in most cases. In one patient there was an apparent deficiency of vitamin D 25-hydroxylase activity (12).

Three types of abnormality have been documented in regulation of $1{,}25(OH)_2D$, all presumably reflecting underlying abnormalities in 25(OH)D 1-alpha-hydroxylase activity. First, serum concentrations of $1{,}25(OH)_2D$ are generally high prior to and during therapy; this is attributable, in part, to normal function of the parathyroid gland/1-hydroxylase axis. Second, serum concentrations of $1{,}25(OH)_2D$ are sometimes disproportionally high even considering the PTH concentration. This was most evident in a patient in remission during treatment with normal concentrations of calcium, phosphate, and PTH; brief administration of $25(OH)D_3$ resulted in endogenous generation of $1{,}25(OH)_2D$ concentrations of 2000 pg/ml (1). This suggested a deficiency of receptor-mediated suppression of 1-hydroxylase activity. Third, in some patients with all the usual activators of 1-hydroxylation functioning (i.e., high PTH and low phosphate in serum), serum concentrations of $1{,}25(OH)_2D$ have been normal or minimally elevated prior to therapy. While this phenomenon is not understood, it could result from the effects of severe hypocalcemia on the 1-hydroxylase system (13). One implication is that serum $1{,}25(OH)_2D$ levels are, prior to therapy, a poor predictor of the degree of underlying resistance to $1{,}25(OH)_2D$ (Fig. 3A).

Since $1{,}25(OH)_2D$ is a potent inducer of $25(OH)D_3$ 24-hydroxylase in vivo and in vitro, low serum concentrations of $24{,}25(OH)_2D$ might be predicted to arise from deficient function of $1{,}25(OH)_2D$ response mechanisms. Serum concentrations of $24{,}25(OH)_2D$ have generally been reported as normal. They were low only in one patient (14). However, low concentrations of $24{,}25(OH)_2D$ are, in fact, difficult to document because the techniques that have been applied to date have not ensured that other cross-reacting metabolites had been completely eliminated.

Other Possible Target Tissues. Hochberg and co-workers evaluated regulation of secretion of insulin, thyroid-stimulating hormone (TSH), prolactin, growth

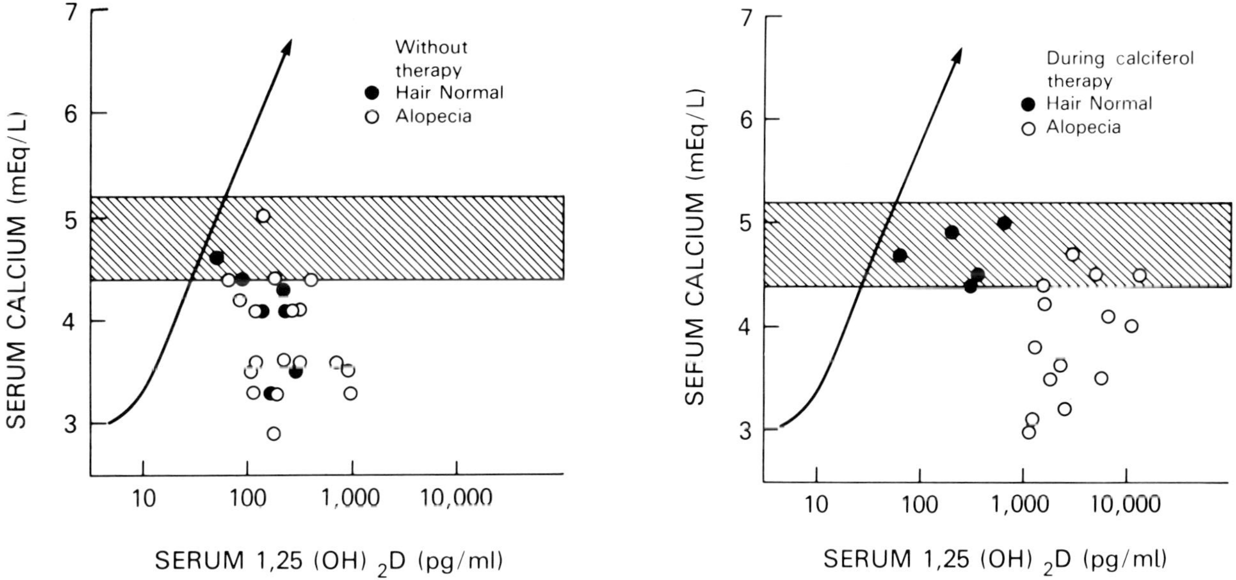

Figure 3 Serum calcemic response as function of serum $1,25(OH)_2D$. Stippled zone indicates normal serum calcium; solid line is normal response (assuming baseline of $1,25(OH)_2D$ deficiency and constant calcium intake). Each point represents one patient (from Ref. 11). Left panel. Data obtained before administration of calciferol therapy. Right panel. Data obtained during long-term administration of high doses of calciferol. Plotted points are from times of therapy with maximal doses required without signs of toxicity.

hormone, and testosterone in six children with alopecia and resistance to 1,25(OH)$_2$D (15). They noted mild deficiencies in provoked secretion only of insulin and TSH, but these abnormalities were correctable by restoration of eucalcemia with calcium infusion.

Temporal Variation in Degree of Resistance. With the indirect indices available, it is difficult to assess the possibility that general resistance may vary over time. For example, several patients have shown striking radiographic improvement without therapy. We believe that the minimum criterion to support the possibility of a change in degree of resistance should be a clear change in the steady-state relation between 1,25(OH)$_2$D and calcium in serum without a causative change in calcium flux between serum and bone or between intestine and serum. Thus, a decrease in skeletal growth rate or an increase of oral calcium intake could easily result in confusion. Even with these caveats, at least one patient has shown unexplained changes in degree of resistance to 1,25(OH)$_2$D (14). This patient, cited above as showing low concentrations of 24,25(OH)$_2$D, showed a dramatic rise in serum calcium levels and a drop towards normal of serum 1,25(OH)$_2$D concomitant with 24,25(OH)$_2$D therapy.

Relation to Osteopetrosis. Osteopetrosis (marble-bones disease) is a process of increased bone mass that usually results from deficient function of osteoclasts (16). Osteopetrosis can be a hereditary disturbance and several variants have been developed in a number of species of animal. The underlying defects of osteoclasts differ widely, from deficiency numbers of osteoclasts to increased numbers with deficient action. Many features of osteopetrosis resemble generalized resistance to 1,25(OH)$_2$D, including mild hypocalcemia, mineralization defects in bone, and high circulating levels of 1,25(OH)$_2$D. One patient with osteopetrosis has been treated with extraordinary dosages of 1,25(OH)$_2$D and a low-calcium diet, with documented improved function of osteoclasts and monocytes (17). However, two other patients showed no benefit from similar therapy (18). Thus in some variants of osteopetrosis the abnormal osteoclast or osteoclast precursor might benefit from treatment with high dosages of calcitriol. It seems unlikely that the majority of 1,25(OH)$_2$D target tissues are resistant to calcitriol in osteopetrosis. Consequently cells other than osteoclasts may develop unpredictable dysfunctions from exposure to high levels of this hormone.

2. *Cellular Defects in Hereditary Resistance to 1,25(OH)$_2$D*

Methods to Study 1,25(OH)$_2$D Interactions in Vitro. Hereditary defects in the 1,25(OH)$_2$D response pathway can be analyzed in vitro because of the presence of this response pathway in almost all cultured cells. Cultured dermal fibroblasts can be used to assess most of the steps in hormone action, from cellular uptake to induction of a bioresponse. We summarize here the general techniques that have been applied.

Hormone Binding to "Cytosol." Cells are extracted with hypertonic KCl (0.3 M); the supernate after centrifugation at 100,000 × g is termed soluble extract. On occasion, such soluble extracts have been called "cytosol"; this term is not accurate because the cellular locaton of unbound hormone receptors is not known as hypertonic KCl can clearly extract receptors from all cell compartments including the nucleus. Soluble extract is incubated for 15 hr at 4°C with graded concentrations of $[^3H]\ 1{,}25(OH)_2D_3$; bound and unbound hormone are then separated and counted. The affinity and maximal capacity of hormone binding can then be derived (19).

Hormone Uptake by Intact Cells. Intact cells in suspension are incubated with $[^3H]\ 1{,}25(OH)_2D_3$ for 1 hr at 37°C. Internalized hormone associated with receptors is then extracted with a lysing buffer, and bound and unbound hormone are then separated and measured. (20).

Hormone Localization to Nucleus. Dispersed intact cells are incubated at 37°C with $[^3H]\ 1{,}25(OH)_2D_3$ for 45 min. The plasma membrane is dissolved with detergent and nucleus-associated hormone is then measured. This assay is simultaneously an index of hormone binding to receptor, receptor sites for nuclear uptake, and cellular processes outside the receptor that help localize the receptor to the nucleus (21).

Receptor Interaction with Nonspecific DNA. Occupied receptor is obtained by incubating soluble extract with $[^3H]\ 1{,}25(OH)_2D_3$. This is then adsorbed to DNA-cellulose and eluted with a linear gradient of KCl. Normal occupied receptors show high affinity for heterologous DNA (from calf thymus) and elute at approximately 0.22 *M* KCl (22,23).

$1{,}25(OH)_2D_3$ Induction of $25(OH)D_3$ 24-Hydroxylase Activity. Cell monolayers are incubated with graded concentrations of $1{,}25(OH)_2D_3$ for 16 hr and then extensively washed; the wash procedure is critical because residual $1{,}25(OH)_2D_3$ at high concentration competes with $25(OH)D_3$ as an effective substrate for the 24-OHase enzyme. Dispersed cells or cell homogenate is incubated with $[^3H]\ 25(OH)D_3$. After brief incubation; $[^3H]\ 24{,}25(OH)_2D_3$ is isolated and measured (24,25). The normal maximal response to $1{,}25(OH)_2D_3$ is at least 40-fold over baseline.

Heterogeneous Defects in $1{,}25(OH)_2D_3$ Interaction with Cultured Skin Fibroblasts. There has been a striking heterogeneity in the cellular defects associated with hereditary resistance to $1{,}25(OH)_2D$ (Fig. 4). We review here published and unpublished studies, in many cases, not all relevant assays have been performed, while in others additional specialized techniques have been applied (e.g., analysis of immunoreactive receptor in hormone-binding-negative cases).

Hormone-Binding-Negative Cases. The most common abnormality documented has been absence of detectable hormone binding with soluble extract. When nuclear localization of hormone has been tested, it too has been unmeas-

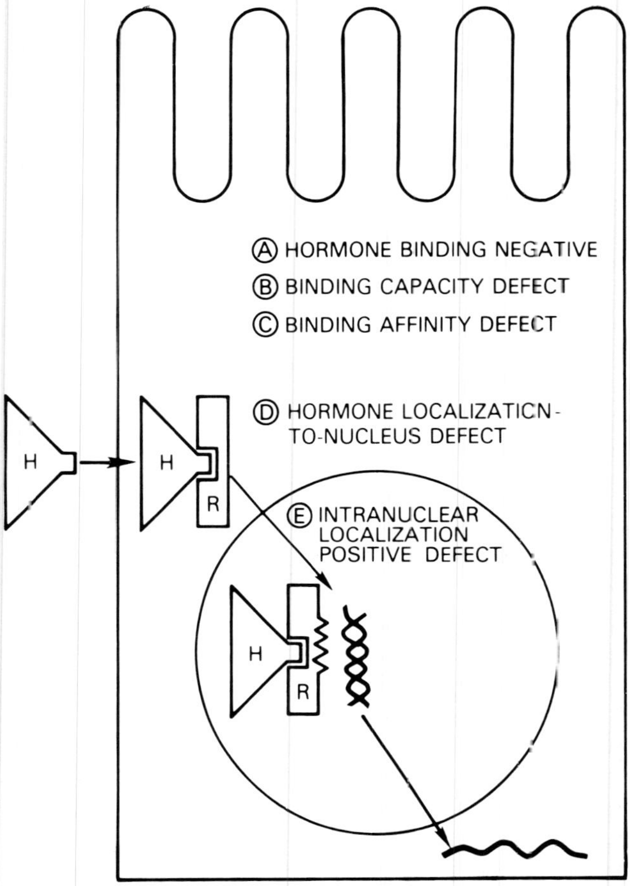

Figure 4 Five classes of defect in cellular interactions with $1,25(OH)_2D_3$ associated with hereditary resistance to $1,25(OH)_2D$. This is a diagrammatic formulation that is not intended to prejudge the issue of the normal location of unoccupied receptors and the question of whether some or all the mutations affect structure of the receptor (from Ref. 5). Type E is a DNA-binding defect (22,23).

urable in these kindreds. With cell extracts from three of these kindreds, receptor was measured by immunoassay and cross-reacting protein was found in normal amounts, furthermore, the protein showed normal sedimentation in a sucrose density gradient (26). This suggests that most, if not all, hormone-binding-negative mutants represent focal abnormalities in the hormone binding domain of the receptor and not absence of receptor protein.

Subnormal Capacity for Hormone Binding. We have observed a binding capacity 10% of normal in two kindreds. In both there was a normal binding affinity. In one kindred, an identical deficiency in capacity for nuclear localization of hormone was documented (19).

Subnormal Affinity for Hormone Binding. Two kindreds have shown a probable 20-30-fold reduction in hormone-binding affinity but a normal binding capacity with soluble extract (27).

Undetectable Hormone Localization to Nucleus. With cells from two kindreds, hormone binding to soluble extract was normal or near normal, yet there was no detectable hormonal localization to the nucleus of intact cells. An identical defect was demonstrated with dermal fibroblasts and osteoblastlike cells cultured from bone of one patient (28).

Isolation of the gene for the $1,25(OH)_2D$ receptor (23B, 23C) allowed confirmation that the DNA-binding defect results from mutations in the DNA-binding ("zinc finger") region of the protein (23C).

Normal or Nearly Normal Hormone Localization to Nucleus. Four kindreds have shown this pattern (22-25). In all three that were evaluated further, receptor elution from DNA-cellulose was abnormal, which suggested that the mutation involved the structure of a DNA-binding domain of the receptor (22,23).

Relation of Defect Type to Clinical Features. The type of defect detected with fibroblasts has provided no uniform correlation with clinical features. For example, at least one patient with unmeasurable hormone binding to soluble extract showed a transient calcemic response to calciferols in vivo (we have speculated that a severe defect in receptor affinity for hormone could account for these findings) (7). For another example, two kindreds showed unmeasurable hormone localization to nucleus, however, both showed calcemic responses to high dosages of calciferols (1). Lastly, normal or near-normal hormone localization to the nucleus was associated with alopecia and no response to calciferols in two kindreds but with a calcemic response and no alopecia in another (24, 25). It seems likely that each type of defect can produce a spectrum of severity of clinical features.

Assays of Response to Calciferols in Vitro. A wide spectrum of human cells is amenable to sampling for assessment of calciferol responsivity; osteoblastlike cells from bone, epidermal keratinocytes, circulating monocytes (differentiation and multinucleation response), B lymphocytes (inhibition of proliferation and of immunoglobulin secretion), and T lymphocytes (inhibition of proliferation and of interleukin-2 secretion).

Dermal fibroblasts have been tested most extensively. The peak response of 24-hydroxylase in dermal fibroblasts (25) occurs after exposure to 10^{-7} *M* $1,25(OH)_2D_3$ (Fig. 5); the half-maximal response occurs after exposure to 3×10^{-9} *M* $1,25(OH)_2D_3$. The minimal dose for a detectable response is 3×10^{-10}

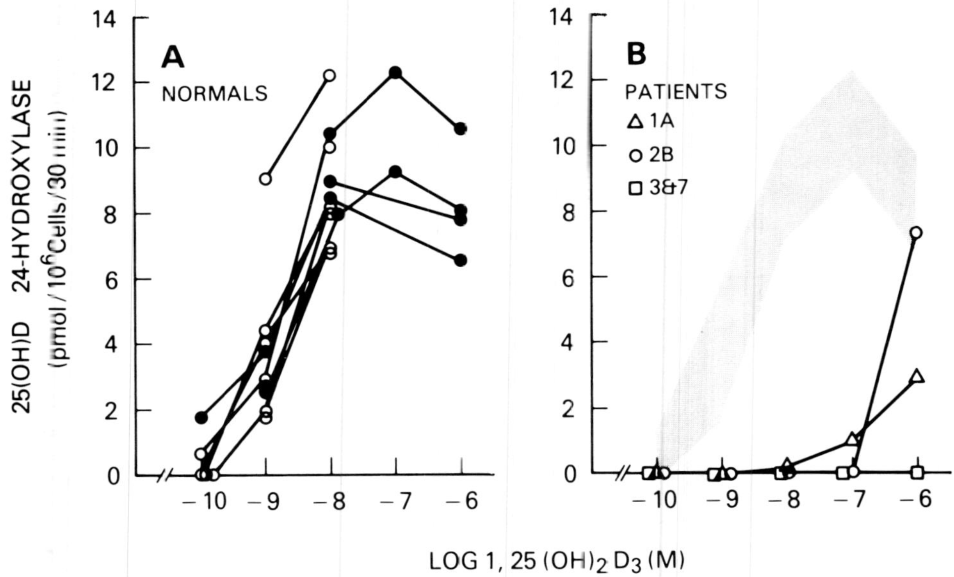

Figure 5 25(OH)D_3 24-Hydroxylase response to 1,25$(OH)_2D_3$ in cultured dermal fibroblasts. Patients 1A and 2B both show normal hormone binding to soluble extract but unmeasurable hormone localization to nucleus. Both showed calcemic responses to high doses of 1,25$(OH)_2D_3$ in vivo. Patients 3 and 7 both show receptors with a DNA-binding defect. Neither showed a calcemic response to high doses of calciferols (from Ref. 25).

M. 24-Hydroxylase induction by 1,25$(OH)_2D_3$ has been abnormal in cells from every case of hereditary resistance to 1,25$(OH)_2D$ tested to date. Our own studies have shown unmeasurable induction even at 10^{-6} *M* 1,25$(OH)_2D_3$ in two kindreds; in both kindreds there was no calcemic response to high doses of calciferols. We have found measurable induction in two other kindreds but at half-maximal doses of 1,25$(OH)_2D_3$ more than 100-fold higher than normal (Fig. 5). In both of these kindreds, there were also calcemic responses to high doses of 1,25$(OH)_2D_3$ in vivo. Studies from other laboratories have confirmed this overall pattern with two other kindreds showing responses in vitro and in vivo and four other kindreds lacking responses in vivo and in vitro.

Osteoblast-like cells can be cultured from bone biopsies and used to demonstrate resistance to at least two actions of 1,25$(OH)_2D_3$ induction of 24-hydroxylase activity and stimulation of osteocalcin secretion (29).

Koren et al. have shown that 1,25$(OH)_2D_3$ inhibits DNA synthesis in lectin-stimulated peripheral mononuclear cells from normals, but this inhibition is not observed in cells from patients with hereditary resistance to 1,25$(OH)_2D_3$.

This assay may have wide utility since it does not require long-term cell culture (30).

Hormonal inhibition of proliferation has also been tested as an index of bioresponse in cultured dermal fibroblasts (31). While deficient response was documented in the one kindred tested, the normal response was too small for wide application.

E. Resistance to 1,25(OH)$_2$ D$_3$ in New World Primates

Osteomalacia associated with high concentrations of 1,25(OH)$_2$ D has been reported in marmosets and tamarins (32–34), two closely related groups of New World monkey. Furthermore, serum concentrations of 1,25(OH)$_2$ D were found to be high in all members of these groups without osteomalacia (mean serum concentration in the marmoset is approximtely 10-fold the human mean). Unusual features in metabolism of the true steroids have previously been studied among New World primates compared to Old World primates, the latter of which humans are a member (35). The New World primates show higher serum concentrations of cortisol (20-fold for total hormone and 100-fold for free hormone), aldosterone (twofold), peak luteal phase progesterone (10-fold), and peak preovulatory estradiol (five-fold). This resistance has been associated with abnormalities in transport proteins and target receptors for these steroids. Whereas "resistance" to any one of these hormones has deleterious consequences (testosterone, aldosterone, cortisol) or is undocumented (estradiol resistance may be lethal) in humans, it seems to be well tolerated by these animals. However, when studied in captivity on an artificial diet with a high content of vitamin D$_3$, some marmosets show histological and radiographic signs of osteomalacia (36). Abnormal interactions with 1,25(OH)$_2$ D$_3$ have been demonstrated with intestinal extracts, dermal fibroblasts, and transformed B lymphocytes from marmosets; the abnormalities have included deficient hormone-binding capacity, deficient hormone-binding affinity, and deficient receptor binding to DNA-cellulose (33,37,38). To date there has been no satisfactory answer to the fascinating question of what beneficial role steroid and secosteroid hormone resistance might have in the natural selection of these animals. Resistance to 1,25(OH)$_2$ D could cause tolerance or even dependence upon dietary components rich in bioactive calciferols, the recent recognition of glycosides of 1,25(OH)$_2$ D in certain plants, illustrates one potential source.

F. Resistance to 1,25(OH)$_2$ D in Cell Lines

Kuribayashi et al. have developed variant strains from HL-60 human promyelocytic leukemia cells (39). Cells from the parental strain show a dramatic differentiation towards mature macrophages after incubation with 1,25(OH)$_2$-D$_3$. As a component of this response, 1,25(OH)$_2$ D$_3$ also inhibits proliferation of these cells, and this feature has been used to select for cells not inhibited by $1,25(OH)_2D_3$ in culture. Two variant cell strains were described. In each case, $1,25(OH)_2D_3$ binding with soluble extract showed normal affinity but decreased capacity. In the parental strain, several classes of agents induce a similar program of differentiation; one variant strain showed selective deficiency of response to $1,25(OH)_2D_3$ while another showed global deficiency of response to all classes of inducer.

Kelley et al. have documented a receptor variant in LLC-MK2 cells, derived from kdiney of the rhesus (*Macacca mulatta*), an Old World monkey (40). In these cells, 24 hydroxylase induction showed the hormonal specificity expected for mediation by a $1,25(OH)_2D$ receptor, but all analogs were required at 100-fold higher doses than required in control cells. While receptor could not be detected with standard radioligand techniques, it was demonstrable after purification with DNA-cellulose. Presumably, this is a receptor with low hormone-binding affinity. Our own studies of hormone binding with soluble extract from virus-transformed B lymphocytes of the stump-tailed macaque (*Macacca arctoides*), another Old World monkey, have shown normal (i.e., similar to human) affinity and capacity for $1,25(OH)_2D_3$, indicating that $1,25(OH)_2D_3$ binding in the LLC-MK2 strain is not representative of all nonhuman Old World primates (25).

III. CONCLUSIONS

Hereditary resistance to $1,25(OH)_2D$ in humans shows a spectrum of features. The variable features including serum calcium levels (from severe hypocalcemia to normocalcemia), bone status (from infantile rickets to late onset osteomalacia), and hair growth (from absent to apparently normal) form a continuum with direct correlations among these features. One exception to this generalization is osteopetrosis, a hereditary defect in osteoclast function, in which there are features of resistance to $1,25(OH)_2D$ in the osteoclast but presumably not in other calcitriol target tissues.

Analyses of cultured dermal fibroblasts allow one to recognize intracellular steps in which genes determining $1,25(OH)_2D$ interactions are abnormal. At least five classes of defect have been identified. Each might reflect modification of a separate functional domain of the receptor for $1,25(OH)_2D$. However, some could result from mutations outside the receptor gene. There are good correlations between deficiencies in responsivity to high doses of calciferols in vivo and in vitro (measured by induction of $25(OH)D_3$ 24-hydroxylase). The features in vivo and in cultured fibroblasts suggest that the defective gene(s) determine the expression of the $1,25(OH)_2D$ effector pathway similarly in all target tissues.

"Resistance" to $1,25(OH)_2D$ is a feature of normal marmosets and is associated with abnormal hormone binding to the $1,25(OH)_2D$ receptor. Since these animals also show resistance to the true steroids, some events during evolution favored a coordinated modification of effector pathways for these structurally related hormones.

REFERENCES

1. Marx, S. J., Liberman, U. A., Eil, C., Gamblin, G. T., Degrange, D. A., and Balsan, S. Hereditary resistance to 1,25-dihydroxyvitamin D. *Recent Prog. Horm. Res. 40*:589-615 (1984).
2. Tieder, M., Modai, D., Samuel, R., Arie, R., Halabe, A., Bab, I., Gabizon, D., and Liberman, U. A. Hereditary hypophosphatemic rickets with hypercalciuria. *N. Engl. J. Med. 312*:611-617 (1985).
3. Halloran, B. P., and DeLuca, H. F. Appearance of the intestinal cytosolic receptor for 1,25-dihydroxyvitamin D_3 during neonatal development in the rat. *J. Biol. Chem. 256*:7338-7342 (1981).
4. Chen, T. L., Hirst, M. A., Cone, C. M., Hochberg, Z., Tietze, H.-U., and Feldman, D. 1,25-Dihydroxyvitamin D resistance, rickets, and alopecia: Analysis of receptors and bioresponse in cultured fibroblasts from patients and parents. *J. Clin. Endocrinol. Metab. 59*:383-388 (1984).
5. Marx, S. J., Liberman, U. A., Eil, C., DeGrange, D. A., and Bliziotes, M. M. Resistance to 1,25-dihydroxycholecalciferon in man and in other species. In *Vitamin D: Chemical, Biochemical, and Clinical Update*. (A. W. Norman, K. Schaefer, H.-G. Grigoleit, and D. Herrath, eds.). Walter de Gruyter, New York, 1985, pp. 107-116.
6. Marx, S. J., Swart, E. G., Hamstra, A. J., and DeLuca, H. F. Normal intrauterine development of the fetus of a woman receiving extraordinarily high doses of 1,25-dihydroxyvitamin D_3. *J. Clin. Endocrinol. Metab. 51*:1138-1142 (1980).
7. Balsan, S., Garabedian, M., Liberman, U. A., Eil, C., Bourdeau, A., Guillozo, H., Grimberg, R., LeDeunff, M. J., Lieberherr, M., Guimbaud, P., Broyer, M., and Marx, S. J. Rickets and alopecia with resistance to 1,25-dihydroxyvitamin D: Two different clinical courses with two different cellular defects. *J. Clin. Endocrinol. Metab 57*:803-811 (1983).
8. Balsan, S., Garabedian, M., Larchet, M., Groski, A. M., Cournot, G., Tau, C., Bourdeau, A., Silve, C., and Ricour, C. Long-term nocturnal calcium infusions can cure rickets and promote normal mineralization in hereditary resistance to 1,25-dihydroxyvitamin D. *J. Clin. Invest. 77*:1661-1667 (1986).
9. Hochberg, Z., Benderli, A., Levy, J., Vardi, P., Weisman, Y., Chen, T., and Feldman, D. 1,25-Dihydroxyvitamin D resistance, rickets, and alopecia. *Am. J. Med. 77*:805-811 (1984).
10. Fujita, T., Nomura, M., Okajima, S., and Furuya, H. Adult-onset vitamin D-resistant osteomalacia with the unresponsiveness to parathyroid hormone. *J. Clin. Endocrinol. Metab. 50*:927-931 (1980).

11. Marx, S. J., Bliziotes, M. M., and Nanes, M. Analysis of the relation between alopecia and resistance to 1,25-dihydroxyvitamin D. *Clin. Endocrinol. 25*:373–381 (1986).
12. Zerwekh, J. E., Glass, K., Jowsey, J., and Pak, C. Y. C. An unique form of osteomalacia associated with end organ refractoriness to 1,25-dihydroxyvitamin D and apparent defective synthesis of 25-hydroxyvitamin D. *J. Clin. Endocrinol. Metab. 49*:171-175 (1979).
13. Tanaka, Y., and DeLuca, H. F. Stimulation of 1,25-dihydroxyvitamin D3 production by 1,25-dihydroxyvitamin D3 in the hypocalcemic rat. *Biochem. J. 214*:893-897 (1983).
14. Liberman, U. A., Samuel, R., Halabe, A., Kauli, R., Edelstein, S., Weisman, Y., Papapoulos, S. E., Clemens, T. L., Fraher, L. J., and O'Riordan, J. I. H. End-organ resistance to 1,25-dihydroxycholecalciferol. *Lancet 1*:504–507 (1980).
15. Hochberg, Z., Borochowitz, Z., Benderli, A., Vardi, P., Oren, S., Spirer, Z., Heyman, I., and Weisman, Y. Does 1,25-dihydroxyvitamin D participate in the regulation of hormone release from endocrine glands? *J. Clin. Endocrinol. Metab. 60*:57–61 (1985).
16. Castells, S. Osteopetrosis. Chapter 12, this volume.
17. Key, L., Carnes, D., Cole, S., Holtrop, M., BarShavit, Z., Shapiro, F., Arceci, R., Steinberg, J., Gundberg, C., Kahn, A., and Anast, C. S. Treatment of congenital osteopetrosis with high-dose calcitriol. *N. Engl. J. Med. 310*: 409-415 (1984).
18. Blazar, B. R., Fallon, M. D., Teitelbaum, S. L., and Ramsay, N. K. C. Calcitriol for congenital osteopetrosis (Letter to the Editor). *N. Engl. J. Med. 311*:55 (1984).
19. Liberman, U. A., Eil, C., and Marx, S. J. Resistance to 1,25-dihyroxyvitamin D: Association with heterogeneous defects in cultured skin fibroblasts. *J. Clin. Invest. 71*:192-200 (1983).
20. Adams, J. S., Gacad, M. A., and Singer, F. R. Specific internalization and action of 1,25-dihydroxyvitamin D_3 in cultured dermal fibroblasts from patients with X-linked hypophosphatemia. *J. Clin. Endocrinol. Metab. 59*: 556-560 (1984).
21. Eil, C., and Marx, S. J. Nuclear uptake of $[^3H]$-1,25-dihydroxycholecalciferol in dispersed fibroblasts cultured from normal human skin. *Proc. Natl. Acad. Sci. 78*:2562-2566 (1981).
22. Hirst, M., Hochman, H., and Feldman, D. Vitamin D resistance and alopecia: A kindred with normal 1,25-dihydroxyvitamin D binding, but decreased receptor affinity for deoxyribonucleic acid. *J. Clin. Endocrinol. Metab. 60*:490–495 (1985).
23a. Liberman, U. A., Eil, C., and Marx, S. J. Receptor positive hereditary resistance to 1,25-dihydroxyvitamin D: Chromatography of hormone-receptor complexes on deoxyribonucleic acid-cellulose shows two classes of mutation. *J. Clin. Endocrinol. Metab. 62*:122-126 (1986).
23b. Haussler, M. R., Mangelsdorf, D. J., Komm, B. S., et al. Molecular biology of the vitamin D hormone. *Rec. Progr. Horm. Res. 44*:263–296 (1988).

23c. Hughes, M. R., Malloy, P. J., Kieback, D. G., Kesterson, R. A., Pike, J. W., Feldman, D., O'Malley, B. W., Point mutations in the human vitamin D receptor gene associated with hypocalcemic rickets. *Science 242*:1702-1705 (1988).

24. Griffin, J. E., Chandler, J. S., Haussler, M. R., and Zerwekh, J. E. Receptor-positive resistance to 1,25-dihydroxyvitamin D: A new cause of osteomalacia associated with impaired induction of 24-hydroxylase in fibroblasts. *J. Clin. Invest. 72*:1190-1199 (1983).

25. Gamblin, G. T., Liberman, U. A., Eil, C., Downs, R. W., Jr., DeGrange, D. A., and Marx, S. J. Vitamin D dependent rickets type II: Defective induction of 25-hydroxyvitamin D_3-24-hydroxylase by 1,25-dihydroxyvitamin D_3 in cultured skin fibroblasts. *J. Clin. Invest. 75*:954-960 (1985).

26. Pike, J. W., Dokoh, S., Haussler, M. R., Liberman, U. A., Marx, S. J., and Eil, C. Vitamin D_3-resistant fibroblasts have immunoassayable 1,25-dihydroxyvitamin D_3 receptors. *Science 224*:879-891 (1984).

27. Castells, S., Greig, F., Fusi, M., Finberg, L., Yasumura, S., Liberman, U. A., Eil, C., and Marx, S. Severely deficient binding of 1,25-dihydroxyvitamin D to its receptors in a patients responsive to high doses of this hormone. *J. Clin. Endocrinol. Metab. 63*:252-256 (1986).

28. Liberman, U. A., Eil, C., Holst, P., Rosen, J. F., and Marx, S. J. Hereditary resistance to 1,25-dihydroxyvitamin D: Defective function of receptors in cells cultured from bone. *J. Clin. Endocrinol. Metab. 57*:958-961 (1983).

29. Silve, C., Grosse, B., Tau, C., Garabedian, M., Fritsch, J., Delmas, P. D., Cournot-Witmer, G., and Balasan, S. Response to parathyroid hormone and 1,25-dihydroxyvitamin D_3 of bone-derived cells isolated from normal children and children with abnormalities in skeletal development. *J. Clin. Endocrinol. Metab. 62*:583-590 (1986).

30. Koren, R., Ravid, R., Liberman, U. A., Hochberg, Z., Weisman, Y., and Novogrodsky, A. Defective binding and function of 1,25-dihydroxyvitamin D_3 receptors in peripheral mononuclear cells of patients with end-organ resistance to 1,25-dihydroxyvitamin D. *J. Clin. Invest. 76*:2012-2015 (1985).

31. Clemens, T. L., Adams, J. S., Horiuchi, N., Gilchrist, E. A., Cho, H., Tsuchiya, Y., Matsuo, N., Suda, T., and Holick, M. F. Interaction of 1,25-dihydroxyvitamin D_3 with keratinocytes and fibroblasts from skin of normal subjects and a subject with vitamin D-dependent rickets, type II: A model for the study of the mode of action of 1,25-dihydroxyvitamin D_3. *J. Clin. Endocrinol. Metab. 56*:824-830 (1983).

32. Shinki, T., Shiina, Y., Takahashi, N., Tanioka, Y., Koizumi, H., and Suda, T. Extremely high circulating levels of 1a,25-hydroxyvitamin D_3 in the marmoset, a new world moneky. *Biochem. Biophys. Res. Commun. 114*:452-457 (1983).

33. Adams, J. S., Gacad, M., Baker, A. J., Kheun, G., and Rude, R. K. Diminished internalization and action of 1,25-dihydroxyvitamin D_3 in dermal fibroblasts cultured from new world primates. *Endocrinology 116*:2523-2527 (1985).

34. Adams, J. S., Gacad, M. A., Baker, A. J., Gonzales, B., and Rude, R. K. Serum concentrations of 1,25-dihydroxyvitamin D_3 in Platyrrhini and Catarrhini: A phylogenetic appraisal. *Am. J. Primatol. 9*:219-224 (1985).
35. Lipsett, M. B., Chrousos, G. P., Tomita, M., Brandon, D. D., and Loriaux, D. L. The defective glucocorticoid receptor in man and nonhuman primates. *Recent Prog. Horm. Res. 41*:199-241 (1985).
36. Yamaguchi, A., Kohno, Y., Yamazaki, T., Takahashi, N., Shinki, T., Horiuchi, N., Suda, T., Koizumi, H., Tanioka, Y., and Yoshiki, S. Bone in the marmoset: A resemblance to vitamin D-dependent rickets, type II. *Calcif. Tissue Int. 39*:22-27 (1986).
37. Liberman, U. A., DeGrange, D., and Marx, S. J. Low affinity of the receptor for 1a,25-dihydroxyvitamin D_3 in the marmoset, a new world monkey. *FEBS Lett. 182*:385-388 (1985).
38. Takahashi, N., Suda, S., Shinki, T., Horiuchi, N., Shiina, Y., Tanioka, Y., Koizumi, H., and Suda, T. The mechanism of end-organ resistance to 1a,25-dihydroxycholecalciferol in the common marmoset. *Biochem. J. 227*:555-563 (1985).
39. Kuribayashi, T., Tanaka, H., Abe, E., and Suda, T. Functional defect of variant clones of a human myeloid leukemia cell line (HL-60) resistant to 1a,25-dihydroxyvitamin D_3. *Endocrinology 113*:1992-1998 (1983).
40. Kelly, M. A., Marion, S. L., Donaldson, C. A., Pike, J. W., and Haussler, M. R. A variant form of the 1,25-dihydroxyvitamin D_3 receptor with low apparent hormone affinity in cultured monkey kidney cells (LLC-MK2). *J. Biol. Chem. 260*:1545-1549 (1985).

8

Hyperresponsiveness to Vitamin D

Harold E. Harrison

The Johns Hopkins University School of Medicine, Baltimore, Maryland

When Steenbock (1) developed the method of producing vitamin D by the ultraviolet irradiation of ergosterol, highly concentrated preparations of vitamin D became available for the first time. Physicians began giving patients large doses of vitamin D not only for the prevention and treatment of rickets but also for unrelated disorders such as rheumatoid arthritis. It was soon learned that large doses of vitamin D given over a period of weeks to several months would produce toxic manifestations, namely hypercalciuria, hypercalcimia, renal calcinosis, renal insufficiency, extraskeletal calcification in a variety of sites, and, in some cases, death due to extreme hypercalcemia or renal failure (2). An alarming observation was that the hypercalcemia and consequent toxicity of hypervitaminosis D persisted sometimes for months after vitamin D was discontinued. The studies by Joseph Warkany (3) showed that the concentration of vitamin D determined by bioassay in the serum of such individuals remained extremely high for prolonged periods of time. The explanation for this finding only became apparent following the major contribution of De Luca and his colleagues (4) on the metabolism of vitamin D.

The toxic dosages of vitamin D were several magnitudes greater than the amount needed to prevent vitamin-D-deficiency rickets. In most studies, as much as 5000 units/kg in infants and 2000 units/kg in older children and adults had to be given daily for weeks to produce hypercalcemia. It was therefore thought that moderately large dosages of vitamin D could be given safely, even though they were greater than the amount needed to prevent vitamin D deficiency. In the United States, because of the leadership of Dr. Philip C. Jeans, Professor of Pediatrics at University of Iowa School of Medicine, and the American Medical Association Council of Food, the fortification with vitamin D of evaporated milk, homogenized cow's milk, or infant feeding preparations at the level of 400 units/equivalent quart was instituted which was highly successful in the prevention of rickets. This dosage had been derived from Jeans' studies of the amount of vitamin D needed to maintain maximum calcium retentions in infants fed cows milk (5). The amount of vitamin D was also the recommended daily dosage provided in vitamin D preparations sold over the counter. In other countries, however, milk was not fortified with vitamin D and the prevention of rickets was dependent on administration of vitamin D preparations. Often much larger dosages than those recommended by Jeans were used. In the case of prematurely born infants who were thought to be at special risk for rickets, doses of 5000 units/day were routinely given on some services. In Germany, the idea of vitamin D stosstherapy of rickets developed, It was thought that daily administration of a vitamin D preparation was not being complied with by many mothers, so that a single large dose of vitamin D (600,000 units) was given in the well baby clinic to maintain adequate vitamin D levels for many months. In some instances intramuscular injection of vitamin D was recommended. There was clearly confidence that the ratio of toxic to therapeutic doses of vitamin D was sufficiently great that moderately large amounts could be given without concern.

The confidence that vitamin D dosages of several thousand units per day could be given safely to infants on a routine basis was shaken by events in the 1940s and 1950s. During World War II, the British government was worried about the nutrition of infants and children and particularly about the possibility of an increase in the incidence of rickets, which had always been significant in the British Isles. A dried milk preparation fortified with vitamin D at the presumed level of 1800 units/equivalent quart was distributed free of charge for the feeding of infants and children. Because vitamin D prepared from irradiated ergosterol was cheap, the manufacturers of this product added more than this amount to the milk product to be sure that loss of vitamin D during storage did not result in vitamin D concentrations less than the required amount. In addition, many infants and children were given the standard cod liver oil preparation, which had been customary prior to the development of the fortified dried milk feed. As a result, many infants and children were receiving daily vitamin D doses of 3,000 or 4,000 units. When cases of a hitherto unrecognized entity–idiopathic hypercalcemia of infancy–began to appear, British pediatricians and nutritionists became concerned about the possibility that overdose of vitamin D might be the basis of this disorder. Approximately 200 cases of idiopathic hypercalcemia of infancy were collected within a few years (6). Since hundreds of thousands of children had received the vitamin-D-fortified preparation, it was evident that the affected infants had a special hyperresponsiveness to vitamin D, the basis of which had yet to be determined. Nevertheless, the routine vitamin D intake of infants was reduced by reducing the level of fortification of the special milk preparation. The incidence of idiopathic hypercalcemia decreased, which suggested that excessive response to moderately high dosages of vitamin D was the problem.

The infants with severe idiopathic hypercalcemia often showed a common pattern of physical abnormalities described as the Williams syndrome: facial dysmorphism: the elfin facies, consisting of a small triangular face with a depressed nasal bridge and upturned nose, a long upper lip, and micrognathia; retarded linear growth; developmental delay; and congenital heart defects, particularly supravalvular aortic stenosis and peripheral pulmonic stenosis. Whether these physical abnormalities are secondary to intrauterine or early neonatal hypercalcemia remains to be determined. Not all patients with the physical findings of Williams syndrome have hypercalcemia, at least at the time that the cardiac lesion is recognized. Hyperresponsiveness to vitamin D can be but it is not necessarily uniformly present in children with Williams syndrome. It must also be noted that the hypercalcemia of infants with Williams syndrome can be transitory and usually does not persist after the first few years of life.

The unusually high incidence of idiopathic hypercalcemia in Britain was presumably related to the routine use of a milk preparation heavily fortified with vitamin D. However, once the syndrome was recognized, cases were observed in other European countries as well as in the United States. Fellers and Schwartz, at the Boston Children's Hospital, determined vitamin D by bioassay in the serum of a patient with idiopathic hypercalcemia and found an elevated concentration, that is, one much higher than would have been expected with the patient's routine of vitamin D intake (7). We also made such measurements in a child with a very severe form of idiopathic hypercalcemia and found a serum vitamin D concentration of 23 units/ml, over 10 times the normal value, which might be seen in a child receiving doses of vitamin D in the toxic range (8). This child's sibling was also studied and was initially hypercalcemic. The serum calcium concentration decreased on a vitamin-D-free diet, but both serum calcium and vitamin D concentrations rose to abnormally high levels when an ordinary vitamin D intake, 400 units/day, was resumed. Such findings suggested either metabolism of vitamin D to a biologically very potent metabolite or failure of the normal mechanism of inactivation of vitamin D.

Before discussing the possible metabolic basis of the hyperresponsiveness to vitamin D in Williams syndrome, it is pertinent to mention other varieties of such hyperresponsiveness. In the 1950s, the Finnish pediatricians, Hallman and Yipoö reported a high incidence of hypercalcemia in premature infants with "interstitial plasma cell pneumonia," which was epidemic in their nursery.

Although the premature infants in their nursery were receiving relatively high doses of vitamin D, the hypercalcemia was confined to the infants with this infection, which may have been *Pneumocystis carinii* pneumonitis.

An even more striking example of a chronic inflammatory disease associated with hyperresponsiveness to vitamin D is sarcoidosis. The hypercalcemia of some patients with sarcoid was shown to be associated with increased intestinal absorption of calcium and was controlled by suppressive doses of glucocorticoid. Further connection with vitamin D was supplied by the seasonal incidence. Serial studies of patients with sarcoid showed higher concentrations of serum calcium at the end of the summer than in the early spring. When the metabolic conversion of vitamin D to physiologically active metabolites was discovered as described in the paper by De Luca (4), the solution of the problem became possible. The formation of the first metabolic product, 25-OH D, by liver enzymes is not under negative feedback control and is the basis of the toxicity of hypervitaminosis D. The concentration of this compound in serum can rise to 10-15 times the normal value in subjects receiving excessively large doses of vitamin D, as shown by Haussler and his colleagues (10). However, the formation of 1,25-dihydroxyvitamin D by a renal tubule cell enzyme is under close negative feedback control and is not elevated by a vitamin D high intake. In patients with sarcoid, however, concentrations of 1,25-dihydroxyvitamin D in serum were found to be above the normal range despite normal or low concentrations of 25-OH D. Elevated concentrations of this extremely potent vitamin D metabolite were found in a patient with sarcoid who was anepheric, indicating extrarenal production of this metabolite (11). Subsequent studies demonstrated 1.25-dihydroxyvitamin D synthesis by sarcoid lymph node homogenates, thus confirming the extrarenal source of this metabolite in these patients. Production of 1,25-dihydroxyvitamin D by some lymphomas was also demonstrated, thus explaining the hypercalcemia occasionally seen in patients with this tumor. Granulomas induced by a foreign body, silicone, were also shown to be associated with hypercalcemia and elevated concentrations of 1,25-dihydroxyvitamin D, suggesting that phagocytic cells of the mononuclear series may be the source of the extrarenal metabolism of 25-OH D (12).

Such extrarenal production of 1,25-dihydroxyvitamin D by chronic inflammatory tissue may explain the combination of subcutaneous fat necrosis and hypercalcemia seen in the neonatal period. As yet, to my knowledge, no measurements of serum 1,25-dihydroxyvitamin D have been made in such a patient. The x-ray findings of submetaphyseal bone resorption in such a patient are compatible with hypervitaminosis D, as is the response of these patients to suppressive doses of glucocorticoids. The hypercalcemia spontaneously resolves concomitantly with resolution of the foreign body reaction in the subcutaneous fat.

Measurement of the concentrations of 25-OH D and 1,25-dihydroxyvitamin D in serum of patients with Williams syndrome was obviously indicated. Recently, Garabedian and her colleagues (13) reported such determinations in three patients and found excessively high concentrations of 1,25-dihydroxyvitamin D, although those of 25-OH D were in the normal range. The concentrations of 1,25-dihydroxyvitamin D in serum gradually decreased, explaining the eventual restoration of a eucalcemic state. The site of the 1,25-dihydroxyvitamin D formation has not been specifically studied, but is presumably renal since no tumor or inflammatory tissue is present of the type associated with uncontrolled production of 1,25-dihydroxyvitamin D.

I. CASE STUDY

The findings of Garabedian et al. are at variance with those of other investigators, who have not found elevated concentrations of 1,25-diOH D in the serum of patients with idiopathic hypercalcemia (14). The following patient illustrates this phenomenon of hypercalcemia due to hyperresponsiveness to vitamin D but without increased serum concentrations of 1,25-dihydroxyvitamin D.

This male infant was born at term weighing 2850 g. The pregnancy was uneventful. The infant had respiratory difficulties in the first weeks of life and cardiac studies revealed a narrowing of the aorta at the ductal site. Eventually, surgical correction of this coarctation was necessary at 18 months of age. Although the surgery was successful, the infant fed poorly, failed to grow or gain weight satisfactorily, and was markedly delayed in his development. Several serum calcium measurements had been normal. However, at age 36 months he was found to be markedly hypertensive and the serum calcium concentration was 15 mg/dl. Subsequent studies are summarized in Table 1. The serum calcium concentration at the start of the study was 14.3 mg/dl, the serum 25-OH D concentration was in the normal range of adequate vitamin D intake (42 ng/ml), but that of 1,25-dihydroxyvitamin D was extremely low (8 pg/ml). He was placed on prednisone, 2 mg/kg per day, which resulted in a rapid drop in the serum calcium level to 11.5 mg/dl. When steroids were discontinued, the serum calcium concentration rose to 14.9 mg/dl despite a serum 1,25-dihydroxyvitamin concentration of less than 5 pg/ml. He was restarted on prednisone and a low-calcium, vitamin-D-free diet was prescribed. He was in an institution and adherence to the diet was not successful at first because of his refusal. Eventually, he did accept the diet and the serum 25-OH D concentration decreased to 13 ng/ml. At this time, the serum calcium level was 10.0 mg/dl and the serum 1,25-dihydroxyvitamin D rose into the normal range of 28 pg/ml for the first time. The prednisone dosage was gradually tapered and after 2 years he is normocalcemic without steroid treatment. The serum 25-OH D concentration has increased somewhat because of relaxation of the diet and the 1,25-diOH D concentration is now at a normal value of 66 pg/ml.

Table 1 Vitamin D Metabolites in Serum of a 3-year-old Patient with Idiopathic Hypercalcemia

Date	Ca (mg/dl)	P (mg/dl)	25-OHD (ng/ml)	1,25-diOHD (pg/ml)
6/18/83	14.3	4.3	41	8
		Prednisone 15 mg/day		
6/28/83	11.5			
		Prednisone discontinued		
7/12/83	14.9			
		Prednisone 15 mg/day, low-Ca, low-vitamin-D diet		
7/28/83	11.1			
		Prednisone 10 mg/day		
8/8/83	11.6	5.1		
9/17/83	11.2	6.0	40	<5
12/6/83	11.1	5.1	44	–
1/31/84	11.0	4.6	38	<5
		Prednisone 10 mg on alternate days		
3/27/84	10.0	6.4	13	28
10/23/84	10.5	5.8		
		Prednisone 5 mg on alternate days		
1/29/85	9.8	4.6		
		Prednisone 1 mg/day		
5/28/85	10.1	–	27	66
		Prednisone discontinued		
7/30/85	9.6		42	15
12/3/85	10.2	4.5	–	–
3/4/86	9.8	6.4	28	71

II. DISCUSSION

Hyperresponsiveness to vitamin D can be due to unregulated extrarenal production of 1,25-dihydroxyvitamin D, as in chronic granulomatous diseases such as sarcoid or in tumors including lymphoma. Despite the report by Garabedian et al. (13), idiopathic hypercalcemia in the majority of reported instances is not associated with increased concentrations of 1,25-dihydroxyvitamin D in serum. The data described in this paper suggest that the production of 1,25-OH D was inhibited by the hypercalcemia; only when the serum 25-OH D concentration was reduced by a vitamin-D-free diet was the hypercalcemia brought under control and serum 1,25-dihydroxyvitamin D levels returned to normal value. This suggests that abnormal responsiveness to 25-OH D might be the basis for the hyperabsorption of calcium and resultant hypercalcemia. 1,25-dihydroxyvitamin D binds in target cells to an intracellular receptor that is either intranuclear or migrates into the nucleus after forming a complex with 1,25-dihydroxyvitamin D. This 1,25-dihydroxyvitamin D receptor complex activates DNA segments, resulting in the synthesis of proteins that mediate the action of 1,25-dihydroxyvitamin D. The specific receptor also binds 25-OH D, but with a much lower affinity than that for 1,25-dihydroxyvitamin D. The physiological concentration of 25-OH D may be, however, as much as 500 times that of 1,25-dihydroxyvitamin D. Since both 25-OH D and 1,25-dihydroxyvitamin D circulate in serum bound to specific vitamin-D-binding protein, the ratios of the free compounds may not be as great as that of the total compounds. The significant finding, however, that hypervitaminosis D results in marked increases of the concentration of 25-OH D in serum that correlates with the toxic manifestations, namely hypercalcemia and hypercalciuria, indicates that excessively high concentrations of 25-OH D can initiate the same sequence of events as an excess of 1,25-dihydroxyvitamin D.

Patients with idiopathic hypercalcemia show the toxic effects of hypervitaminosis D despite concentrations of serum 25-OH within normal limits. A possible explanation might be an increased affinity for 25-OH D by the specific intracellular receptor. This would be compatible with the increased incidence of idiopathic hypercalcemia seen in Great Britain during the period when infants were routinely given a higher intake of vitamin D than is now administered. It would also fit with the therapeutic effect of a low vitamin D intake, which results in reduced concentration of serum 25-OH D but increased concentrations of 1,25-dihydroxyvitamin D. A somewhat puzzling finding is the apparent increased tolerance for vitamin D shown by these infants and children after they have been on a restricted vitamin D intake for several years. Further studies of the response of target cells to 25-OH D and the specific factors determining the affinity of the receptor for this vitamin D metabolite are needed.

III. SUMMARY AND CONCLUSION

Idiopathic hypercalcemia of infancy may be associated with normal concentrations of 25-OH D and reduced concentrations of 1,25-dihydroxyvitamin D in serum. This suggests that hyperresponsiveness to 25-OH D can be the cause of this disorder. The possibility that such hyperresponsiveness to 25-OH D can be due to an increased affinity of an intracellular receptor for this compound warrants further investigaiton.

REFERENCES

1. Steenbock, H., and Black, A. Fat-soluble vitamin XXIII. The induction of growth-promoting and calcifying properties in fats and their unsaponifiable constituents by exposure to light. *J. Biol. Chem. 64*:263-298 (1925).

2. Bauer, J. M., and Freyberg, R. H. Vitamin-D intoxication with metastatic calcification. *J.A.M.A. 130*:1208-1215 (1946).
3. Warkany, J., and Mabon, H. C. Estimation of vitamin D in blood serum. *Am. J. Dis. Child. 60*:606-614 (1940).
4. De Luca, H. Vitamin D metabolism and function. *Arch. Intern. Med. 138*: 836-847 (1978).
5. Jeans, P. C. Vitamin D. *J.A.M.A. 106*:2066-2069 (1936).
6. Committee Report. Hypercalcemia in infants and vitamin-D. *Br. Med. J. 1*: 149 (1956).
7. Fellers, F. X., and Schwartz, R. Etiology of the severe form of idiopathic hypercalcemia of infancy: A defect in vitamin D metabolism. *N. Engl. J. Med. 259*:1050-1058 (1958).
8. Smith, D. W., Blizzard, R. M., and Harrison, H. E. Idiopathic hypercalcemia: A case report with assays of vitamin D in serum. *Pediatrics 24*: 258-269.
9. Hallman, N., and Ylppo, A. Mental and physical disturbances in children recovered from infantile intestitial plasma cell pneumonia. *Acta Paediatr. 43* Suppl. 100:382-396 (1954).
10. Hughes, M. R., Baylink, D. J., Jones, P. G., and Haussler, M. R. Radioligand receptor assay for 25-hydroxyvitamin in D_2/D_3 and 1α, 25-dihydroxyvitamin D_2/D_3. Application to hyper-vitaminosis D. *J. Clin. Invest. 58*:61-70 (1976).
11. Barbour, G. L., Coburn, J. W., Slatapolsky, E., Norman, A. W., and Horst, R. L. Hypercalcemia in an anephric patients with sarcoidosis: Evidence of extra renal generation of 1,25-dihydroxy vitamin D. *N. Engl. J. Med. 305*: 440-443 (1981).
12. Kozeny, G. A., Barbato, A. L., Bansal, V. K., Vertung, L. L., and Hano, J. E. Hypercalcemia associated with silicone-induced granulomas. *N. Engl. J. Med. 311*:1103-1105 (1984).
13. Garabedian, M., Jacquz, E., Guidlozo, H., Grimberg, R., Guillot, M., Gagnadoux, M. F., Broyer, M., Lenoir, G., and Balsan, S. Elevated plasma 1,25-dihydroxy vitamin D concentrations in infants with hypercalcemia and an elfin facies. *N. Engl. J. Med. 312*:948-952 (1985).
14. Aarskog, O., Aksnes, L., and Markestad, T. Vitamin D metabolism in idiopathic infantile hypercalcemia. *Am. J. Dis. Child. 135*:1021-1024 (1981).

9

Renal Osteodystrophy in Children

William L. Oppenheim, Isidro B. Salusky, Daniel Kaplan, and Richard N. Fine

UCLA Medical Center, Los Angeles, California

I. INTRODUCTION

Renal osteodystrophy refers to the abnormal mineral metabolism and resultant osseous abnormalities that occur as renal function declines. Although the effects of renal failure on the developing skeleton were first described over a century ago (1), recent developments in the treatment of children with end-stage renal disease with dialysis and transplantation have changed the presentation and significance of many of the consequences of renal osteodystrophy. New factors, such as steroid-induced avascular necrosis, aluminum toxicity, and immunosuppressive therapy have expanded and complicated the clinical picture. In spite of such issues, patients with renal osteodystrophy can now expect an increased life expectancy and a more active lifestyle. In this chapter we will discuss the pathophysiology of renal osteodystrophy, describe the various orthopedic manifestations, and discuss some of the treatment modalities.

II. PATHOPHYSIOLOGY

The bone changes of renal osteodystrophy are primarily explained on the basis of secondary hyperparathyroidism induced by the effects of azotemia on vitamin D, calcium, and phosphate metabolites as well as parathormone levels (2-5). The mechanism of increased parathormone secretion resulting in secondary hyperparathyroidism is not completely understood, although hypocalcemia is thought to be an important trigger for increased parathyroid hormone (PTH) secretion (6). This hypocalcemia in turn results from renal phosphate retention, an altered calcemic action of parathormone (7,8), and as a result of abnormal vitamin D metabolism. The later is the result of the failing kidney's inability to synthesize 1,25$(OH)_2$-D3 and 24,25-D3, which are needed to facilitate calcium absorption from the gut (9–12).

Aside from a hypocalcemic stimulus, an elevated serum phosphate level can also act as a direct stimulus to promote parathormone secretion, although the exact mechanism remains obscure (13,14). The "trade off" hypothesis suggests that transient and possibly undetectable hypocalcemia is enhanced by postprandial phosphate retention in the early phase of chronic renal failure (15,15). However, other studies have shown the opposite phenomenon: that fasting patients with early chronic renal failure often have both hypocalcemia and hypophosphatemia (17).

Whatever the initial stimulus, as renal function deteriorates to 25% of the normal glomerular filtration rate (GFR), marked hyperphosphatemia usually occurs (18). At this degree of renal functional impairment, the extent of the hypocalcemia as well as the degree of hyperparathyroidism are directly related to the increase in the serum phosphorus levels (19,20). This picture originally suggested that phosphate retention led to hyperphosphatemia and caused hyperparathyroidism by lowering the ionized calcium level. This classic picture of hyperparathyroidism (HPTH) is complicated by many issues, however.

The kidneys are also a target organ for the actions of parathormone as well as an important route for the excretion and metabolism of the hormone (21). Increased serum phosphate levels seem to have a direct effect on lowering renal alpha-hydroxylation and therefore vitamin D activation. Indeed, Portale et al. (7) have demonstrated increased 1,25$(OH)_2$-D_3 production when phosphate intake is restricted. Moreover, as functioning renal mass decreases, 1-alpha hydroxylation of 25OH-D_3 in the proximal renal tubules declines. Vitamin D may facilitate the action of parathormone on the skeleton, which in established chronic renal failure may become resistant to the actions of parathormone, resulting in a further rise in parathormone levels. In fact, in early renal failure, given the hypocalcemia present, serum 1,25$(OH)_2$-D_3 levels are already inappropriately low. It has recently been shown that the number of receptors for 1,25$(OH)_2$-D_3 in the parathyroid glands are reduced in patients with advanced renal failure (22). These new findings offer a new insight into our understanding of the pathogenesis of secondary hyperparathyroidism in uremic patients. Depressed 25OH-D_3 levels can also result from decreased dietary intake of vitamin D, reduced sun exposure, urinary losses in patients with the neprhotic syndrome, and an increased catabolism by anticonvulsant-induced hepatic P450 enzymes, which are commonly administered to patients with chronic renal failure (23–25).

Serum levels of 24,25-D_3 are also reduced in patients with end-stage renal disease (26). However, there is minimal evidence that this sterol has any specific biological action and it may simply be a biodegradation product.

The development of hyperparathyroidism in patients with end-stage renal disease is thus multifactorial. Hyperphosphatemia and hypocalcemia may act directly on the parathyroid glands, and reduced vitamin D activity may have a further impact indirectly on these minerals, both by effecting absorption and excretion of these minerals and through less well studied relationships dealing directly with the parathyroid glands themselves.

III. SKELETAL RESISTANCE

An interesting observation in patients with end-stage renal disease is the apparent resistance of the skeleton to the calcemic actions of parathormone. This has been demonstrated by observing a subnormal calcemic response to an infusion of parathormone extract in patients with moderate to advanced chronic renal failure and in those undergoing maintenance dialysis (27). Impaired metabolism of parathormone 1-84 to parathormone 1-34 may explain the observed resistance, since the calcemic response to the injection of parathormone 1-34 in uremic patients is normal. Despite the controversy over a specific mechanism of parathormone resistance, it should be noted that administration of calcitriol to dogs with mild renal insufficiency results in resolution of the skeletal resistance to parathormone (28). This suggests that altered vitamin D metabolism has an important role in the genesis of the skeletal resistance.

IV. HISTOLOGICAL CHARACTERISTICS IN RENAL OSTEODYSTROPHY

The determination of bone histological characteristics and tetracycline-labeling-based measurements of bone formation obtained from iliac crest bone biopsies in normal healthy controls has facilitated the classification of the different types of bone disease in uremic patients (14,29,30). Prior to the performance of the biopsy, tetracycline, 10 mg/kg per day, is given on two occasions separated by an interval of 17 days to label bone. The rates of mineralized bone apposition are determined from measurements of the width of separation of double tetracycline labels divided by the time interval between the administration of the two labels (31). In addition, the bone aluminum content is evaluated by both a chemical technique that measures total bone aluminum content and a histochemical technique that indicates the amount of aluminum at the mineralization front. The latter is a more sensitive technique for determining the toxic effect of aluminum on osteoblast function and for the evaluation of treatment with desferioxamine in patients with aluminum toxicity. On the basis of these different variables, the following types of bone disease may be present in patients with chronic failure:

1. Osteitis fibrosa: Osteoid area $< 12\%$, presence of fibrosis and elevated bone formation rate (BFR).
2. Mild lesion: Osteoid area $< 12\%$, no tissue fibrosis and elevated BFR.
3. Normal histological appearance: All the variables are within the limits found in normal healthy controls.
4. Aplastic bone: Osteoid area $< 12\%$, no fibrosis, and decreased BFR.
5. Osteomalacia: Osteoid area $> 12\%$, no fibrosis, and low BFR.
6. Mixed lesion: Osteoid area $> 12\%$, fibrosis present, and BFR diminished.

Parathyroid hormone is the driving force for the development of secondary hyperparathyroidism, that is osteitis fibrosa and mild lesions. These are the predominant lesions seen in patients with renal osteodystrophy. At the present time the low bone turnover disease processes—aplastic and osteomalacia lesions—are mainly seen with aluminum accumulation.

V. ALUMINUM TOXICITY

Although initially thought to occur only in patients receiving hemodialysis with contaminated water, aluminum toxicity is now seen with increasing frequency in patient who have received extensive treatment with aluminum hydroxide prescribed as a phosphate-binding agent (6,32,33). In some patients, excessive aluminum accumulates and is deposited in several organs in the body (34,35). The principal findings of aluminum-related bone disease are the presence of a significant amount of histologically demonstrable aluminum on the bone-forming surfaces at the interface between the osteoid and the calcified matrix and a reduced rate of bone formation (36,37). One possible explanation for the adverse effect of aluminum on collagen synthesis is a reduction in the number and/or cellular activity of osteoblasts. Histologically, however, diminished matrix synthesis can be identified as well. The toxicity of aluminum on bone may thus result from an effect on collagen synthesis as well as on matrix mineralization. The spectrum of histological changes seen in patients treated with maintenance dialysis may also be a reflection of a pre-existing level of bone turn over. It has been suggested that the effect of aluminum on bone formation may depend on the activity level of the bone immediately prior to exposure to aluminum overload (38).

VI. GROWTH AND DEVELOPMENT IN RENAL OSTEODYSTROPHY

It is important to recognize that age has an influence on the clinical manifestations of secondary hyperparathyroidism. Many of the common signs of secondary hyperparathyroidism seen in adults are not present in children with renal osteodystrophy (39). The latter include metastatic calcification, calcium pyrophosphate deposition, tendon rupture, and bursitis (40). Manifestations of secondary hyperparathyroidism that are frequently observed in children with renal osteodsytrophy include myopathy, growth retardation, muscle weakness, osseous deformity, bone pain, slipped epiphyses, and avascular necrosis. The diffuse myopathy is particulary pervasive and frequently overlooked, often being incorrectly attributed to malaise or generalized weakness associated with chronic disease. In addition, young children with uremia often suffer retardation in motor development. By the time end-stage renal disease has developed, one-third of children are below the third percentile for height, and the actual growth rate is reduced in 50% of patients with end-stage renal disease (41,42). Although a number of factors have been documented as potentially harmful to the growth process, the exact mechanism of growth retardation in uremia is poorly understood (43). Metabolic derangements such as acid–base abnormalities, alterations in carbohydrate handling, amino acid synthesis, and hormonal function have been implicated (44). The demonstration of inhibited protein synthesis in the serum of uremic patients and a limited uptake of thymidine in bone marrow suggest that protein metabolism may be markedly depressed. The level of renal insufficiency at which growth is inhibited varies with age, cause of the renal disease, and the associated metabolic abnormalities. A glomerular filtration rate of less than 25 ml/min per 1.73 m^2 has been reported as the point at which growth is clinically affected (45).

Another factor in growth inhibition appears to be somatomedin activity. Bioassay has revealed low somatomedin levels in uremic children, which can be improved acutely by hemodialysis (46). This suggests the presence of a circulating low-molecular-weight inhibitor that is removed by dialysis and may explain why the radioimmunoassay for somatomedin activity yields elevated levels in uremic children in association with low growth rates. The permissive effect of somatomedins on insulin can also explain the relative insulin resistance in the face of high circulating levels of insulin. This insulin resistance may in turn delay linear growth proportionately more than bone maturation, resulting in a permanent loss of growth potential.

Treatment with vitamin D derivatives has a variable influence on growth in patients with renal osteodystrophy. The apparent improvement in observed growth velocity may be a result of straightening of deformities, but other data have shown improvement of growth velocity with the administration of $1,25(OH)_2\text{-}D_3$ in some uremic children who do not have significant deformities (47,48). Bone maturation can also be delayed by vitamin D treatment so that the relationship of linear growth to bone maturation during $1,25(OH)_2\text{-}D_3$ treatment either improves or is unchanged (49). Long-term prospective studies are needed to evaluate further the effect of calcitrol therapy on growth.

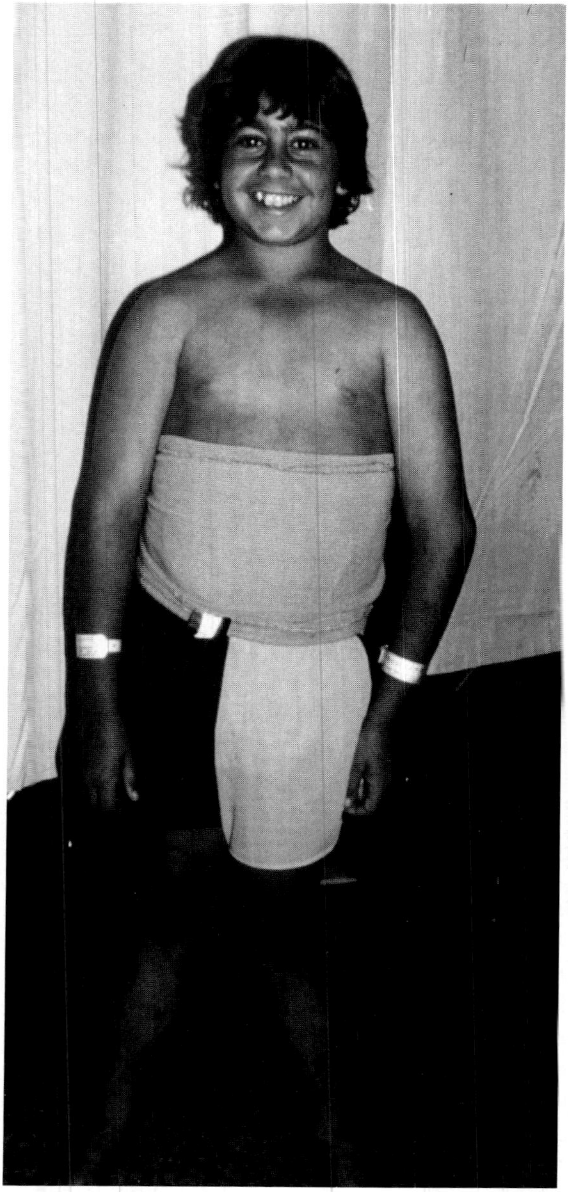

(A)

Figure 1 Startling valgus deformities of the knee are frequently seen in renal osteodystrophy. They may represent an accentuation of the normal patterns of early childhood. A, B. Preoperative appearance in a 10-year-old boy. C, D. Postoperative appearance following distal femoral osteotomies.

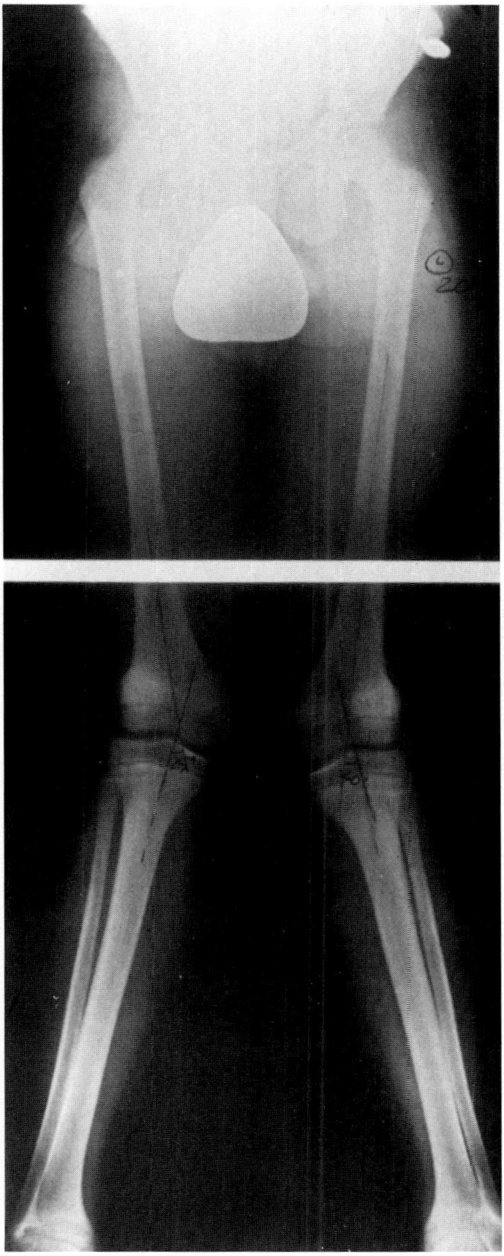

(B)

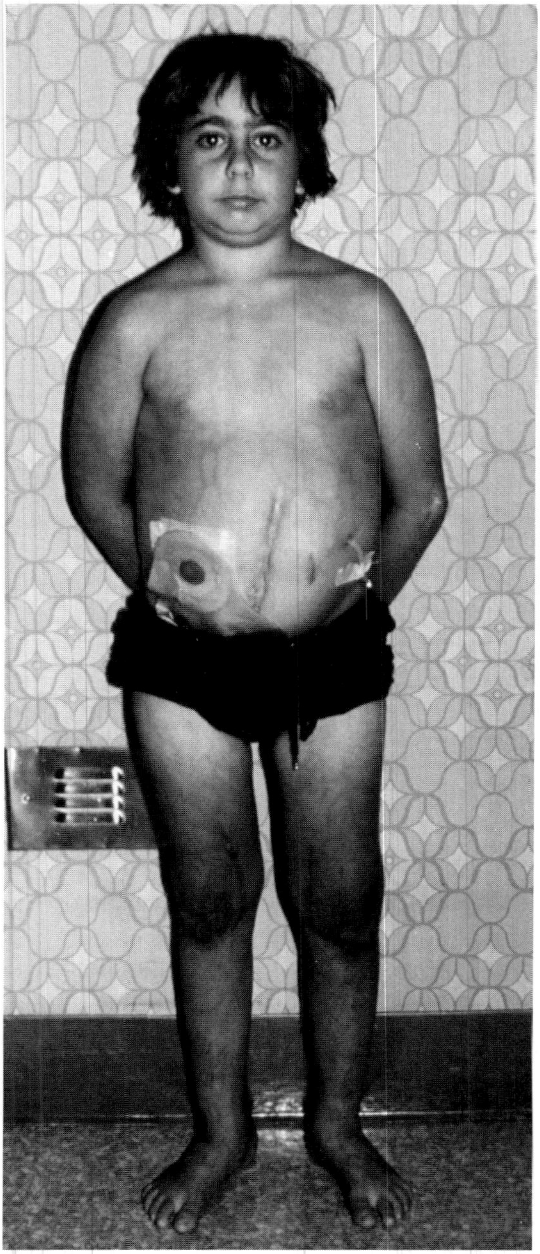

(C)

Figure 1 (continued)

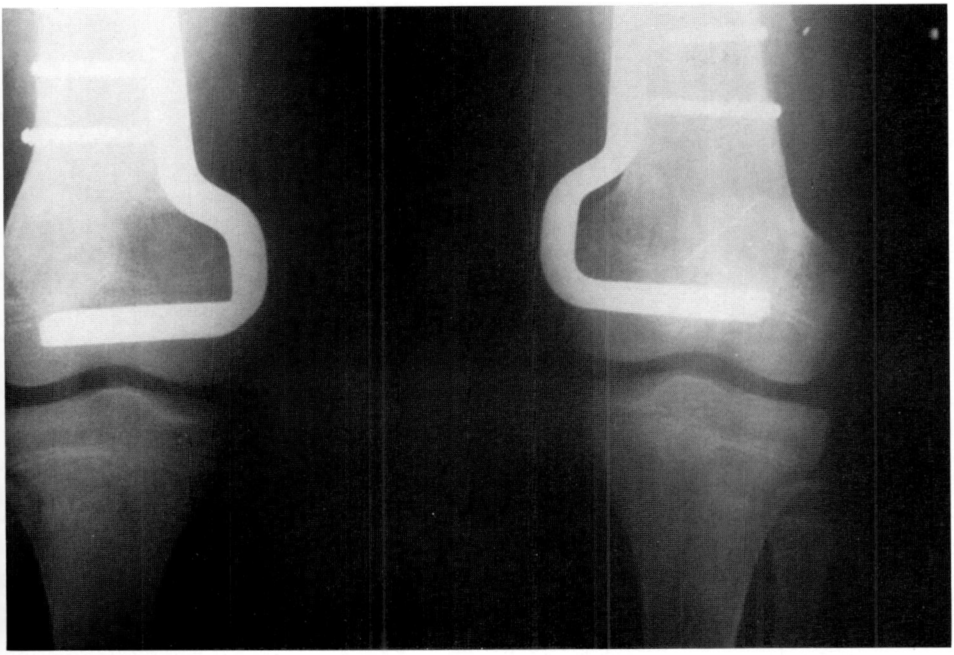

(D)

Dialysis has a variable influence on growth rate: some children have improved growth velocity while the majority have decreased growth rates (50).

Renal transplantation yields marked improvement in the growth velocity of some patients, while others continue to exhibit retarded growth (46). Influential factors include the age at the time of transplantation, the status of graft function, frequency of rejection, and steroid dose (51). Following successful transplantation, somatomedin levels are restored to normal values and a parallel increase in growth rate may be seen.

Angular deformities, particularly about the knees, reflect a common manifestation of epiphyseal distortion and altered growth. Children with renal osteodystrophy suffer from elongation in the columns of cells in the zone of maturation (52), with resultant defective mineralization of the zone of provisional calcification. A widened band of chrondro-osteoid develops associated with disturbed vascular invasion. Angular deformities, such as genu varum or valgum, develop in response to the stresses of applied weight bearing on the growing skeleton. Since children are normally bow-legged prior to the age of 2, but knock-kneed by the age of 3, the timing of the onset of renal osteodystrophy may accentuate these normal patterns and result in progressive deformity (Fig. 1).

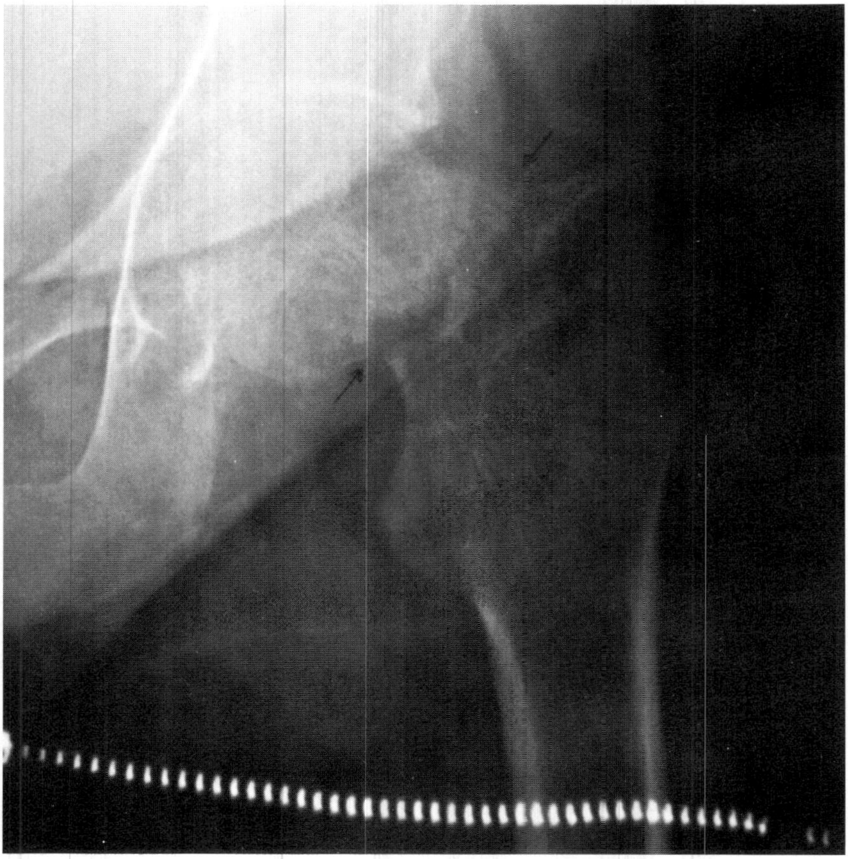

(A)

Figure 2 The types of fractures seen in renal osteodystrophy are analogous to those normally seen in a population 50 years older. A, B. This femoral neck fracture occurred spontaneously in a 15-year-old girl with poorly controlled renal osteodystrophy. C, D. Because of poor bone quality, initial repair could not prevent collapse into varus deformity. E. Reoperation was undertaken following control of hyperparathyroidism.

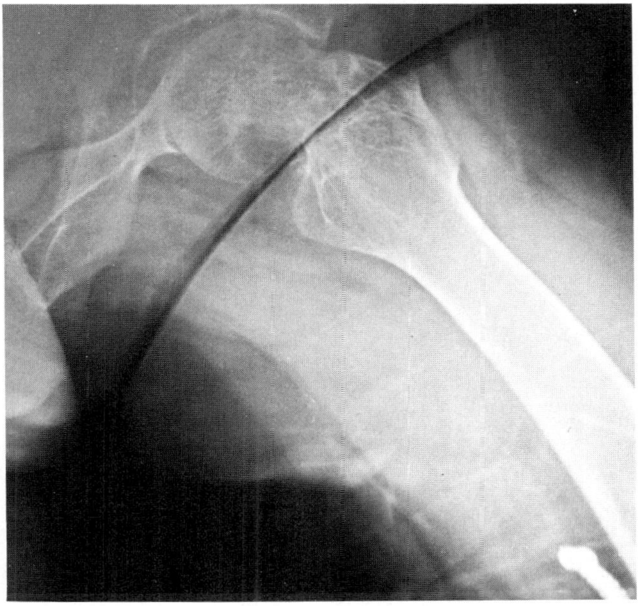

(B)

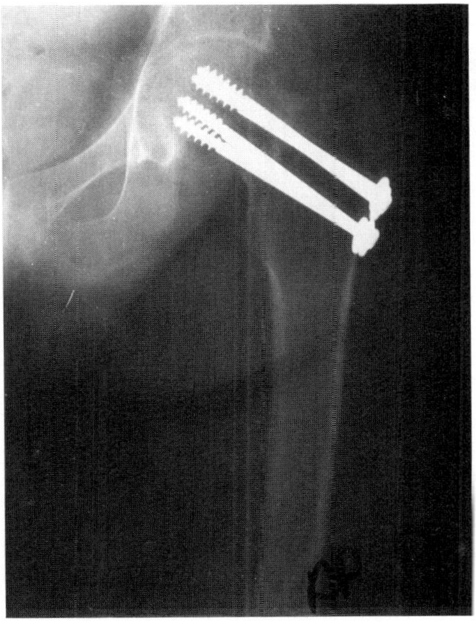

(C)

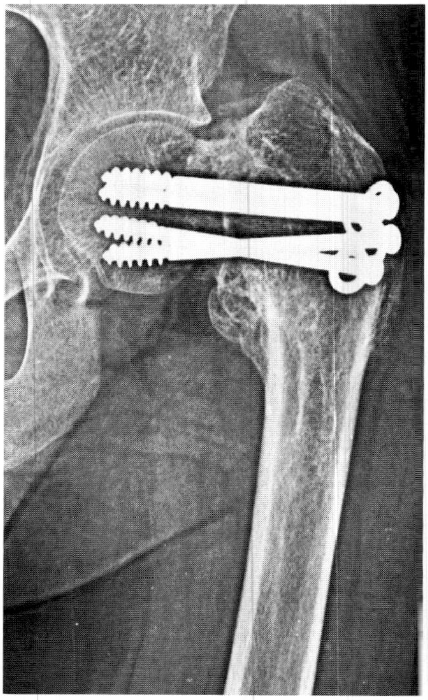
(D)

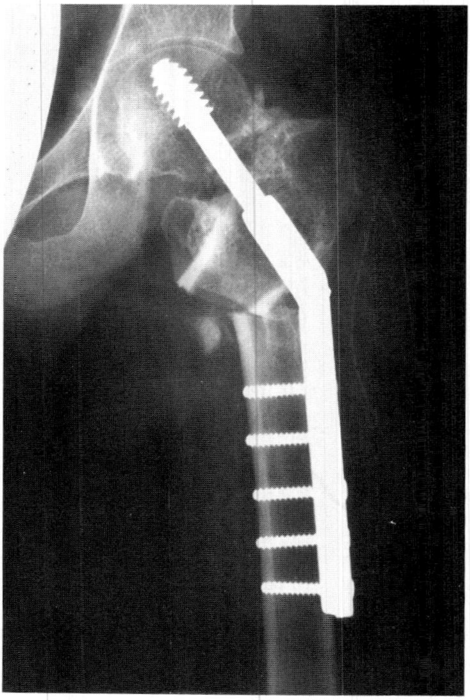
(E)

Figure 2 (continued)

VII. FRACTURES

Acute orthopedic skeletal complaints consequent to renal osteodystrophy may be a result of microfractures that occur in the weakened bone and present as stress fractures. Because of the generally "weakened" bone, traumatic fractures occur at sites generally expected to be seen in a population over 50 years of age (Fig. 2). These fractures include the femoral neck and distal radius. They typically heal in the expected time and are well managed with appropriate open or closed techniques.

VIII. EFFECTS ON THE EPIPHYSIS

Unique to growing children are the changes seen in the epiphyses. Clinical manifestations include epiphyseal slips (epiphysiolysis) and rickettsial widening of the growth plates accompanied by flaring of the metaphyses. Although these two problems are seen in other metabolic derangements, the pathophysiology differs according to the cause. Idiopathic epiphysiolysis most commonly presents in the normal adolescent as slipped capital femoral epiphyses, probably resulting from mechanical distortion involving the layer of hypertrophic cartilage (53,54). In contrast, children with chronic renal failure develop slips at a much earlier age, and in a variety of locations (55,56) (Fig. 3). One explanation is that the secondary hyperparathyroidism seen in children with renal osteodystrophy, with resultant histological findings of osteofibrosis, adversely affects the normal connection between the epiphyses and the metaphyses by the developing spongiosa (59). A weaker tissue plane composed of unossified and distorted cartilage between the epiphyses and metaphyses ensues, through which the slip results due to normal mechanical stresses (58). Another possible mechanism for slipping is micropathological fractures through bone that has been weakened by extensive osteoclastic resorption due to secondary hyperparathyroidism (18). The fact that epiphysiolysis occurs in patients with hyperparathyroidism or in those with secondary hyperparathyroidism as a result of pseudohyperparathyroidism is thought to support this concept (55). It may be that the "microtrauma" hypothesis applies to children with advanced renal osteodystrophy, while the former explanation applies primarily to those with the less severe variety.

Children with severe osteofibrosis can manifest slippage in nearly any epiphysis. The site of the slip seems to be related to the patient's age. Younger children have a predilection for slips in the upper and lower femoral epiphysis and near the distal tibia. Older children have involvement primarily in the upper femur and distal epiphyses of the forearm. Clinical presentations range from mild limping to gross skeletal deformities that are especially evident at the distal forearm or tibia.

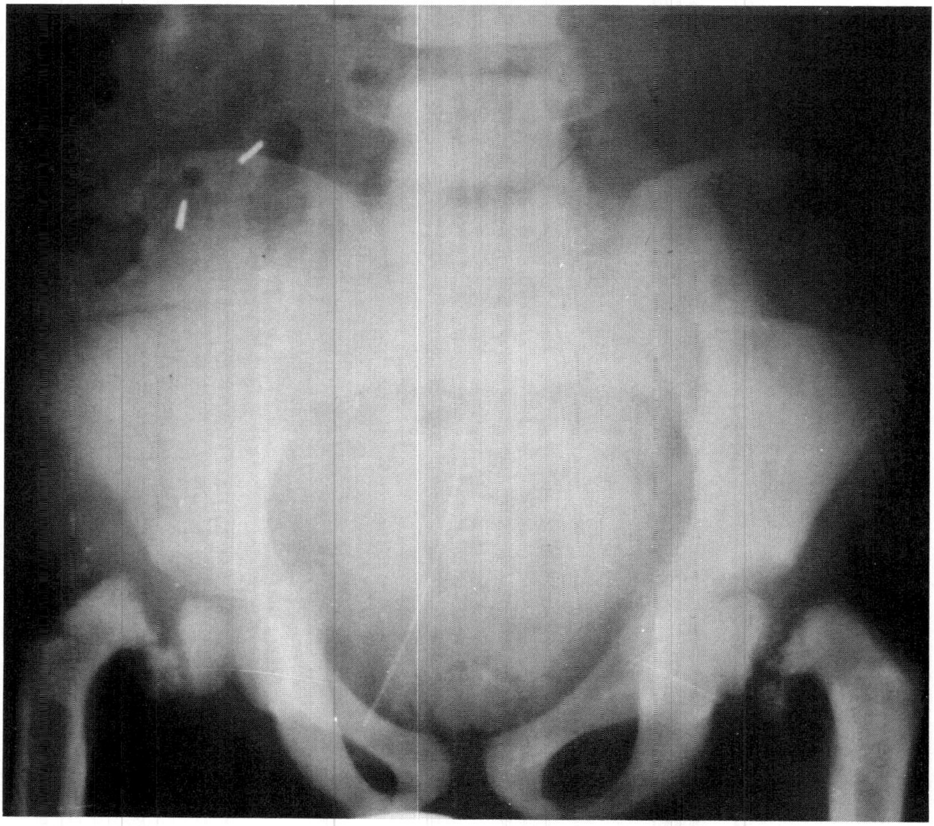

(A)

Figure 3 Slipped epiphyses are common, seen earlier than expected, and in unusual areas in addition to the hips. Slips of the hips (A) and distal radius (B) are shown.

IX. TREATMENT OF RENAL OSTEODYSTROPHY

Treatment of the musculoskeletal abnormalities that develop during the course of chronic renal failure in children must be tailored to the individual patient, while taking into account the severity of deformity and the chronicity and degree of renal failure. Many of the skeletal deformities will improve, if not resolve, with appropriate medical therapy (12,59). Others will require surgical management in spite of apparently adequate medical treatment.

The timing of surgery is important. Secondary hyperparathyroidism should be controlled preoperatively to enhance fixation techniques and to avoid recur-

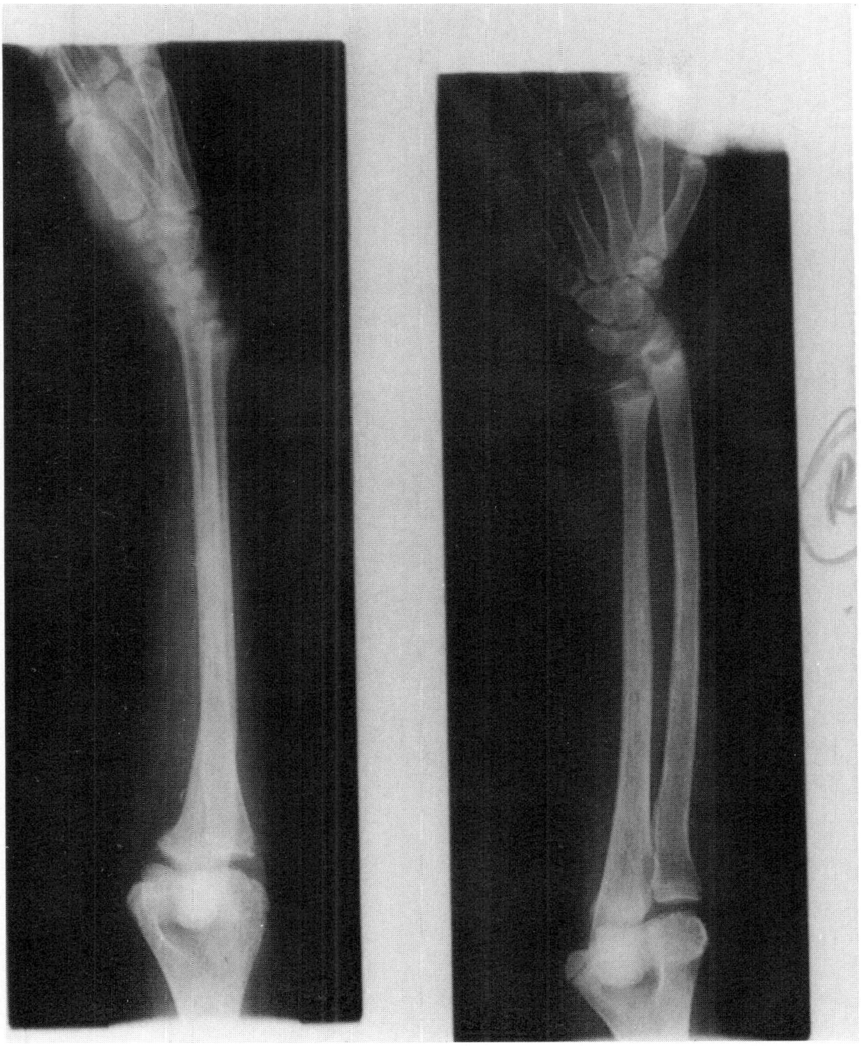

(B)

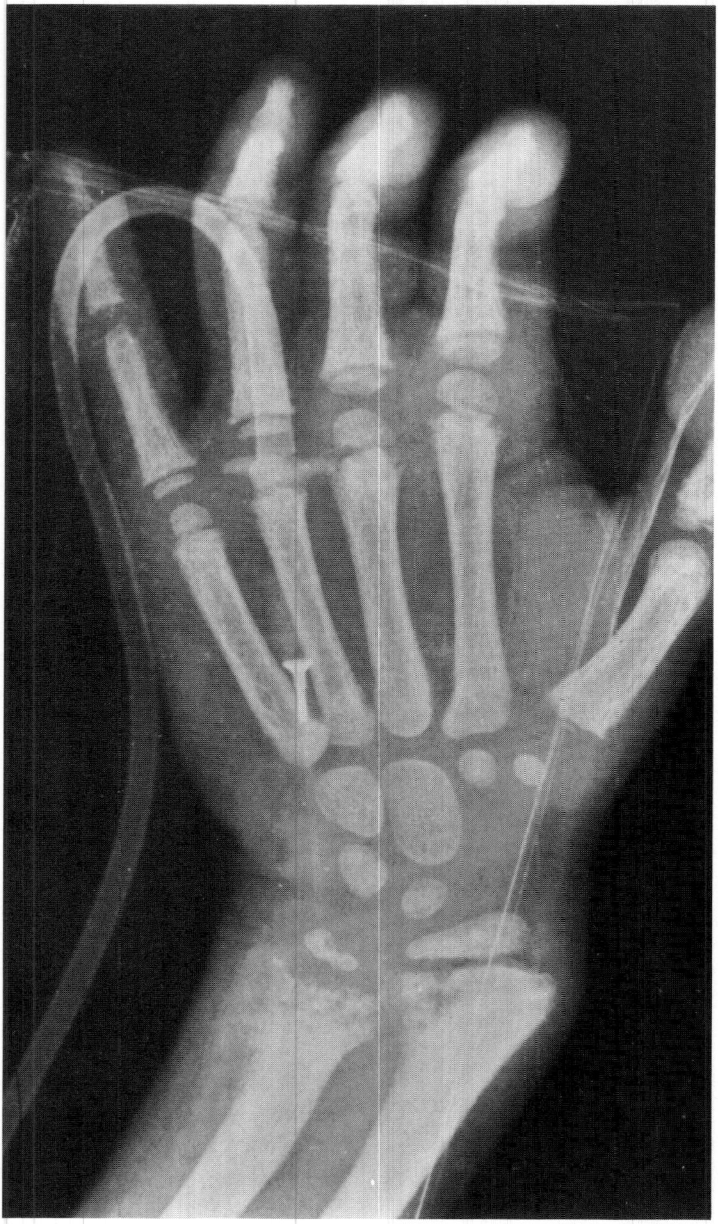

Figure 4A Prior to treatment of hyperparathyroidism.

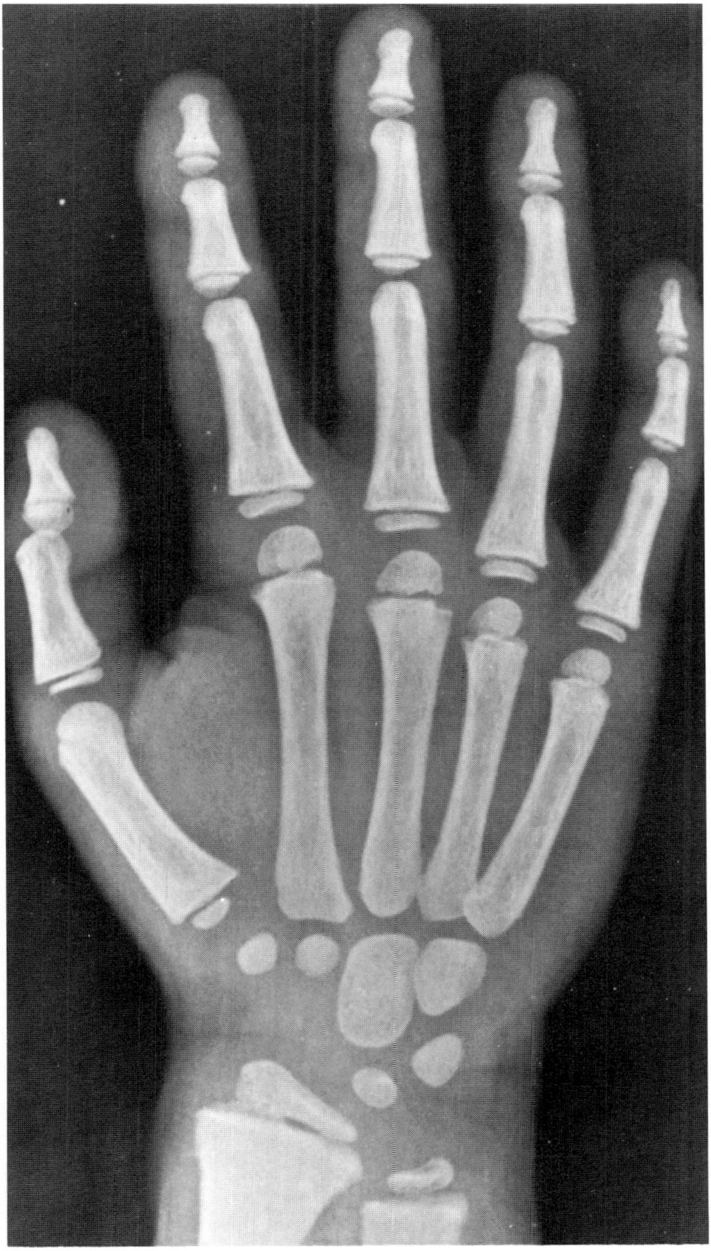

Figure 4B After treatment with vitamin D. Treatment of hyperparathyroidism is a prerequisite for successful orthopedic internal fixation techniques, and may be accomplished both medically and surgically.

rence of the deformity. Preoperative control of the secondary hyperparathyroidism is accomplished by reducing the serum phosphate level, supplemental oral calcium intake, and by administration of $1,25(OH)_2$-D_3 in an effort to reduce parathormone levels (Fig. 4). Since the primary source of phosphate intake is from ingestion of meat and dairy products, the serum phosphate level is reduced by limiting phosphate intake and by the use of phosphate-binding agents, such as calcium carbonate or aluminum-containing gels (60). By adherence to a low-protein diet, phosphate intake can be reduced by up to 50% (61). As renal failure worsens, phosphate binders have a greater role in management. Calcium carbonate has been demonstrated to control adequately the serum phosphate levels in children on dialysis who are receiving a regular diet with an average of 100% of the Recommended Daily Allowance for intake (62). It should be the drug of choice to avoid the aluminum accumulation delineated above.

The benefits of vitamin D in the control of secondary hyperparathyroidism in patients with stable chronic renal failure, those undergoing maintenance hemodialysis, and those on chronic ambulatory peritoneal dialysis is well documented (13,41,63). Despite appropriate treatment, however, 14% of children on dialysis and 35% of children with stable chronic renal failure still will develop progressive bone disease after 2–5 years (64). While it is not clear which children will respond, the dose of vitamin D sterol appears to be quite important. One study focusing on children maintained on continuous ambulatory peritoneal dialysis showed that only 35% of patients receiving low-dose calcitriol or dihydrotachysterol experienced reduced progression of bone disease (59). Children who had worsening of disease had lower serum calcium levels, increased alkaline phosphatase activity, increased serum parathormone levels, and worsening of the roentgenographic findings compared to patients in whom clinical and radiological features of secondary hyperparathyroidism were improved. Subsequent studies indicated that the use of oral "high" doses calcitriol produced healing and/or prevented the development of hyperparathyroidism in the majority of children undergoing continuous ambulatory peritoneal dialysis (65–67). Serum calcium levels were significantly increased while serum alkaline phosphatase levels decreased to normal during treatment. Serum parathormone levels fell significantly or remained within acceptable range in 76% of the patients. These findings are consistent with the in vitro observation of an elevation in the parathormone "set point," which is the serum calcium level that produces a 50% inhibition of parathormone release by isolated parathyroid cells (68,69). It appears that serum calcium levels between 10.5 and 11 mg/dl provide maximal parathormone suppression in this group of patients. This "medical parathyroidectomy" with calcitriol reduces serum parathormone levels, allowing healing of bone lesions, promotes resolution of the myopathy and obviates the need for surgical parathyroidecomy with the attendant complications (70). The major side effect of this therapeutic regimen with calcitrol is asymptomatic hypercalcemia, which was seen in 65% of patients (8). The hypercalcemia resolved in most instances after the dose was decreased or use of calcitrol was stopped briefly until serum calcium levels had returned to normal. Caution must be exercised when treating patients who may have aluminum osteomalacia, because they are susceptible to severe prolonged hypercalcemia during $1,25(OH)_2$-D_3 treatment. The intravenous form of calcitrol was associated with a greater reduction of the parathormone level in adult patients treated with hemodialysis (71). However, the use of this form of calcitrol in children has not been studied.

X. TREATMENT OF ALUMINUM INTOXICATION

Prevention of aluminum-related bone disease is much more effective than treatment. Current recommendations for prevention include maintaining the concentration of aluminum dialysate below 10 μg/L, thus avoiding transfer of aluminum into the circulation. In the United States the principal source of aluminum is by the intestinal absorption of aluminum from the phosphate-binding agents (72–74). One means of reducing the aluminum absorption is by reducing dietary phosphate intake to 800–900 mg/day, with a concomitant limitation of aluminum hydroxide ingestion to 3.0 g/day. However, reduced-phosphate diets are both less palatable and more expensive. The alternative is thus the avoidance of aluminum-containing phosphate binders and the use of calcium carbonate to bind phosphate, especially in children (62,64). Once aluminum toxicity has developed, the aluminum can be removed by chelating agents such as deferoxamine (Fig. 5). However, severe lethal infection (mucormycosis) has recently been described with the use of deferoxamine. Thus, deferoxamine should be used with caution, according to the severity of the total body aluminum burden.

A. Surgery

Surgical management for skeletal problems that develop during end-stage renal disease is appropriate after adequate control of secondary hyperparathyroidism. This objective itself may require surgical parathyroidectomy if medical management fails. Until surgery is undertaken, every effort should be made to keep the child ambulatory. However, if prolonged immobilization occurs, careful monitoring of the serum calcium level should be done, especially in patients receiving vitamin D sterol therapy.

Reconstructive surgery in patients with chronic renal failure used to be discouraged because of the increased postoperative morbidity (75). With improved metabolic management and an increased life span and activity level, a more aggressive approach appears warranted (76,77). Although chronic anemia is often present, uremic patients with markedly lower baseline hematocrits are usually well compensated by alterations in the hemoglobin–oxygen saturation curve.

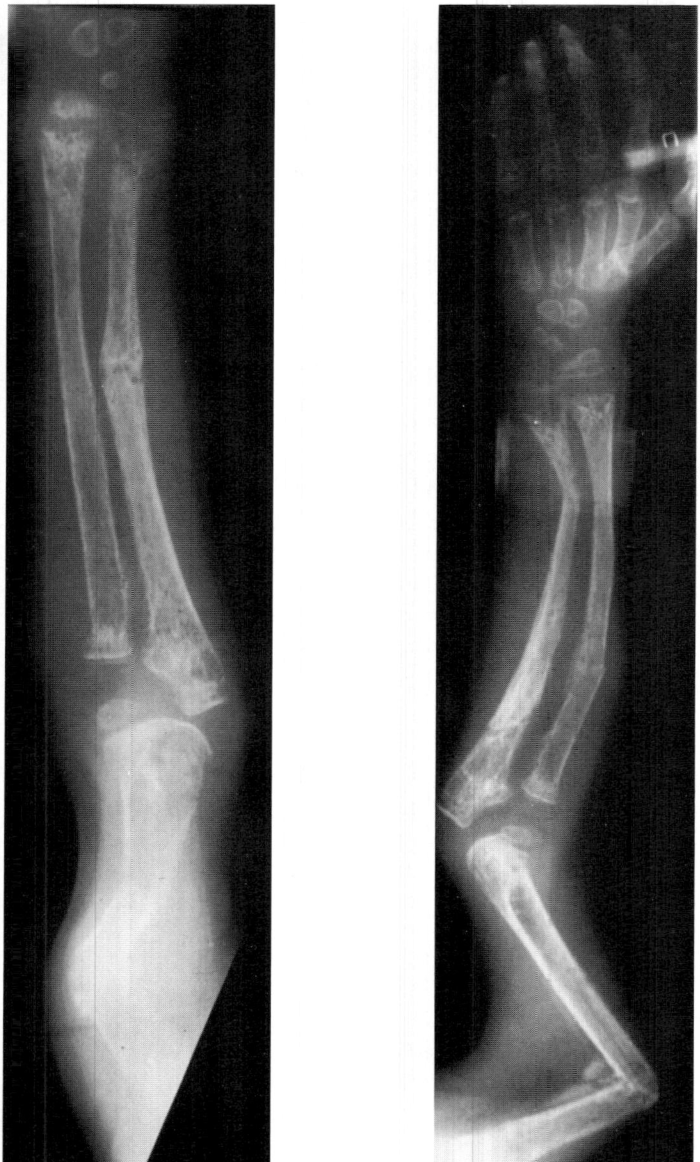

(A) (B)

Figure 5 A–D. Severe aluminum intoxication in an 8-year-old boy. The patient had sustained numerous fractures and had not walked in 3 years. E, F. Resumption of independent ambulation after treatment with deferoxamine and orthopedic procedures. G. Before chelation therapy. H. Three months after institution of chelation therapy.

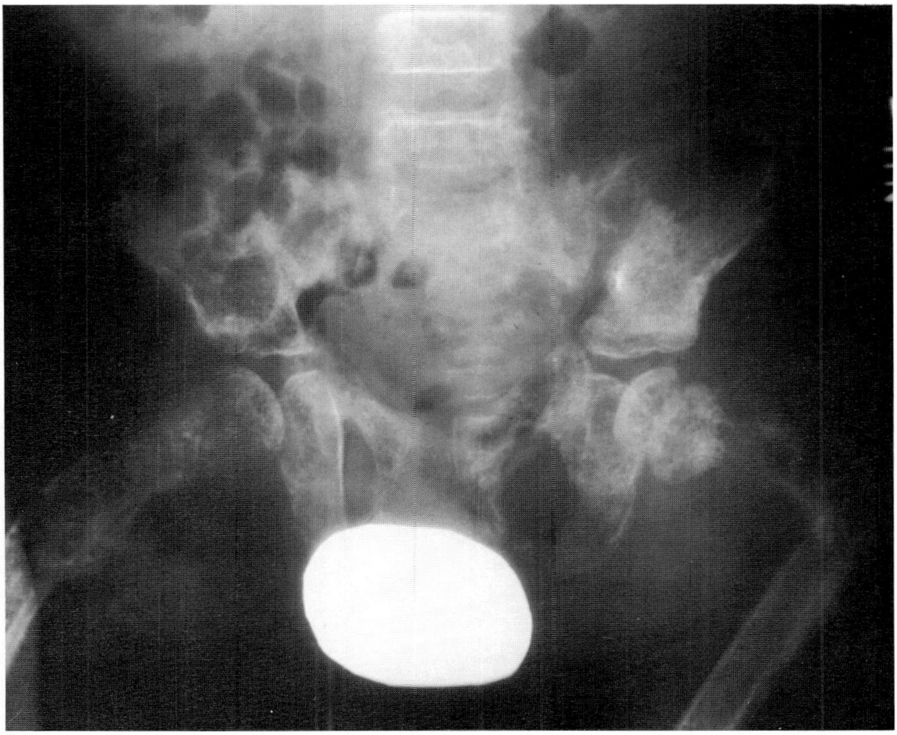

(C)

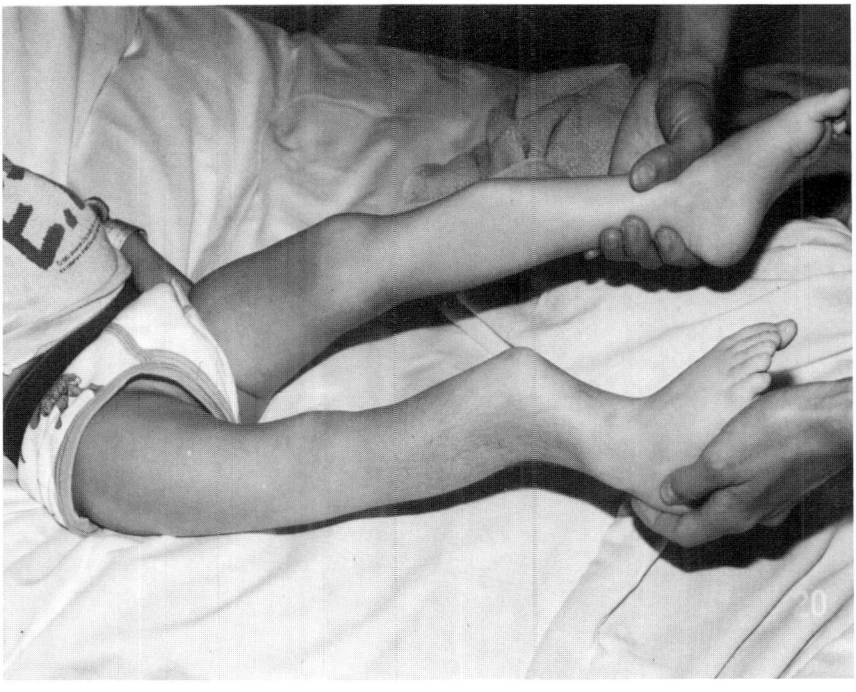

(D)

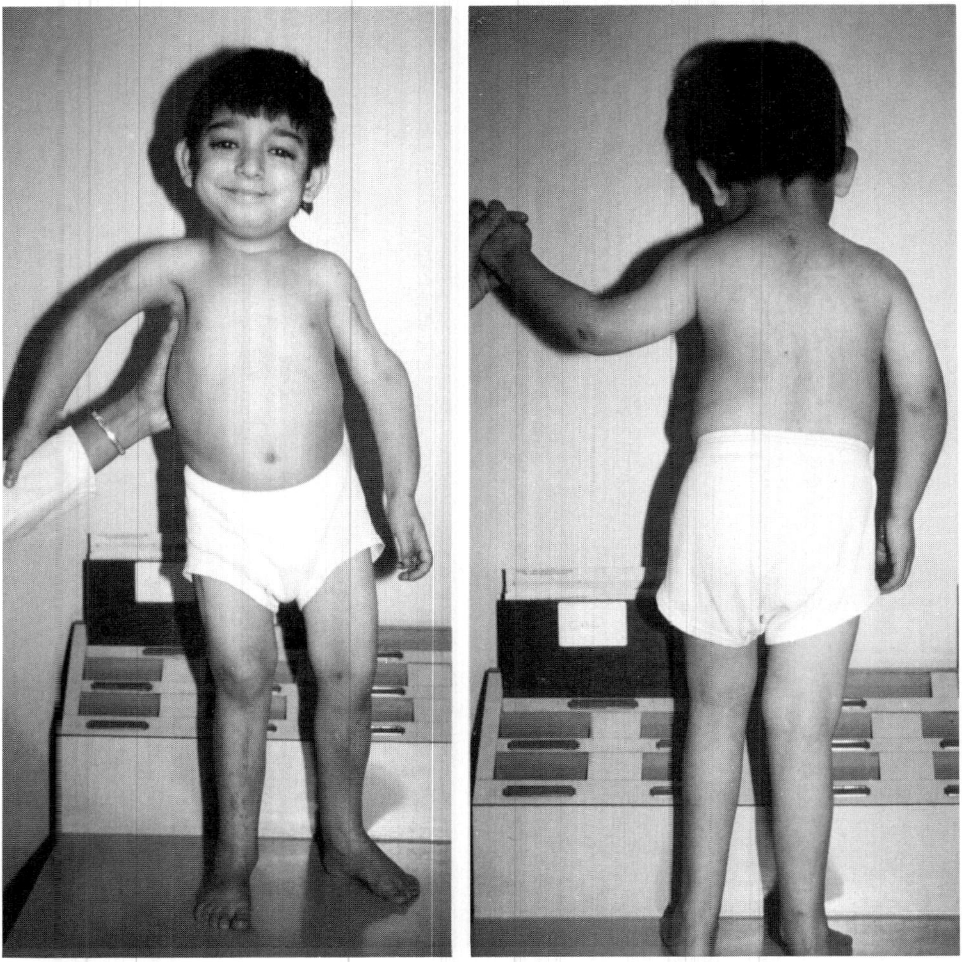

(E) (F)

Figure 5 (continued)

These chronic adaptations allow them to tolerate surgery and anesthesia with lower circulating hemoglobin levels than one might otherwise anticipate.

Because of treatment with immunosuppressive agents (corticosteroids, cyclosporine, azathioprine) renal allograft recipients have an increased risk for postoperative infection of surgical wounds. This potential problem can be minimized by careful handling of tissues during surgery as well as the use of perioperative prophylactic antibiotics.

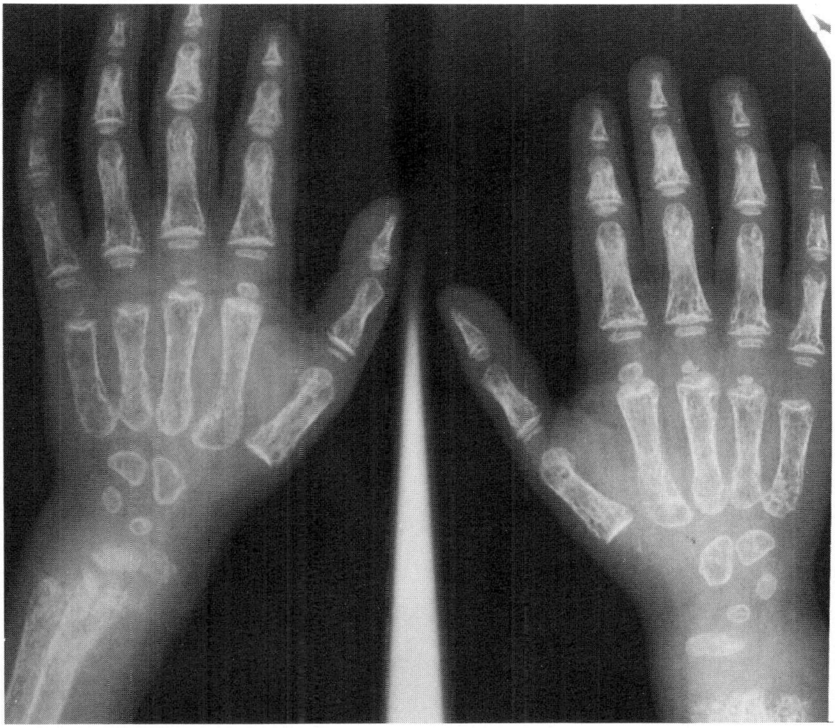

(G)

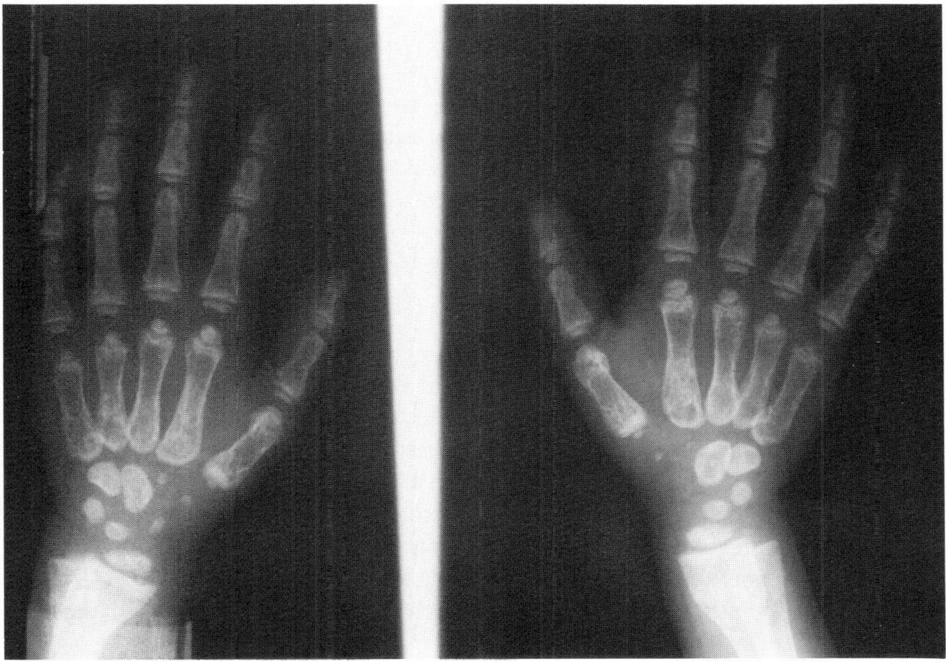

(H)

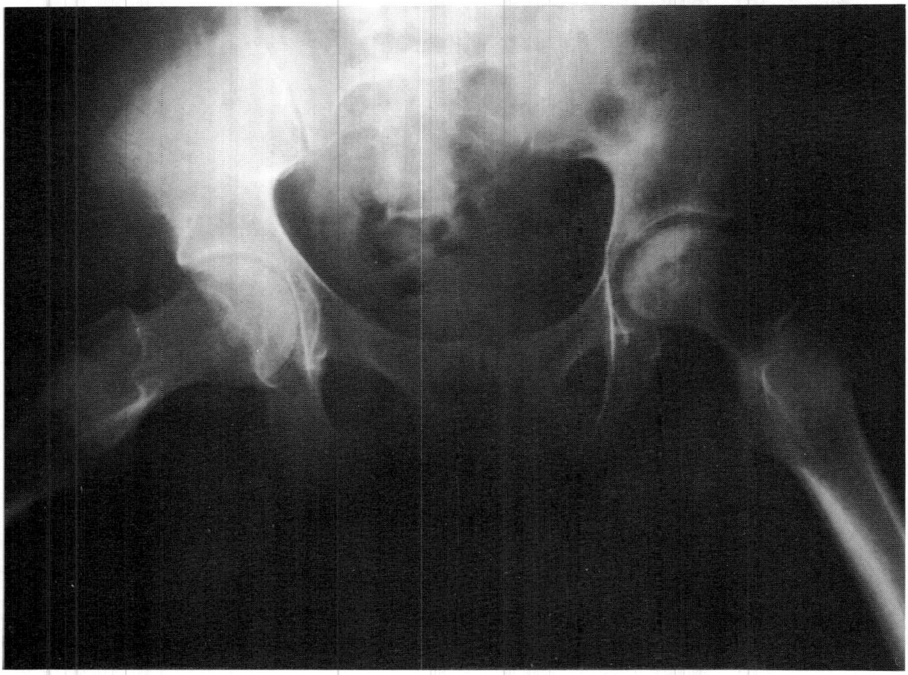

(A)

Figure 6 Avascular necrosis is one of the more difficult complications to treat. Here the femoral head has been replaced with a hemiarthroplasty, anticipating later conversion to a total hip replacement. Because of an inactive lifestyle in this particular patient, the arthroplasty has lasted 8 years to date. Arthrodesis or initial total hip replacement may be appropriate in other cases. A. Avascular necrosis of the femur in a 17-year-old patient. B. Hemiarthroplasty. C. Operative specimen, with extracted piece of necrotic bone that fell out of the cavity is seen just beneath the intact cartilage.

A review of 24 patients with renal osteodystrophy who had undergone 41 orthopedic operations at UCLA between January, 1979, and September, 1985, was performed. We assessed the end result as well as the complication rate for the orthopedic procedures performed. Despite the multiple risk factors, surgery was well tolerated with resultant salutary outcome. There was no significant postoperative would infections and all osteotomies healed within an appropriate time. One patient required repeat pinning for slipped capital femoral epiphyses because of poorly controlled hyperparathyroidism that did not permit epiphyseal fusion, and another poorly controlled patient with a femoral neck frac-

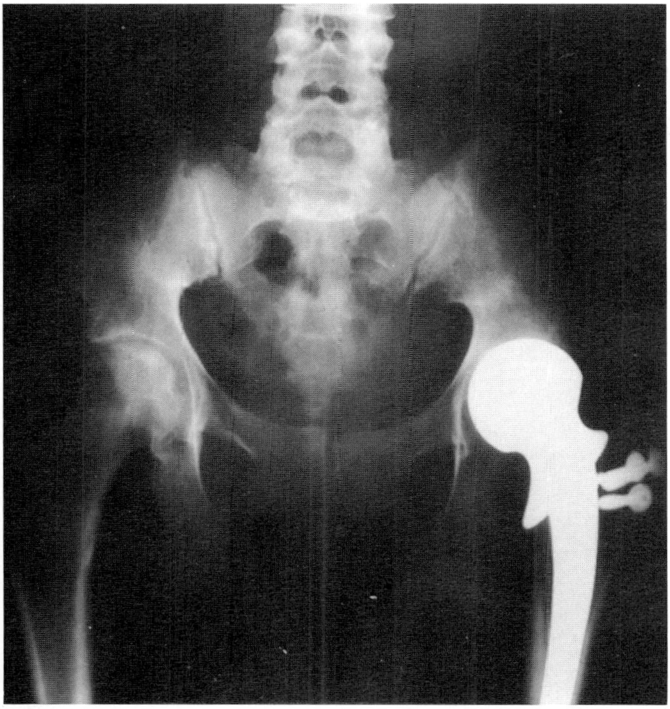

(B)

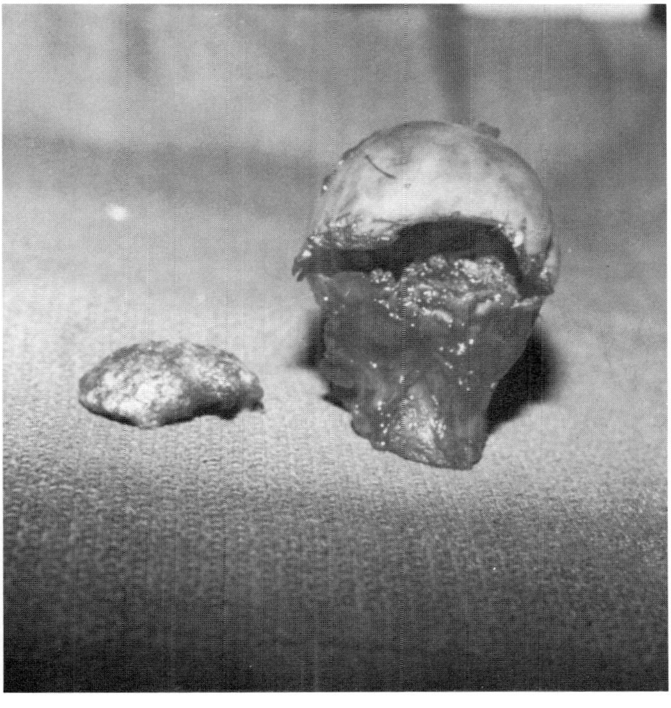

(C)

ture lost reduction due to softened bone in spite of internal fixation. Once the hyperparathyroidism was medically controlled, both patients underwent successful reoperations. The angular deformity seen in aluminum-induced osteomalacia responded well to multiple osteotomies with intramedullary and extramedullary fixation after treatment with deferioxamine.

Given the minimal complication rate in this group of patients, operative treatment appears to yield satisfactory results once secondary hyperparathyroidism is controlled. Although an alternative to early in situ pinning of slipped capital femoral epiphyses could be restriction of activity, this approach may necessitate later proximal femoral osteotomies to prevent arthritis, or may result in further slippage and avascular necrosis. Our success in preventing progression of slips, combined with the low morbidity of percutaneous pinning, demonstrate the utility of this procedure in patients with renal osteodystrophy.

Genu valgum and other angular deformities of the skeleton are said to resolve once the secondary hyperparathyroidism is brought under control. None of the nine patients in our series demonstrated spontaneous improvement. Thus osteotomy was performed in all at either the distal femoral or proximal tibial level, depending on which location would restore alignment while keeping the knee and ankle joints parallel to the ground when the patient stood.

B. The Role of Transplantation

Although transplantation is curative for many of the problems seen in end-stage renal disease, it also can generate new difficulties. A small group of children develop persistent hypophosphatemia following transplantation in the presence of normal serum parathormone levels, probably because of graft ischemia at harvest, which causes tubular damage. Defective phosphate handling by the transplanted kidney results in increased urinary phosphate and hypophosphatemia.

Aseptic necrosis is the most serious osseous change seen after transplantation (Fig. 6). Although corticosteroid treatment appears to be the major predisposing factor, the description of aseptic necrosis in patients who have not received steroids or allografts suggests that hyperparathyroidism itself may be influential (78–80). If hyperparathyroidism does play a role, it is relatively minor, since the majority of the available data implicate steroid administration as the most important influence. The radiographic diagnosis of aseptic necrosis can be difficult, since cancellous bone content is increased in uremia. This resultant osteosclerosis is caused by an increase in the number and size of trabeculae in metaphyseal bone. It must not be confused with increased sensitivity seen in areas of aseptic necrosis (41).

Magnetic resonance imaging has recently improved the time to diagnosis as well as the specificity of diagnosis. The reported frequency of posttransplantation aseptic necrosis (4–48%) varies with the duration of follow-up, number of previous grafts, and steroid dosages. The sites of aseptic necrosis, in descending order, include the femoral head, humeral head, proximal tibia, talus, and scaphoid (81-87). The diagnosis must be kept in mind when patients describe new "aches and pains." Symptoms typically develop within 1 year of transplantation and radiographic changes lag 2 months behind. No direct mechanisms for corticosteroid influence on bone growth has been shown; however, there is much circumstantial evidence for the observed deleterious role. Several authors have shown a lowered incidence of aseptic necrosis with diminished corticosteroid dosage (88). The influence of azathioprine has questionable effects on aseptic necrosis. Cyclosporine, which necessitates a lower corticosteroid dosage, may prove to be more valuable in this respect (56). Long-term follow-up studies are obviously needed in these patients.

XI. CONCLUSION

As the underlying causes of chronic renal failure become more fully appreciated, and the lives of children with end-stage renal disease are prolonged, an ironic increase in the severity of renal osteodystrophy is seen. The control of renal osteodystrophy is brought about partly by prevention using proper dietary restriction; partly by medical management through the judicious use of vitamin D sterol, calcium supplementation, and phosphate binders; and partly by surgery, addressing both the hyperparathyroidism by parathyroidectomy if necessary, as well as any residual deformities by orthopedic reconstruction. The quality of life is markedly improved when the bone disease is addressed aggressively by all of the disciplines involved. As a result, these children are living not only longer lives but also more active ones.

ACKNOWLEDGMENT

This work was supported in party by USPHS grant DK-35423.

REFERENCES

1. Lucas, R. C. On a form of late rickets associated with albuminuria. *Lancet 1*: 993–994 (1883).
2. Albright, F., Drake, T. G., and Sulkowitch, H. W. Rickets resistant to vitamin D therapy. *Am. J. Dis. Child. 54*:529–547 (1937).
3. Follis, R. R. Skeletal changes associated with hyperparathyroidism. *Bull. Johns Hopkins Hosp. 92*:405–421 (1953).
4. Follis, R. H., and Jackson, D. A. Renal osteodystrophy and osteitis fibrosa in adults. *Bull. Johns Hopkins Hosp. 72*:232–241 (1943).
5. Pendras, J. P. Parathyroid disease in long-term maintenance hemodialysis. *Arch. Intern. Med. 11*:302–311 (1951).

6. Andreoli, S. P., Bergstein, J. M., and Sherrard, D. J. Aluminum intoxication from aluminum-containing phosphate binders in children with azotemia not undergoing dialysis. *N. Engl. J. Med. 310*:1079–1084 (1984).
7. Portale, A. A., Booth, B. E., Halloram, B. P., and Morris, R. C. Effect of dietary phosphorus on circulating concentrations of 1,25-dihydroxyvitamin D and immunoreactive parathyroid hormone in children with moderate renal insufficiency. *Clin. Invest. 73*:1580–1589 (1984).
8. Ritz, E., Malluche, H., Krempien, B., Tschope, W., and Massary, S. G. Pathogenesis of renal osteodystrophy: Role of phosphate and skeletal resistance to PTH. *Adv. Exp. Med. Biol. 103*:423–436 (1978).
9. Avioli, L. V., Birge, S., Lee, S. W., and Slatopolsky, E. The metabolic fate of Vitamin $D_3{}^{-3}$H in chronic renal failure. *J. Clin. Invest. 45*:982–983 (1966).
10. Brickman, A. S., Coburn, J. W., and Norman, A. W. Action of 1,25-dihydroxycholecalciferol, a potent kidney produced metabolite of vitamin D-3 in uremic man. *N. Engl. J. Med. 287*:891–895 (1972).
11. Fraser, D. R., and Kodicek, E. Unique biosynthesis by kidney of a biologically active vitamin D metabolite. *Nature 228*:764–766 (1970).
12. Parfitt, A. M. Renal osteodystrophy. *Orthop. Clin. North Am. 3*:681–698 (1972).
13. Langman, C. B., Mazur, A. T., Baron, R., and Norman, M. E. 25-Hydroxyvitamin D3 (calciferol) therapy of juvenile renal osteodystrophy: Beneficial effect on linear growth velocity. *J. Pediatr. 100*:815–820 (1982).
14. Sherrard, D. J., Baylink, D. J., Wergedal, J. E., and Maloney, N. Quantitative histological studies on the pathogenesis of uremic bone disease. *J. Clin. Endocrinol. 39*:119–135 (1974).
15. Bricker, N. S., Slatopolsky, E., Reiss, E., and Avioli, L. V. Calcium, phosphorus, and bone in renal disease and transplantation. *Arch. Intern. Med. 123*:543–553 (1969).
16. Slatopolsky, E., Calgar, S., Gradowska, L., et al. On the prevention of secondary hyperparathyroidism in experimental chronic renal disease using "proportional reduction" of dietary phosphorus intake. *Kidney Int. 2*:147 (1977).
17. Friis, T., Hahnemann, S., and Weeke, E. Serum calcium and serum phosphorus in uremia during administration of sodium phytate and aluminum hydroxide. *Acta Med. Scand. 183*:497 (1968).
18. Kirkwood, J. R., Ozonoff, M. B., and Steinbach, H. L. Epiphyseal displacement after metaphyseal fracture in renal osteodystrophy. *Am. J. Roentgenol. 115*:547–554 (1972).
19. Coburn, J. W.. Popovtzer, M., Massry, S. G., and Kleeman, C. R. The physiochemical state and renal handling of divalent ions in chronic renal failure. *Arch. Intern. Med. 124*:302 (1969).
20. Goldman, R., and Basset, S. H. Phosphorus excretion in renal failure. *J. Clin. Invest. 33*:1623–1628 (1954).
21. Reiss, E., Canterbury, M., and Kanter, A. Circulating parathyroid hormone concentration in chronic renal insufficiency. *Arch. Intern. Med. 124*:417–422 (1969).

22. Korkor, A. B. Reduced binding of [^{3}H] 1,25-dihydroxyvitamin D_3 in the parathyroid glands of patients with renal failure. *N. Engl. J. Med. 316*: 1573–1577 (1987).
23. Genuth, S. M., Klein, L., Rabinovich, S., and King, K. C. Osteomalacia accompanying chronic anticonvulsant therapy. *J. Clin. Endocrinol. Metab. 35*: 378 (1972).
24. Jubiz, W., Haussler, M. R., McCaw, T. A., and Tolman, K. G. Plasma 1,25-dihydroxyvitamin D levels in patients receiving anticonvulsant drugs. *J. Clin. Endocrinol. Metab. 44*:617–620 (1977).
25. Pierides, A. M., Kerr, D. N., Ellis, H. A., O'Riordan, J. L. H., and Deluca, H. F. 1-Alpha-hydroxy-cholecalciferol in hemodialysis renal osteodystrophy. Adverse effects of anticonvulsant therapy. *Clin. Nephrol. 5*:189 (1976).
26. Mawer, E. B., and Taylor, C. M. Vitamin D metabolism in man, the role of the kidney. In *Proceedings of Seventh International Congress of Nephrology, Montreal*. S. Karger, Basel, 1978, p. 469.
27. Evanson, J. M. The response to the infusion of parathyroid extract in hypocalcemic states. *Clin. Sci. 31*:63 (1986).
28. Jacob, A. I., Gavellas, G., Canterbury, J., and Bourgergnie, J. J. Calcemic and phosphaturic response to parathyroid hormone in normal and chronically uremic dogs. *Kidney Int. 22*:21–26 (1982).
29. Hodgson, S. F. Skeletal remodeling and renal osteodystrophy. *Semin. Nephrol. VI*:42–55 (1986).
30. Ritz, E., Malluche, H. H., Krempien, B., and Mehlis, O. Bone histology in renal insufficiency. In: *Perspectives in Nephrology and Hypertension* (David, D. S., ed.). John Wiley, New York, 1977, pp. 197–233.
31. Sedman, A. B., Alfrey, A. C., Miller, N. L., and Goodman, W. G. Tissue and cellular basis for impaired bone formation in aluminum related osteomalacia in the pig. *J. Clin. Invest. 79*:86–92 (1987).
32. Heaf, J. G., Podenphant, J., and Anderson, J. R. Bone aluminum deposition in maintenance dialysis patients treated with aluminum-free dialysate: Role of aluminum hydroxide consumption. *Nephron 42*:210–216 (1986).
33. Sedman, A. B., Miller, N. L., Waredy, B. A., Lum, G. M., and Alfrey, A. C. Aluminum loading in children with CRF. *Kidney Int. 26*:201–204 (1984).
34. Kaehny, W. D., Hegg, A. P., and Alfrey, A. C. Gastrointestinal absorption of aluminum from aluminum-containing antacids. *N. Engl. J. Med. 296*: 1389–1390 (1977).
35. Salusky, I. B., Coburn, J. W., Paunier, L., Sherrard, D. J., and Fine, R. N. Role of aluminum hydroxide in raising serum aluminum levels in children undergoing continuous ambulatory peritoneal dialysis (CAPD). *J. Pediatr. 105*:717 (1984).
36. Hodsman, A. B., Sherrard, D. J., Alfrey, A. C., Ott, S. M., Brickman, A. S., Miller, N. L., Maloney, N. A., and Coburn, J. W. Bone aluminum and histomorphometric features of renal osteodystrophy. *J. Clin. Endocrinol. Metab. 54*:539–546 (1982).

37. Norris, K., Crooks, P. W., Nebeker, H. G., Hertz, G., Milliner, D. S., Gerszi, K., Slatapolsky, E., Andress, D. L., Sherrard, D. J., and Coburn, J. W. Clinical and laboratory features of aluminum-related bone disease: Differences between sporadic and "epidemic" forms of the syndrome. *Am. J. Kidney Dis. 6*:342–347 (1985).
38. Coburn, J., Norris, K., Salusky, I., et al. Renal osteodystrophy: Views on pathogenesis and management. In *Vitamin D: Chemical, Biochemical and Clinical Update* (Annaman et al., eds.). De Gruyter, Berlin, 1985, pp. 926–934.
39. Ritz, E., Mehls, O., Bomner, J., et al. Vascular Ca^{++} under maintenance hemodialysis. *Klin. Wochenschr. 55*:375–378 (1977).
40. Fournier, A. E., Arnaud, C. D., Johnson, W. J., Taylor, W. F., and Goldsmith, R. S. Etiology of hyperparathyroidism and bone disease during chronic hemodialysis: II. Factors affecting serum immunoreactive parathyroid hormone. *J. Clin. Invest. 50*:599 (1971).
41. Mehls, O., Ritz, E., Gilli, G., and Kreusser, W. Growth in renal failure. *Nephron. 21*:237–247 (1978).
42. Scharer, K., Chantler, C., Brunner, R. P., et al. Combined report on regular dialysis and transplantation of children in Europe, 1975. *Proc. Eur. Dialysis Transplant. Assoc. 13*:59 (1976).
43. Broyer, M. Growth in children with renal insufficiency. *Pediatr. Clin. North Am. 4*:991–1003 (1982).
44. DeLuca, N. F. Metabolism and molecular mechanics of action of Vitamin D: 1981. *Biochem. Soc. Trans. 10(3)*:147–158 (1982).
45. Geary, D. F., Fennell, R. S., Braylan, A., et al. Hyperparathyroidism and anemia in chronic renal failure. *Eur. J. Pediatr. 139(4)*:296–298 (1982).
46. Saenger, P., Wiedman, E., Schwartz, E., Korthz-Schultz, S., Lewy, J. E., Riggio, R. R., Rubin, A. L., Steinzel, K., and New, M. I. Somatomedin and growth after renal transplantation. *Pediatr. Res. 8*:163 (1974).
47. Chesney, R. W., Dabbagh, S., Uehling, D. T., and DeLuca, H. F. The importance of early treatment of renal bone disease in children. *Kidney Int. 28*: S75–S78 (1985).
48. Pennisi, A. J., Phillips, L. S., Uittenbogaart, C., et al. Nutritional intake, somatomedin activity and linear growth in children undergoing hemodialysis. *Proc. Dialysis Transplant. Forum* p. 181, 1976.
49. Pennisi, A. J., Wang, M., and Kopple, J. D. Effects of protein and amino acid diets in chronically uremic and control rats. *Kidney Int. 13*:472 (1978).
50. Von Lilien, T., Salusky, I. B., Boechat, I., Ettinger, R. B., and Fine, R. N. Five year's experience with continuous ambulatory or continuous cycling peritoneal dialysis in children. *J. Pediatr. 111*:513–518 (1987).
51. Cundy, T., Hand, D. J., Oliver, D. O., and Kanis, J. A. Who gets renal bone disease before beginning dialysis? *Br. Med. J. 290*:271–275 (1985).
52. Mankin, H. J. Rickets, osteomalacia, osteodystrophy. *J. Bone Joint Surg. 56A*:352–386 (1974).

53. Martin, W. D., and Riddervold, H. O. Epiphysiolysis in rickets. *Va Med. 107(8)*:566–567 (1980).
54. Nixon, J. R., and Douglas, J. F. Bilateral slipping of the upper femoral epiphysis in end-stage renal failure. A report in two cases. *J. Bone Joint Surg. 62B*:18–21 (1980).
55. Tebor, G. B., Ehrlich, M. G., and Herrin, J. Slippage of the distal tibial epiphysis in end-stage failure. A report of two cases. *J. Bone Joint*
56. Bone, L. B., Roach, J. W., Wad, T., and Warthen, H. G. Slipped capital femoral epiphysis associated with hyperparathyroidism. *J. Pediatr. Orthop. 3*:589–592 (1985).
57. Mehlis, O., Ritz, E., Krempien, B., et al. Slipped epiphyses in renal osteodystrophy. *Arch. Dis. Child. 50*:545–554 (1975).
58. Goldman, A. B., Lane, J. M., and Salvat, E. Slipped capital femoral epiphysis complicating renal osteodystrophy; report of three cases. *Radiology 126*:333–339 (1978).
59. Paunier, L., Salusky, I. B., Hall, T., et al. Renal osteodystrophy in children undergoing continuous ambulatory peritoneal dialysis. Am. Soc. Bone Mineral Research (ABST), San Francisco, June 1982.
60. Makoff, D. L., Gordon, A., Franklin, S. S., Gerstein, A. R., and Maxwell, M. H. Chronic calcium carbonate therapy in uremia. *Arch. Intern. Med. 123*:15–21 (1969).
61. Salusky, I., Coburn, J. W., Foley, J., Nelson, P., and Fine, R. N. Effects of oral calcium carbonate on control of serum phosphorus and changes in plasma aluminum levels after discontinuation of aluminum-containing gels in children receiving dialysis. *J. Pediatr. 108*:767–770 (1986).
62. Fournier, A., Moriniere, P. H., Sebert, J. L., Dkhissi, H., Atik, A., Leflon, P., Renaud, H., Gueris, J., Gregoire, I., Idrissi, A., and Garabedian, M. Calcium carbonate, an aluminum-free agent for control of hyperphosphatemia, hypocalcemia and hyperparathyroidism in uremia. *Kidney Int. 29* Suppl. 18:S-114–S-119 (1986).
63. Chan, J. C. M., and De Luca, H. F. Growth velocity in a child on prolonged hemodialysis: Beneficial effect of 1-alpha-hydroxyvitamin D3. *J.A.M.A. 238*:2053–2054 (1977).
64. Mak, R. H. K., Turner, C., Thompson, T., Powell, H., Haycock, G. B., and Chantler, C. Suppression of secondary hyperparathyroidism in children with chronic renal failure by high dose phosphate binders: Calcium carbonate versus aluminium hydroxide. *Br. Med. J. 291*:623–626 (1985).
65. Dabbagh, S., and Chesney, R. W. Treatment of renal osteodystrophy during childhood. In *End-Stage Renal Disease in Children*. (R. M. Fine and A. B. Gruskin, eds.). W. B. Saunders, Philadelphia, 1984, pp. 251–270.
66. Salusky, I. B., Fine, R. N., Kangarloo, H. K., Gold, R., Paunier, L., Goodman, W. G., Brill, J. E., Gilli, G., Slatopolsky, E., and Coburn, J. W. High dose calcitriol for control of renal osteodystrophy in children on CAPD. *Kidney Int. 32*:89–95 (1987).
67. Slatopolsky, E., Weerts, C., Thielan, J., Horst, R., Harter, H., and Martin, K. J. Marked suppression of secondary hyperparathyroidism by intravenous

administration of 1,25-dihydroxy-cholecalciferol in uremic patients. *J. Clin. Invest. 74*:2136–2143 (1984).

68. Brown, E. M., Wilson, R. E., Eastman, R. C., et al. Abnormal regulation of parathyroid hormone release by calcium in secondary hyperparathyroidism due to chronic renal failure. *J. Clin. Endocrinol. Metab. 54*:172–179 (1982).
69. Brown, E. M. Set point for calcium: Its role in normal and abnormal secretion. In *Hormonal Control of Calcium Metabolism*. (D. V. Cohen, R. V. Talmage, and J. L. Matthews, eds.). Excerpta Medica, Amsterdam, 1981, p. 35.
70. Salusky, I. B., Paunier, L., Slatopolsky, E., Kagarloo, H., Coburn, J. W., and Fine, R. N. Use of "high" dose calcitriol in pediatric patients undergoing continuous ambulatory peritoneal dialysis (CAPD). In *Calcitriol: A Clinical Update*. (J. W. Coburn, ed.). Excerpta Medica, Princeton, NJ, 1984, p. 36.
71. Slatopolsky, E., and Bricker, N. S. The role of phosphorus restriction in the prevention of secondary hyperparathyroidism in chronic renal disease. *Kidney Int. 4*:141 (1973).
72. Cournot-Witmer, J., Plachot, J. J., Bourdeau, A., Lieberherr, M., Jorgetti, V., Mendes, V., Halpern, S., Hemmerle, J., Drueke, T., and Balsan, S. Effect of aluminum on bone and cell localization. *Kidney Int. 29*:S37 (1986).
73. Meyer, J. L., and Thomas, W. C. Aluminum and aluminum complexes. Effects on calcium phosphate precipitation. *Kidney Int. 29*:S20–S23 (1986).
74. Posner, A. A., Blumenthal, N. C., and Boskey, A. L. Model of aluminum-induced osteomalacia: Inhibition of apatite formation and growth. *Kidney Int. 29*:S17–S19 (1986).
75. Shea, D., and Mankin, H. J. Slipped capital femoral epiphysis in renal failure; report of three cases. *J. Bone Joint Surg. 48A*:349–355 (1966).
76. Cattel, H. S., Levin, S., Kopits, S., and Lyne, E. D. Reconstructive surgery in children with azotemic osteodystrophy. *J. Bone Joint Surg. 52A*:216–228 (1971).
77. Recker, R., Schoenfeld, P., Letteri, J., Slatopolsky, E., Goldsmith, R., and Brickman, A. S. The efficiency of calcifediol in renal osteodystrophy. *Arch. Intern. Med. 138*:857–863 (1978).
78. Bailey, G. L., Griffiths, H. L., Mocelin, A. J., et al. Avascular necrosis of the femoral head in patients on chronic hemodialysis. *Trans. Am. Soc. Artif. Intern. Organs 18*:401 (1972).
79. Hall, M. C., Elmore, E. M., Bright, R. W., et al. Skeletal complications in a series of human renal allografts. *J.A.M.A. 208*:1825–1829 (1969).
80. Mehls, O., Ritz, E., Oppermann, H. C., et al. Femoral head necrosis in uremic children without steroid treatment or transplantation. *J. Pediatr. 6*:926–929 (1981).
81. Arbus, G. S., Galiwango, J., De Maria, J. E., and Churchill, B. M. The first ten years of the dialysis treatment program at the Hospital for Sick Children, Toronto. *Can. Med. Assoc. J. 122*:659–664 (1980).
82. Cruess, R. L., Blennerhassett, M. B., et al. Aseptic necrosis after renal transplantation. *J. Bone Joint Surg. 50A*:1577–1588 (1968).

83. Harrington, K. D., Murray, W. R., et al. Avascular necrosis of bone after renal transplant. *J. Bone Joint Surg. 53A*:203–215 (1971).
84. Sinclair, N. R., et al. A randomized trial of cyclosporin in cadveric renal transplantations. *N. Engl. J. Med. 314*:1219–1225 (1986).
85. Stern, P., and Watts, H. G. Osteonecrosis after renal transplant in children. *J. Bone Joint Surg. 61A*:851–856 (1979).
86. Uttenbogaart, C. H., et al. Aseptic necrosis after renal transplantation in children. *Am. J. Dis. Child. 132*:765–767 (1978).
87. Venderhoof, G. A., and Coleman, S. S. Reversal of skeletal changes in renal osteodystrophy following partial parathyroidectomy and renal allotransplantation. *Clin. Orthorp. Rel Res. 88*:113–118 (1972).
88. Elmstedt, E., and Syahn, T. Skeletal complications following renal transplantation. *Acta Orthop. Scand. 52*:279–286 (1981).

10

Aluminum and Bone Diseases in Children

Sharon P. Andreoli

James Whitcomb Riley Hospital for Children, Indiana University Medical Center, Indianapolis, Indiana

I. INTRODUCTION

Aluminum intoxication has become a major cause of morbidity and mortality, not only in patients with end-stage renal disease but also in nondialyzed patients with chronic renal failure who are exposed to aluminum. Aluminum accumulation has been implicated in the pathogenesis of dementia, microcytic anemia, and a severe form of osteomalacia that is relatively resistant to vitamin D therapy (1–4). Since aluminum is excreted by the kidney, the patient with renal insufficiency is at risk of intoxication once exposed to aluminum (5). The major sources of aluminum are dialysate that is prepared from water high in aluminum content and the gastrointestinal absorption of aluminum from aluminum-containing phosphate binders (1–6).

Although their toxic effects were unknown, increased serum and bone levels of aluminum were demonstrated as early as 1970 and 1971, respectively (7,8). Aluminum contaminated dialysate and gastrointestinal absorption of aluminum from aluminum hydroxide and aluminum-cycle resins used for treatment of hyperkalemia were implicated as the source of aluminum. That aluminum retention was detrimental was suggested in 1976, when Alfrey demonstrated high levels of aluminum in brain gray matter from patients dying with an encephalopathy syndrome compared to those who died without encephalopathy (1). Additional studies demonstrated that patients with dementia frequently had a severe form of osteomalacia that was resistant to vitamin D therapy (9). Epidemiological studies demonstrated that the osteomalacia and encephalopathy syndromes occurred primarily in certain dialysis centers that used softened water with a high aluminum content (10). Later studies demonstrated that aluminum was transferred from dialysate to blood when the dialysate's aluminum content was high (11).

Bone biopsies from patients with the osteomalacia syndrome showed a high correlation between the histological pattern of osteomalacia and elevated bone aluminum levels, as measured by flameless atomic absorption spectrophotometry (12). Additional morphometric studies using a histochemical stain, electron microprobe, and ion microscopy demonstrated that aluminum was deposited at the bone–osteoid interface, which suggested that aluminum accumulation is associated with abnormal mineralization of bone (3,4,13). These studies have helped to characterize and differentiate bone disease due to aluminum intoxication from that due to osteitis fibrosa as a result of secondary hyperparathyroidism.

II. ALUMINUM INTOXICATION

A. Aluminum-Induced Bone Disease

The characteristic clinical features of aluminum-induced bone disease include bone pain, muscle weakness that is primarily proximal, nonhealing pathological fractures, and a poor response to vitamin D therapy (3,4,13). These disabling symptoms are in contrast to the relative lack of symptomatic bone disease in patients with secondary hyperparathyroidism. Previous reports from chronic dialysis patients noted a weak association between symptomatic bone disease and the biochemical, radiological, and histological findings of hyperparathyroidism but a strong association between bone pain and histological features of osteomalacia (14). Recent studies have confirmed the high frequency of symptomatic bone disease in patients with aluminum-induced osteomalacia, as demonstrated by histomorphometric analysis of bone biopsy samples (15,16). Several patients with aluminum-induced osteomalacia were asymptomatic at the time of biopsy but subsequently developed the characteristic clinical symptoms of the osteomalacia syndrome (16). Thus, aluminum-induced osteomalacia appears to be asymptomatic in its early stages and symptoms of bone pain, pathological fractures, and muscle weakness occur as late manifestations.

The characteristic biochemical features of aluminum-induced bone disease include hypercalcemia (spontaneous or with low doses of vitamin D analogs), relatively low levels of parathyroid hormone and alkaline phosphatase activity, and higher serum aluminum levels than in patients without aluminum-induced bone disease. Hypercalcemia may result from decreased calcium entry into bone

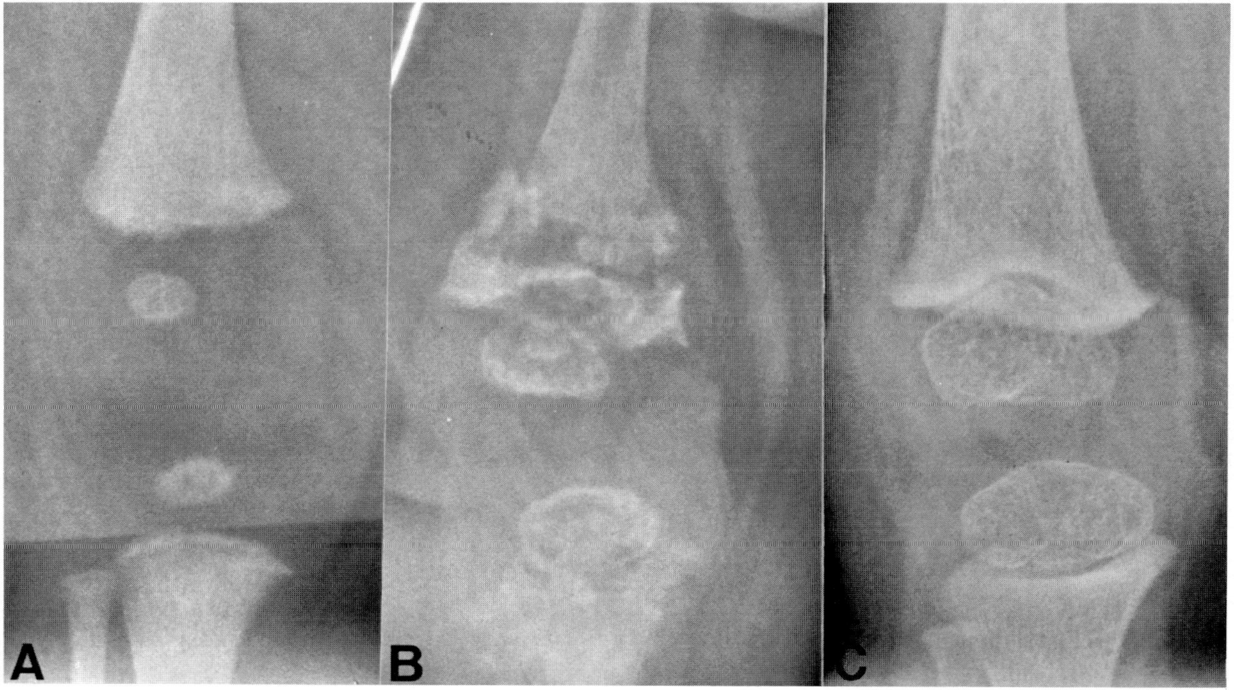

Figure 1 Serial knee radiographs in an infant with chronic renal failure and severe aluminum bone disease. A. Radiograph taken at 5 months of age while patient was consuming aluminum hydroxide demonstrates fraying of the metaphysis and widened physis. B. Radiograph at 13 months of age, 3 months after aluminum hydroxide was stopped, showin lucent defects in the metaphysis of femur and in the epiphysis. C. Radiograph at 2 years of age demonstrates normal knee with complete healing of aluminum bone disease (from Ref. 27).

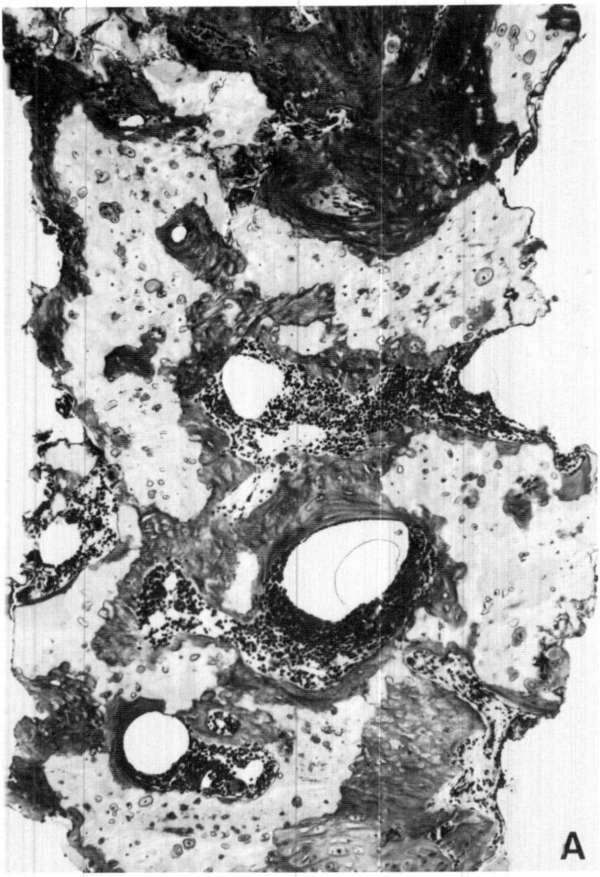

Figure 2 Goldner (A) and Aluminon (B) stains of bone from a patient with severe aluminum-induced bone disease. With the Goldner stain, the mineralized bone appears light grey, while the excess osteoid appears dark grey. With the Aluminon stain, the aluminum is demonstrated by the heavy black staining at the bone(b)–osteoid(o) junction (from Ref. 6).

as a result of the aluminum-induced mineralization defect. Hypercalcemia in turn results in lower parathyroid hormone and alkaline phosphatase levels (18). Additional causes of reduced parathyroid hormone levels in aluminum-intoxicated patients may include direct suppression of parathyroid hormone secretion by aluminum and aluminum accumulation in the parathyroid gland with resultant parathyroid failure (19,20). Since many parathyroid hormone assays use an antibody that recognizes carboxyterminal and other inactive fragments

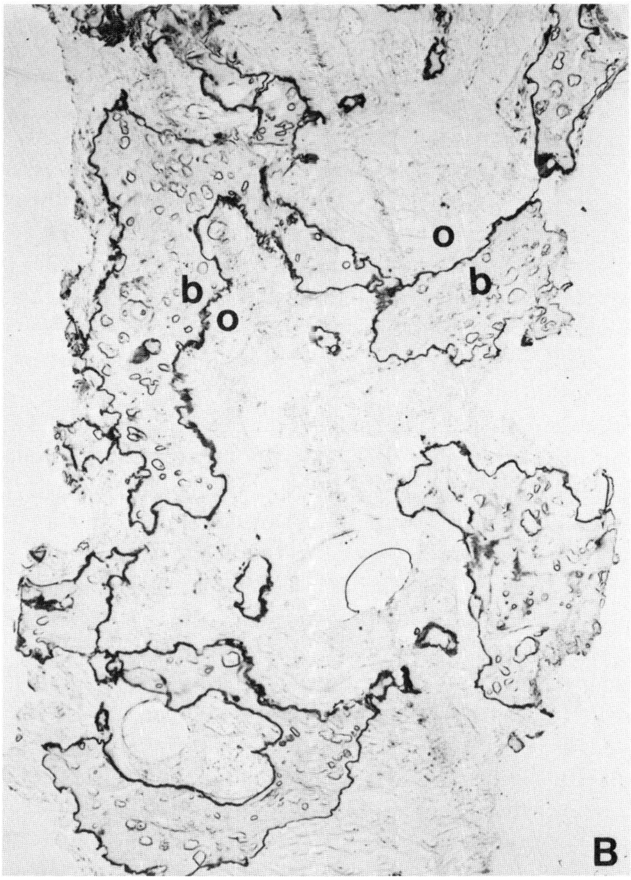

that are excreted by the kidneys (21), elevated parathyroid hormone levels (although inappropriately low for the degree of bone disease) may be frequently seen in aluminum-induced osteomalacia and an elevated parathyroid hormone level should not exclude consideration of aluminum-induced bone disease.

Although not of diagnostic value in individual cases due to overlap, several studies in adults have demonstrated that serum aluminum levels are higher in patients with aluminum-induced bone disease than in those with osteitis fibrosa or mild bone disease (16,22,23). In children with aluminum-induced bone disease, serum aluminum levels are usually greater than 100 ng/ml (6,24,25). In a study of 31 children with chronic renal failure receiving aluminum hydroxide, bone aluminum deposition correlated with the serum aluminum level and five of six children with serum aluminum levels greater than 100 ng/ml had bone aluminum deposition detected by the aurin tricarboxylic stain techniques (26). Use of the deferoxamine challenge test, frequently used in adults to evaluate for aluminum-induced bone disease, has not been evaluated in children.

The radiographic features of aluminum-induced bone disease include osteopenia, nonhealing pathological fractures, and the absence of subperiosteal resorption or other changes suggestive of hyperparathyroidism (4,12). Additional features found in children with aluminum-induced bone disease include fraying of the metaphysis of the long bones and markedly widened physis (Fig. 1A) (27). Although these findings are nonspecific and can be seen in other forms of renal osteodystrophy and metabolic bone disease, the absence of features of hyperparathyroidism may suggest aluminum-related bone disease in a susceptible patient.

Although clinical, biochemical, and radiographic evidence may suggest aluminum bone disease, the diagnosis can be made with certainty only with a bone biopsy. Single or preferably double tetracycline labels should be administered prior to bone biopsy so that bone formation rates can be determined. In aluminum-induced bone disease, bone histomorphometry typically demonstrates excess unmineralized osteoid, a paucity of osteoblasts and osteoclasts, minimal or no features of osteitis fibrosis (Fig. 2A), and in a low bone formation rate as demonstrated by reduced tetracycline uptake (3,4,13). In some instances, bone histomorphometry demonstrates an aplastic lesion characterized by little cellular activity, greatly reduced tetracycline uptake, and only slightly increased or normal amounts of osteoid (3). Aluminum is deposited predominately at the bone–osteoid junction at the mineralization front; in addition, some aluminum may also be found in cement lines within bone (Fig. 2B) (3,4,13).

Although aluminum is involved in the pathogenesis of the osteomalacia lesion, the precise mechanism of the toxicity is unknown. Some studies suggest that aluminum directly interferes with the physiochemical precipitation of calcium apatite and calcium phosphate and directly inhibits hydroxyapatite proliferation (28,29). Aluminum, particularly citrated complexes of aluminum, have been shown to inhibit the crystal growth of calcium phosphate (28). Heavy aluminum deposition at the mineralization front and the lack of tetracycline uptake as a marker of bone formation rate at areas of aluminum deposition support this concept. It has also been suggested that aluminum is an osteoblast toxin and that mineralization is inhibited as a result of aluminum interference with osteoblast metabolism (30,31). Aluminum-mediated osteoblast dysfunction then results in reduced collagen synthesis, osteoid formation, and a low bone formation rate at the mineralization front. The absence of cellular activity and aluminum localization in the mitochondria of osteoblasts suggests that high intracellular levels of aluminum may modulate cellular activity of the osteoblast (31). It is likely that aluminum-induced bone disease is multifactorial, mediated in part by each of these and perhaps additional mechanisms.

The role of parathyroid hormone in the pathogenesis of aluminum-induced osteomalacia is also complex and unclear. It has been suggested that absorption of orally administered aluminum is increased in the presence of elevated levels of parathyroid hormone (32). However, most patients with aluminum-induced bone disease have reduced parathyroid hormone levels and bone accumulation of aluminum appears to be enhanced following parathyroidectomy (33,34). It seems that normal parathyroid hormone levels exert a permissive role in bone aluminum deposition at the mineralization front, while high levels of parathyroid hormone may have a protective effect possibly because the high bone formation rate typical of osteitis fibrosa prevents critical amounts of aluminum from localizing at the mineralization front. Animal studies suggest that the parathyroid hormone level at the time of aluminum exposure may have an effect on the compartmentalization of aluminum in the body (35). As previously discussed, aluminum may also modulate parathyroid function through hypercalcemia, the direct inhibition of parathyroid hormone secretion, and the accumulation of aluminum in the parathyroid gland (18-20). Although the role of parathyroid hormone in the pathogenesis of the osteomalacia syndrome is unclear, reduced levels are usually detected once the syndrome of aluminum-induced bone disease is established.

B. Additional Features of Aluminum Intoxication

Because the central nervous system signs of aluminum intoxication were first observed in patients maintained by hemodialysis, the encephalopathy syndrome was called dialysis encephalopathy (1). However, a number of children with chronic renal failure not yet on dialysis have developed encephalopathy while consuming high doses of aluminum hydroxide (36-38). The typical central nervous system manifestations of aluminum intoxication include dementia, generalized or focal seizures, myoclonus, dysarthria, asterixis, and personality changes (1,39). The electroencephalogram (EEG) shows multifocal bursts of slow and spike wave activity with either normal or slow background rhythms; these EEG abnormalities frequently precede clinical signs of the encephalopathy syndrome by several months. Computer tomography scans are either normal or may show cerebral atrophy (39). This symptom complex has been seen in older children and adults. In infants, signs of dementia, speech disturbance, asterixis, and personality changes cannot be evaluated and infants with aluminum intoxication frequently demonstrate delayed attainment or regression of developmental milestones (26). Although the mechanism of aluminum-induced CNS abnormalities is uncertain, it has been suggested that aluminum forms complexes with ATP, inhibits hexokinase activity, which is important in maintaining glycolytic metabolism, and interferes with calcium metabolism, as a result of impaired calmodulin function (40,41).

Aluminum intoxication may also result in a microcytic, hypochromic anemia not due to iron deficiency (2,42). In 1978, Elliott and MacDougall reported that a microcytic anemia often preceded signs and symptoms of dialysis encephalopathy and osteomalacia (42). Aluminin-induced bone disease in children is frequently accompanied by a microcytic anemia; in one study, three of four children with aluminum intoxication had a mean corpuscular volume (MCV) below the lower limit of normal for their age (6). Recently, it has been demonstrated that aluminum is bound to transferrin, suggesting that aluminum interferes with iron utilization and/or transport (43). In some aluminum-intoxicated patients, aluminum deposits have been found in bone marrow macrophages, suggesting that aluminum may interfere with normal medullary iron processing provided by macrophages (44,45). In addition to interfering with iron utilization, aluminum may inhibit delta aminolevulinic acid dehydratase, a rate-limiting enzyme in heme biosynthesis.

III. SOURCES OF ALUMINUM

Early epidemiological studies demonstrated that encephalopathy and osteomalacia occurred much more frequently in dialysis centers in cities whose water contained high levels of aluminum (9,10). In centers that utilized deionized water and water made by reverse osmosis, the incidence of dialysis encephalopathy and osteomalacia was much less. Later studies demonstrated that aluminum was transferred to the patient when the dialysate aluminum content was elevated (11). Because aluminum in plasma is highly protein bound and because all aluminum in dialysate is free, aluminum can be transferred from the dialysate to the patient whenever the patient's free plasma aluminum level is less than the dialysate aluminum level. Therefore, dialysate aluminum content should be kept as low as possible and certainly less than 10 μg/L. Since deionized and reverse osmosis water are commonly used now, dialysate should no longer be a source of aluminum to the patient on chronic dialysis. Although most peritoneal dialysate fluids are low in aluminum (46,47), an occasional contaminated batch has resulted in transfer of aluminum to the patient with resultant disease (18).

Recently, gastrointestinal absorption of aluminum from aluminum-containing phosphate binders has been found to result in aluminum intoxication in patients with chronic renal failure. As early as 1970, elevated serum aluminum levels were detected in patients with chronic renal failure who were consuming oral aluminum (7). In 1977, renal excretion of aluminum following an oral aluminum load was demonstrated in normal people (5). Reports of dementia, osteomalacia, and microcytic anemia in nondialyzed patients receiving aluminum-containing phosphate binders demonstrated that gastrointestinal absorption of aluminum could result in aluminum intoxication (6,25,37,38,48,49).

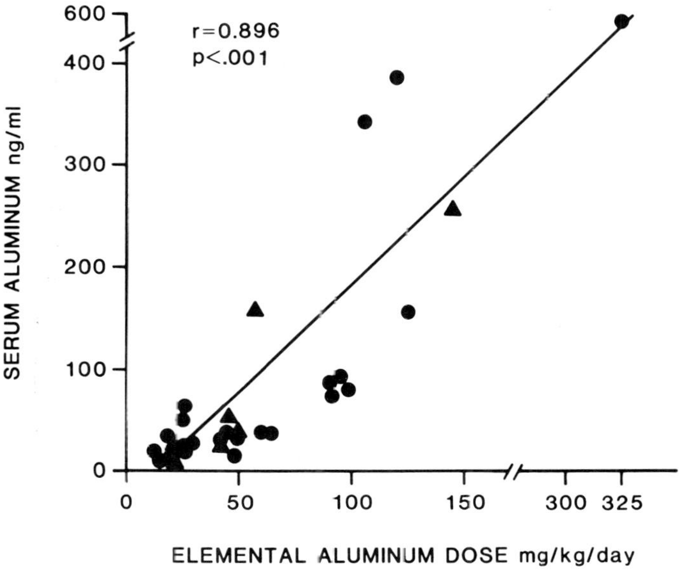

Figure 3 Correlation between serum aluminum level and elemental aluminum dosage in mg/kg per day in 31 children with chronic renal failure who were consuming aluminum hydroxide. Twenty-four children (●) were not receiving dialysis therapy while seven (▲) were maintained by continuous ambulatory peritoneal dialysis.

Children, especially infants, appear to be particularly susceptible to aluminum intoxication from the gastrointestinal absorption of aluminum. Several studies in children have demonstrated a direct correlation between the serum aluminum level and the mg/kg per day dosage of elemental aluminum (Fig. 3) (6,24–26). Weight and age have also been found to be significantly inversely correlated with the serum aluminum level (6,24,26). In these studies, the children with the highest serum aluminum levels frequently demonstrated osteomalacia with heavy bone aluminum deposition detected by a histochemical stain or flameless atomic absorption spectrophotometry. Thus, the small child consuming large amounts of aluminum hydroxide appears to be at the greatest risk for the development of aluminum intoxication. The rapid development of severe aluminum-induced bone disease in infants and young children suggests that once the aluminum is absorbed, a rapidly growing skeleton seems to be particularly susceptible to aluminum accumulation.

There are several potential explanations for these findings. Since infants and small children obtain the majority of their caloric and fluid requirements from milk products that have a high phosphorus content, these children require higher doses of aluminum hydroxide to maintain serum phosphorus in the normal range. In addition, the immature gastrointestinal tract of the newborn and small infant may absorb an increased fractional dose of orally administered aluminum. Although the mechanism for the gastrointestinal absorption of aluminum is unknown, it has been suggested that aluminum absorption is active via mucosal transferrin as iron is absorbed (50). Since most infants and small children have high iron requirements to meet growth demands, aluminum ingestion at a young age could result in increased absorption. In addition, dietary citric acid has been shown to substantially enhance aluminum absorption. Thus, children receiving sodium citrate therapy for chronic acidosis may be at greater risk for aluminum loading (17). Other factors that can influence the amount of aluminum absorbed include the solubility of the aluminum compound ingested and the gastric pH (5,51). In an acid environment, aluminum is in the soluble, free form and is presumably more available for absorption. Some studies suggest that the parathyroid hormone level and administration of vitamin D analogs may also modulate aluminum absorption (51).

Casein hydrolysate amino acids, albumin solutions, and some components of intravenous fluids have been found to be contaminated with aluminum (52–54). When these aluminum-contaminated parenteral products are administered to adults, children, and infants, elevated serum, urine, and bone levels of aluminum have been detected (52–54). Although aluminum loading via parenteral fluids has not resulted in signs or symptoms of intoxication in the majority of cases, prolonged exposure, particularly in association with renal insufficiency, places such patients at risk for aluminum toxicity.

IV. TREATMENT OF ALUMINUM INTOXICATION

Treatment of the child with established aluminum intoxication consists of ensuring that the dialysate aluminum concentration is less than 10 μg/L if the patient is undergoing dialysis therapy. In addition, use of aluminum-containing phosphate binders should be discontinued. After aluminum hydroxide is stopped, serum aluminum levels fall in both nondialyzed and dialyzed children (Fig. 4) (5,55,56). When the child has sufficient residual renal function and is able to excrete aluminum, severe aluminum-induced osteomalacia can resolve and bone aluminum deposition can decrease by simply withdrawing the exposure to aluminum (6).

Depending on the severity of the intoxication and the amount of residual renal function, additional therapy with deferoxamine is indicated in some patients. Since aluminum is tightly protein bound, very little is removed during dialysis in the absence of deferoxamine (57,58). Deferoxamine forms a chelate with aluminum with a molecular weight of about 587, and the aluminum-deferoxamine chelate is freely diffusible. Deferoxamine therapy also decreases the

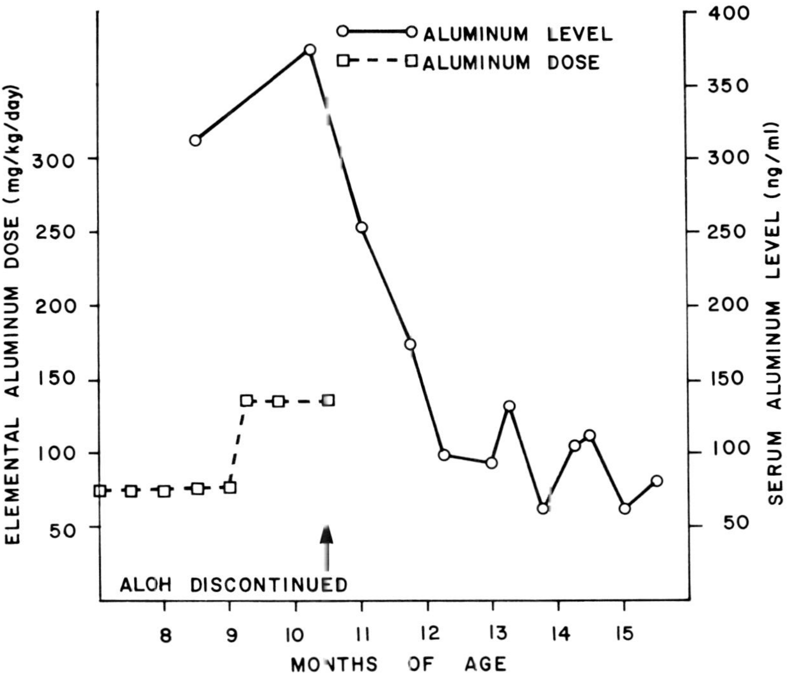

Figure 4 Serum aluminum level in relation to the dosage of aluminum hydroxide in an infant with chronic renal failure. When aluminum hydroxide was discontinued, the serum aluminum level fell (from Ref. 6).

protein bound portion of aluminum from 80% to 70% or less and increases the serum level as aluminum is mobilized from tissue stores so that more aluminum is available to be removed during dialysis (57,58). Deferoxamine administered intravenously has been used successfully to treat aluminum-induced encephalopathy and osteomalacia in adults maintained by hemodialysis and continuous ambulatory peritoneal dialysis (59,60). Deferoxamine therapy in adults with aluminum-induced osteomalacia has resulted in resolution of symptomatic bone disease, reduction of bone aluminum levels, and improved bone histological findings on repeat biopsy (60). Deferoxamine administered by the intraperitoneal route resulted in resolution of encephalopathy in one adult patient maintained by continuous ambulatory peritoneal dialysis (61).

Experience in treating children with deferoxamine is limited. In one child treated with intraperitoneal deferoxamine, encephalopathy improved, microcytic anemia reversed, and bone histological findings improved following a 3 month course of therapy (62). Aluminum removal from peritoneal dialysate increased from 87 μg/24 hr prior to deferoxamine therapy to 690 μg/24 hr after intraperitoneal deferoxamine therapy was initiated. Comparison of bone biopsies before and after therapy demonstrated a decrease in osteoid volume and surface area and an increase in mineralized bone, indicating improvement of the osteomalacia. The stainable bone aluminum decreased from 4.36 mm of aluminum/mm^2 of tissue before therapy to 2.39 m/mm^2 tissue after therapy; in addition, 85% of the stainable aluminum was located in cement lines after therapy, whereas 86% of the aluminum was previously located at the mineralization front (62). Because deferoxamine therapy has been associated with ophthalmological and otological toxicity, periodic hearing tests and eye examinations are indicated in children receiving deferoxamine therapy (63,64).

The radiographic appearance of the bones during healing of aluminum-induced bone disease is children is unusual (27). In two children with aluminum intoxication, cessation of exposure to aluminum (both children) and deferoxamine therapy (one child) resulted in dramatically increased calcification of the bones. Calcification of the long bones began at the most recently formed osteoid of the metaphysis, leaving a radiolucent area between newly calcified and previously calcified bone (Fig. 1B). Calcification of the epiphysis also appeared to begin in the periphery and proceed centrally. This pattern of calcification transiently created a "bone within a bone" appearance. With continued healing, the radiolucent zones were calcified and abolished (Fig. 1C). A similar pattern of bone mineralization has been observed in rats after cessation of exposure to aluminum an in some children during healing from nutritional rickets (65,66). It is interesting, that a bone biopsy from a 14-year-old boy following treatment with deferoxamine for aluminum induced bone disease showed partially mineralized osteoid surrounded by unmineralized woven osteoid, which was then encircled by apparently newly mineralized bone (67).

V. PREVENTION

Aluminum-induced encephalopathy, osteomalacia, and microcytic anemia are iatrogenic diseases and, therefore, are preventable. Since the major cause of aluminum intoxication in children is gastrointestinal absorption of aluminum from aluminum hydroxide, alternative phosphate binders are needed. By demonstrating that infants consuming high doses of aluminum hydroxide (greater than 100 mg/kg per day of elemental aluminum) are at greatest risk for aluminum intoxication does not imply that consuming lower doses is benign. Indeed, significantly elevated aluminum levels have been detected in children receiving 26–50 and 51–100 mg/kg per day of elemental aluminum compared to children with chronic renal failure not receiving aluminum hydroxide (26). Thus, chronic aluminum loading in lower doses may eventually result in adverse effects and alternative phosphate binders are needed.

Calcium carbonate has been demonstrated to be an effective phosphorus binder in adults and children with chronic renal failure (55,56,68-70). The major difficulty noted with calcium carbonate therapy has been the development of hypercalcemia or an inability to normalize the serum phosphorus level. Hypercalcemia frequently followed an increase in the vitamin D analog or calcium carbonate dose and usually quickly resolved following adjustment of the dosage. Although most studies have reported good results with calcium carbonate, one recent study reported that calcium carbonate was effective in controlling the serum phosphorus without side effects in only 50% of patients (71). Calcium- and iron-charged polymers of heteropolyuronic acid have been tested as phosphate binders, with encouraging preliminary results (72).

By using calcium carbonate as the initial phosphate binder in children with renal failure, ensuring that the dialysate aluminum concentration is less than 10 μg/L, and avoiding parenteral products high in aluminum content, aluminum-induced bone disease should disappear as cause of morbidity and mortality in children with renal failure.

ACKNOWLEDGMENTS

Dr. Donald J. Sherrard performed the histomorphometric analysis of the bone biopsies.

REFERENCES

1. Alfrey, A. C., LeGender, Z. R., and Kaehny, W. D. The dialysis encephalopathy syndrome: Possible aluminum intoxication. *N. Engl. J. Med. 294*:184-188 (1976).
2. O'Hare, J. A., and Murnaghan, D. J. Reversal of aluminum induced hemodialysis anemia by a low-aluminum dialysate. *N. Engl. J. Med. 306*:654-656 (1982).
3. Ott, S. M., Maloney, N. A., Coburn, J. W., Alfrey, A. C., and Sherrard, D. J. The prevalence of bone aluminum deposition in renal osteodystrophy and its relation to the response to calcitriol therapy. *N. Engl. J. Med. 307*:709-713 (1982).
4. Ihle, B., Buchanan, M., Stevens, B., Marshal, A., Plomley, R., d'Apice, A., and Kincaid-Smith, P. Aluminum associated bone disease: Clinico-pathologic correlation. *Am. J. Kidney Dis. 2*:255-263 (1982).
5. Kaehny, W. D., Hegg, A. P., and Alfrey, A. C. Gastrointestinal absorption of aluminum from aluminum-containing antacids. *N. Engl. J. Med. 296*:1389-1390 (1977).
6. Andreoli, S. P., Bergstein, J. M., and Sherrard, D. J. Aluminum intoxication from aluminum containing phosphate binders in children with azotemia not undergoing dialysis. *N. Engl J. Med. 310*:1079-1083 (1984).

7. Berlyne, G. M., Pest, D., Ben-Ari, J., Weinberger, J., Stern, M., Gilmore, G. R., and Levine, R. Hyperaluminaemia from aluminum resins in renal failure. *Lancet 2*:494–496 (1970).
8. Parsons, V., Davies, C., Good, C., Ogg, C., and Siddiqui, J. Aluminin in bone from patients with renal failure. *Br. Med. J. 4*:273–275 (1971).
9. Ward, M. K., Ellis, H. A., Feest, T. G., Parkinson, I. S., and Kerr, D. N. S. Osteomalacic dialysis osteodystrophy: Evidence for a water-borne etiologic agent, probably aluminum. *Lancet 1*:841–845 (1978).
10. Parkinson, I. S., Ward, M. K., Feest, T. G., Fawcett, R. W. P., and Kerr, D. N. S. Fracturing dialysis osteodystrophy and dialysis encephalopathy. *Lancet 1*:406–409 (1979).
11. Kaehny, W. D., Alfrey, A. C., Holman, R. E., Shorr, W. J. Aluminum transfer during hemodialysis. *Kidney Int. 12*:361–365 (1977).
12. Hodsman, A. B., Sherrard, D. J., Wong, E. G. C., Brickman, A. S., Lee, D. B., Alfrey, A. C., Singer, F. R., Norman, A. W., and Coburn, J. W. Vitamin-D-resistant osteomalacia in hemodialysis patients lacking secondary hyperparathyroidism. *Ann. Intern. Med. 94*:629–637 (1981).
13. Cournot-Witmer, G., Zingraff, J., Plachot, J. J., Escaig, R. L., Lefevre, R., Boumati, P., Bourdeau, A., Garabedian, M., Galle, P., Bourbon, R., Dueke, T., and Balsan, S. Aluminum localization in bone from hemodialysis patients: Relation to matrix mineralization. *Kidney Int. 20*:375–385 (1981).
14. Alvarez-Ude, F., Feest, T. G., Ward, M. K., Pierides, A. M., Ellis, H. A., Peart, K. M., Simpson, W., Weightman, D., and Kerr, D. N. S. Hemodialysis bone disease: Correlation between clinical, histologic and other findings. *Kidney Int. 14*:68–73 (1978).
15. Ihle, B. U., Becker, G. J., and Kincaid-Smith, P. S. Clinical and biochemical features of aluminum-related bone disease. *Kidney Int. 29*(Suppl. 18): S80–S86 (1986).
16. Llach, F., Felsenfeld, A. J., Coleman, M. D., Keveney, J. J., Pederson, J. A., and Medlock, T. R. The natural course of dialysis osteomalacia. *Kidney Int. 29*(Suppl. 18):S74–S79 (1986).
17. Slanina, P., French, W., Ekstrom, L. G., Loof, L., Slorach, S., Cedergren, A. Dietary citric acid enhances absorption of aluminum in antacids. *Clin. Chem. 32*:539 (1986).
18. Cannata, J. B., Briggs, J. D., Junor, B. J. R., Fell, G. S., and Beastall, G. Effect of acute aluminum overload on calcium and parathyroid-hormone metabolism. *Lancet 1*:501–503 (1983).
19. Morrissey, J., Rothstein, M., Mayor, G., and Slatopolsky, E. Suppression of parathyroid hormone secretion by aluminum. *Kidney Int. 23*:699–704 (1983).
20. Cann, C. E., Prussin, S. G., and Gordan, G. S. Aluminum uptake by the parathyroid glands. *J. Clin. Endocrinol. Metab. 49*:543–545 (1979).
21. Freitag, J., Martin, K. J., Hruska, K. A., Anderson, C., Conrades, M., Ladenson, J., Klahr, S., and Slatopolsky, E. Impaired parathyroid hormone metabolism in patients with chronic renal failure. *N. Engl. J. Med. 298*:29–32 (1978).

22. Charhon, S. A., Chavassieux, P. M., Meunier, P. J., and Accominotti, M. Serum aluminum concentration and aluminum deposits in bone in patients receiving hemodialysis. *Br. Med. J. 290*:1613–1614 (1985).
23. Hodsman, A. B., Hood, S. A., Brown, P., and Cordy, P. E. Do serum aluminum levels reflect underlying skeletal aluminum accumulation and bone histology before and after chelation by deferoxamine? *J. Lab. Clin. Med. 106*:674–681 (1985).
24. Salusky, I. B., Coburn, J. W., Paunier, L., Sherrard, D. J., and Fine, R. N. Role of aluminum hydroxide in raising serum aluminum levels in children undergoing continuous ambulatory peritoneal dialysis. *J. Pediatr. 105*:717–720 (1984).
25. Sedman, A. B., Miller, N. L., Warady, B. A., Lum, G. M., and Alfrey, A. C. Aluminum loading in children with chronic renal failure. *Kidney Int. 26*: 201–204 (1984).
26. Trompeter, R. S., Polinsky, M. S., Andreoli, S. P., and Fennell, R. S. Neurologic complications of renal failure. *Am. J. Kidney Dis. 7*:318–323 (1986).
27. Andreoli, S. P., Smith, J. A., and Bergstein, J. M. Aluminum bone disease in children: Radiographic features from diagnosis to resolution. *Radiology 156*:663–667 (1985).
28. Meyer, J. L., and Thomas, W. C. Aluminum and aluminum complexes. Effect on calcium phosphate precipitation. *Kidney Int. 29*(Suppl. 18):S20–S23 (1986).
29. Posner, A. S., Blumenthal, N. C., and Boskey, A. L. Model of aluminum-induced osteomalacia: Inhibition of apatite formation and growth. *Kidney Int. 29*(Suppl. 18):S17–S19 (1986).
30. Goodman, W. G. Bone disease and aluminum: Pathogenic considerations. *Am. J. Kidney Dis. 6*:330–335 (1985).
31. Cournot-Witmer, G., Plachot, J. J., Bourdeau, A., Lieberherr, M., Jorgetti, V., Mendes, V., Halpern, S., Hemmerle, J., Drueke, T., and Balsan, S. Effect of aluminum on bone and cell localization. *Kidney Int. 29*(Suppl. 18): S37–S40 (1986).
32. Major, G. H., Keiser, J. A., Makdani, D., and Ku, P. K. Aluminum absorption and distribution: Effect of parathyroid hormone. *Science 197*:1187–1189 (1977).
33. Andress, D. L., Ott, S. M., Maloney, N. A., and Sherrard, D. J. Effect of parathyroidectomy on bone aluminum accumulation in chronic renal failure. *N. Engl. J. Med. 312*:468–473 (1985).
34. de Vernejoul, M. C., Marchais, S., London, G., Morieux, C., Bielakoff, J., and Miravet, L. Increased bone aluminum deposition after subtotal parathyroidectomy in dialyzed patients. *Kidney Int. 27*:785–791 (1985).
35. Alfrey, A. C., Sedman, A. B., and Chan, Y-L. The compartmentalization and metabolism of aluminum in uremic rats. *J. Lab. Clin. Med. 105*:227–233 (1985).
36. Baluarte, H. J., Gruskin, A. B., Hines, L. B., Foley, A. N., and Grover, W. D. Encephalopathy in children with chronic renal failure. *Proc. Clin. Dialysis Transplant. Forum 7*:95 (1977).

37. Nathan, E., and Pederson, S. E. Dialysis encephalopathy in a non-dialyzed uraemic boy treated with aluminum hydroxide orally. *Acta Paediatr. Scand. 69*:793–796 (1980).
38. Sedman, A. B., Wilkening, G. N., Warady, B. A., Lum, G. M., and Alfrey, A. C. Encephalopathy in childhood secondary to aluminum toxicity. *J. Pediatr. 105*:836–838 (1984).
39. Alfrey, A. C. Dialysis encephalopathy. *Kidney Int. 29*(Suppl. 18):S53–S57 (1986).
40. Siegel, N. Aluminum interaction with biomolecules: The molecular basis for aluminum toxicity. *Am. J. Kidney Dis. 6*:353–357 (1985).
41. Trapp, G. A. Interaction of aluminum with cofactors, enzymes, and other proteins. *Kidney Int. 29*(Suppl. 18):512–516 (1986).
42. Elliott, H. L., Dryburgh, F., Fell, G. S., Sabet, S., and MacDougall, A. I. Aluminum toxicity during regular haemodialysis. *Br. Med. J. 1*:1101–1103 (1978).
43. Trapp, G. A. Plasma aluminum is bound to transferrin. *Life Sci. 33*:311–316 (1983).
44. Kaye, M. Bone marrow aluminum storage in renal failure. *J. Clin. Pathol. 36*:1288–1291 (1983).
45. Drueke, T. B., Lacour, B., Touam, M., Jucquel, J. P., Plachot, J. J., Cournot-Witmer, G., and Galle, P. Effects of aluminum on hematopoiesis. *Kidney Int. 29*(Suppl. 18):S45–S48 (1986).
46. Rottembourg, J., Gallego, J. L., Jaudon, M. C., Clavel, J. P., and Legrain, M. Serum concentration and peritoneal transfer of aluminum during treatment by continuous ambulatory peritoneal dialysis. *Kidney Int. 25*:919–924 (1984).
47. Stummvoll, H. K., and Graf, H. Aluminum kinetics during renal replacement therapies. *Am. J. Kidney Dis. 6*:293–296 (1985).
48. Felsenfeld, A. J., Gutman, R. A., Llach, F., and Harrelson, J. M. Osteomalacia in chronic renal failure: A syndrome previously reported only with maintenance dialysis. *Am. J. Nephrol. 2*:147–154 (1982).
49. Griswold, W. R., Reznik, V., Mendoza, S. A., Trauner, D., and Alfrey, A. C. Accumulation of aluminum in a nondialyzed uremic child receiving aluminum hydroxide. *Pediatrics 71*:56–58 (1983).
50. Cannata, J. B., Suarez, C. S., Cuesta, V., Roza, R. R., Allende, M. T., Herrera, J., and Llanderal, J. P. Gastrointestinal aluminum absorption: Is it modulated by the iron absorptive mechanism. *Proc. Eur. Dialysis Transplant Assoc. 21*:354–359 (1984).
51. Ihle, B. U., and Becker, G. J. Gastrointestinal absorption of aluminum. *Am. J. Kidney Dis. 6*:302–305 (1985).
52. Ott, S. M., Maloney, N. A., Klein, G. L., Alfrey, A. C., Ament, M. E., Coburn, J. W., and Sherrard, D. J. Aluminum is associated with low bone formation in patients receiving chronic parenteral nutrition. *Ann. Int. Med. 98*:910–914 (1983).
53. Milliner, D. S., Shinaberger, J. H., Shuman, P., and Coburn, J. W. Inadvertent aluminum administration during plasma exchange due to aluminum con-

tamination of albumin-replacement solutions. *N. Engl. J. Med. 312*:165–167 (1985).

54. Sedman, A. B., Klein, G. L., Merritt, R. J., Miller, N. L., Weber, K. O., Gill, W. L., Anand, H., and Alfrey, A. C. Evidence of aluminum loading in infants receiving intravenous therapy. *N. Engl. J. Med. 312*:1337–1343 (1985).
55. Salusky, I. B., Coburn, J. W., Foley, J., Nelson, P., and Fine, R. N. Effects of oral and calcium carbonate on control of serum phosphorus and changes in plasma aluminum levels of the discontinuation of aluminum-containing gels in children receiving dialysis. *J. Pediatr. 108*:767–770 (1986).
56. Andreoli, S. P., Dunson, J. W., and Bergstein, J. M. Calcium carbonate is an effective phosphorus binder in children with chronic renal failure. *Am. J. Kidney Dis. 9*:206–210 (1987).
57. Stummvoll, H. K., Graft, H., and Meisinger, V. Effect of desferrioxamine on aluminum kinetics during hemodialysis. *Miner. Electrolyte Metab. 10*:263–266 (1984).
58. Leung, F. Y., Hodsman, A. B., Muirhead, N., and Henderson, A. R. Ultrafiltration studies in vitro of serum aluminum in dialysis patients after deferoxamine chelation therapy. *Clin. Chem. 31*:20–23 (1985).
59. Ackrill, P., Ralston, A. J., Day, J. P., and Hodge, K. C. Successful removal of aluminum from patient with dialysis encephalopathy. *Lancet 2*:692 (1980).
60. Malluche, H. H., Smith, A. J., Abreo, K., and Faugere, M. C. The use of deferoxamine in the management of aluminum accumulation in bone in patients with renal failure. *N. Engl. J. Med. 311*:140–144 (1984).
61. Payton, C. D., Junor, B. J. R., and Fell, G. S. Successful treatment of aluminum encephalopathy by intraperitoneal desferrioxamine. *Lancet 1*: 1132 (1984).
62. Andreoli, S. P., Dunn, D., DeMyer, W., Sherrard, D. J., and Bertstein, J. M. Intraperitoneal deferoxamine therapy for aluminum intoxication in a child undergoing continuous ambulatory peritoneal dialysis. *J. Pediatr. 107*:760–763 (1985).
63. Borgna-Pignatti, C., Stefano, P. D., and Broglia, A. M. Visual loss in patient on high-dose subcutaneous desferrioxamine. *Lancet 1*:681 (1984).
64. Olivieri, N. F., Buncic, J. R., Chew, E., Gallant, T., Harrison, R. V., Keenan, N., Logan, W., Mitchell, D., Ricci, G., Skarf, B., Taylor, M., and Freedman, M. H. Visual and auditory neurotoxicity in patients receiving subcutaneous deferoxamine infusions. *N. Engl. J. Med. 314*:869–873 (1986).
65. Ellis, H. A., McCarthy, J. H., and Herrington, J. Bone aluminum in haemodialyzed patients and in rats injected with aluminum chloride: Relationship to impaired bone mineralization. *J. Clin. Pathol. 32*:832–844 (1979).
66. Caffey, J. Metabolic abnormalities of the skeleton. In: *Pediatric X-Ray Diagnosis*, (J. McCaffrey and F. N. Silverman, eds.). 8th ed. Year Book, Chicago, 1985, pp. 666–674.
67. Ott, S. M., Andress, D. L., Nebeker, H. G., Milliner, D. S., Maloney, N. A., Coburn, J. W., and Sherrard, D. J. Changes in bone histology after treatment with desferioxamine. *Kidney Int. 29*(Suppl. 18):S108–S113 (1986).

68. Mak, R. H. K., Turner, C., Thompson, T., Powell, H., Haycock, G. B., and Chantler, C. Suppression of secondary hyperparathyroidism in children with chronic renal failure by high dose phosphate binders: Calcium carbonate versus aluminum hydroxide. *Br. Med. J. 291*:623–627 (1985).
69. Moriniere, P., Roussel, A., Tahiri, Y., deFremont, J. F., Maurel, G., Jaudon, M. C., Gueris, J., and Fournier, A. Substitution of aluminum hydroxide by high doses of calcium carbonate in patients on chronic haemodialysis: Disappearance of hyperaluminemia and equal control of hyperparathyroidism. *Proc. Eur. Dialysis Transplant. Assoc. 19*:784–787 (1982).
70. Addison, J. F., and Foulks, C. J. Calcium carbonate: An effective phosphorus binder in patients with chronic renal failure. *Curr. Ther. Res. 38*: 241–249 (1985).
71. Fournier, A., Moriniere, P., Sebert, J. L., Dkhissi, H., Atik, A., Leflon, P., Renaud, H., Gueris, J., Geogeoire, I., Idrissi, A., and Garabedian, M. Calcium carbonate, an aluminum free agent for control of hyperphosphatemia, hypocalcemia, and hyperparathyroidism in uremia. *Kidney Int. 29*(Suppl. 18):S114–S119 (1986).
72. Schneider, H. W., Kalke, K. D., Weber, H., and Streicher, E. In vitro and in vivo studies with a non-aluminum phosphate-binding compound. *Kidney Int. 29*(Suppl. 18):S120–S123 (1986).

11

Osteopetrosis

Brenda Kohn

Long Island College Hospital and SUNY Health Science Center at Brooklyn, Brooklyn, New York

William Bastian and Salvador Castells

SUNY Health Science Center at Brooklyn, Brooklyn, New York

I. INTRODUCTION

Osteopetrosis is a disease characterized by generalized skeletal involvement. The bone sclerosis observed in X-rays is the feature that prompts its name but other organ systems are frequently involved. Hematological, neurological, and immunological complications are part of the spectrum of clinical presentation. Juvenile and adult forms with dominant or recessive autosomal inheritance have been described. Each of these variants of osteopetrosis can present with variable degrees of severity.

The initial description of osteopetrosis was made by Albers-Schonberg in 1904 (1). Since then, more than 300 reports have appeared in the literature under the names of osteopetrosis, marble bone disease, osteosclerosis fragilis generalisata, and osteopetrosis generalisata (2).

The prevalence of all the variants of osteopetrosis has been estimated to be between 1:100,000 and 1:500,000 inhabitants (3). A recent epidemiological study reveals that the prevalence for the benign autosomal dominant form of osteopetrosis is 5.5:100,000 inhabitants (4). For this variant of osteopetrosis, Johnston et al. report a 1:1 male–female ratio and a 75% penetrance (3).

The histological studies on the osteopetrotic bone suggest that different conditions can produce the characteristic bone sclerosis by a common mechanism of decreased rate of bone resorption.

In this chapter we review some of the recent clinical reports on osteopetrosis with emphasis on the genetic, histological, and biochemical characteristics. An overview of the present knowledge of osteoclast biology and its relevance to osteopetrosis is presented. We believe that a heterogeneous group of disorders has been classified under the term osteopetrosis. With the advent of new therapeutic modalities such as high-dose calcitriol and bone marrow transplantation, a complete characterization of each individual patient will be necessary to develop a rational therapeutic approach.

II. CLINICAL PRESENTATION

A. Malignant Osteopetrosis

Malignant osteopetrosis, inherited as an autosomal recessive trait, represents the most severe form of osteopetrosis. Skeletal sclerosis and bone fractures have been detected in utero (5). Affected infants have progressive leukoerythroblastic anemia and marked hepatosplenomegaly secondary to extramedullary erythropoiesis (6). Deficiencies in immune function and neurological abnormalities are also present.

The skeletal abnormalities that may be found in the osteopetrotic skeleton include macrocephaly (due to thickening of the cranial foramina and associated hydrocephalus) (6), trapezoidal head (due to thickening of the frontal and parietal bones) (7), frontal bossing, hypertelorism, proptosis, flattened nasal bridge, choanal atresia (8), hypoplastic or hyperplastic mandible and maxilla, delayed linear growth, delayed dentition, and rickets (9).

Pathological fractures are common, because of brittle nature of the osteopetrotic bone (10–13). Bone fragility is attributed in part to the persistence of a cartilaginous matrix and to the lack of orderly constructed lamellar bone (14). Since the growth defect is mainly confined to sites of endochondral bone growth, membranous growth tends to be unaffected.

Roentgenographic findings generally include increased density of all bones, decreased remodeling with evidence of increased cortical thickness, widened shafts, and decreased marrow space in long bones (Table 1). The base of the skull, being formed of cartilage, is thickened and sclerotic (7,15). Cranial nerve foramina are narrowed. The disease may wax and wane, with periods of normal bone modeling and density alternating with periods of abnormal growth. This explains the bone-within-bone appearance, that is, alternating bands of dense and normal bone in the long bones, ilia, and vertebral bodies. While conventional radiography is more sensitive in describing the density of bone (16), magnetic resonance imaging (MRI) can depict the status of the bone marrow space. Now that the MRI characteristics of osteopetrosis have been established (Table 1), sequential MRI studies of the bone marrow space may be useful for following

Table 1 Radiological Findings in Osteopetrosis

Plain Films	Magnetic Resonance Imaging (MRI)
Generalized bony sclerosis	Lack of signal from the marrow in the short and long repetition time (TR)/echo time (TE) images
Transverse bands in the metaphyseal region	Black bones, since the signal intensity from the marrow match that of the cortex
Longitudinal striations in the shaft	Higher signal intensity in the intervertebral disk than in the vertebra produce a stepladder sign
Flask-shape configuration at the end of long bones	The ribs are broad and lack magnetic resonance signal
Sclerotic foci termed endobones or "bone-within-bone"	Decreased signal intensity of the liver and spleen relative to the intensity of the kidneys on short TR/TE images
Thickening of the skull (the base more affected than the calvaria) with narrowing of neural foramina and underdevelopment of paranasal sinuses	Decreased signal intensity of the spleen relative to the liver on long TR/TE images
Thickening of the vertebral end plates with the "rugger jersey" or "sandwich" appearance	
Concentric layers of increased density in the developing pelvic bones	
Pathological fractures	

up the effects of the new therapeutic modalities, such as bone marrow transplantation and high-dose calcitriol treatment (17).

Hematological derangements are very common in malignant osteopetrosis, since the skeletal sclerosis is associated with obliteration of the marrow cavities and increasing marrow fibrosis. The fibrosis promotes extramedullary erythropoiesis with hepatosplenomegaly and subsequent hypersplenism. The patients develop a leukoerythroblastic or myelophthisic anemia with macrocytosis, reticulocytosis, erythroblastosis, and leukocytosis of immature myeloid cells (18). The increased number of erythroid and granulocyte-macrophage precursors in the peripheral circulation is similar to that found in adults with myeloproliferative disorders. Hypersplenism is associated with decreased red cell survival, hemolytic anemia, thrombocytopenia, and leukopenia. Functional abnormalities in circulating phagocytes may reflect a primary defect in a common stem cell precursor to both osteoclasts and monocyte/macrophages (19). These hematological derangements have their clinical expression in the increased incidence of hemorrhage and overwhelming sepsis noted in these patients.

Neurological impairment is frequent in patients with malignant osteopetrosis (20). Progressive bony encroachment on cranial nerve foramine causes direct compression of the nerve, vascular occlusion, and gradual deterioration of neural function. The optic nerve, vestibulocochlear nerve, facial nerve (unilateral or bilateral) (21), and trigeminal nerve (mandibular division) are the most frequently affected.

Optic nerve atrophy and blindness result from bony narrowing of the optic canal with direct pressure on the optic nerve and ophthalmic artery. Obstruction of the retinal veins in association with papilloedema and elevation in intracranial pressure is another possible mechanism.

Sensorineural hearing loss results from bony constriction of the cochlear nerve in the internal auditory canal and compression of its vascular supply. Conductive hearing loss is due to encroachment of the bony walls of the epitympanum on the ossicles, narrowing of the external auditory meatus, and narrowing of the oval and round windows.

The causes of hydrocephalus in these patients is unclear. Impaired venous drainage due to overgrowth of cranial foramina, inhibition of cerebrospinal fluid flow due to internal compression of the foramina of Luschka and Magendie, an and compression in the volume of the posterior cranial fossa are possible contributing factors.

1. Case Report

A 3370 g female infant was born by normal spontaneous vaginal delivery to a 26-year-old class A diabetic Arabic woman (gravida 7, para 6). Several years earlier, a 7-month-old infant sibling had died of malignant (congenital) osteopetrosis. In our patient, films taken on the first day of life showed markedly increased density of all the long bones of the upper and lower extremities, the pelvic bones, ribs, and spine. A diagnosis of malignant osteopetrosis was made. Although parental consanguinity could not be confirmed, both parents had lived and grown up in the same village in Jerusalem.

On the fourth day of life, the infant was noted to be tremulous. At that time, laboratory studies revealed a serum calcium level of 5.3 mg/dl; phosphorus, 3.3 mg/dl; magnesium, 1.6 mg/dl; total protein, 7.4 g/dl; albumin, 5.2 g/dl; alkaline phosphatase, 309 g/dl; intact PTH, 62 pg/ml (normal, 10–55); mid-PTH 305 pg/ml (normal, 61–315) with simultaneous serum calcium, 9.1 mg/dl; phosphorus, 2.5 mg/dl (on calcium supplementation). There was no evidence

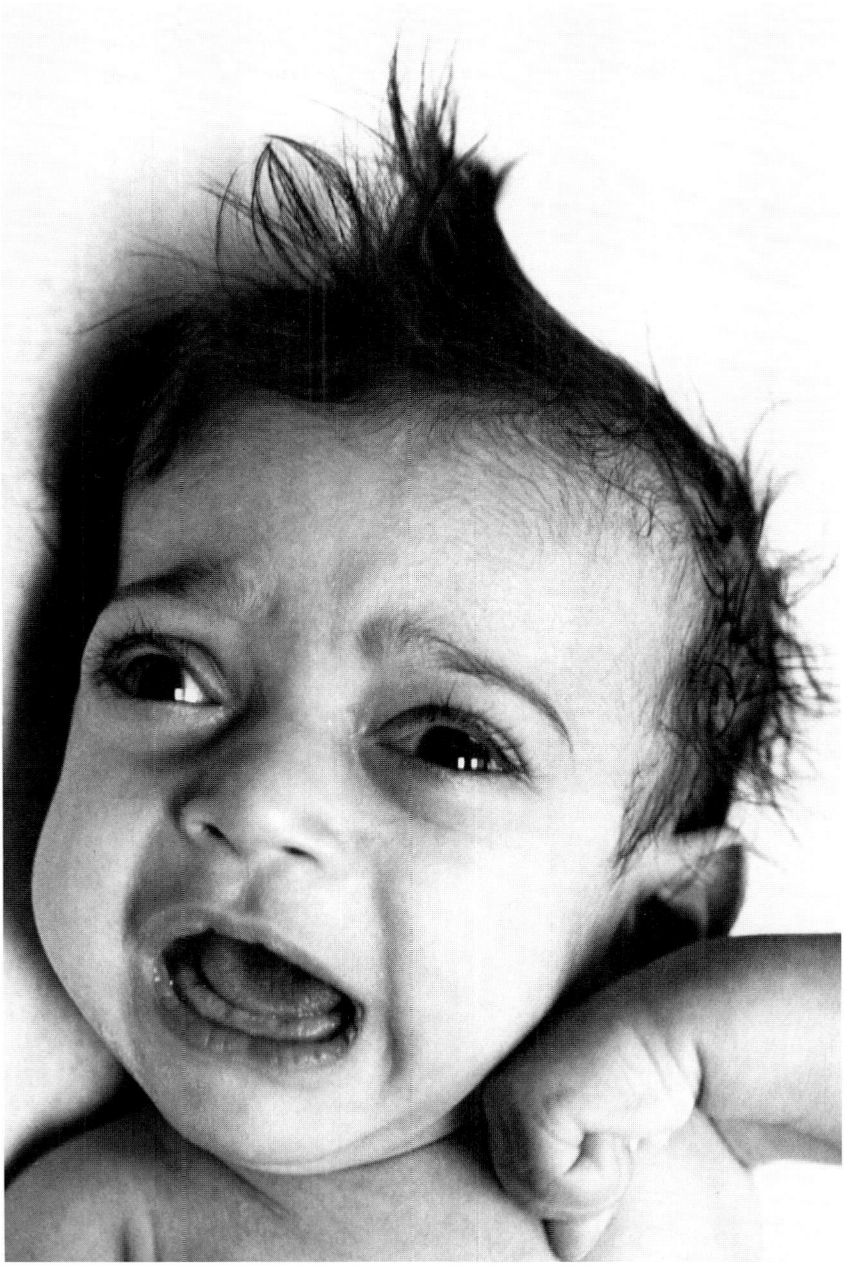

Figure 1 Patient at 4 months of age. Bilateral proptosis, frontal bossing, and trapezoidal shape of the head are present.

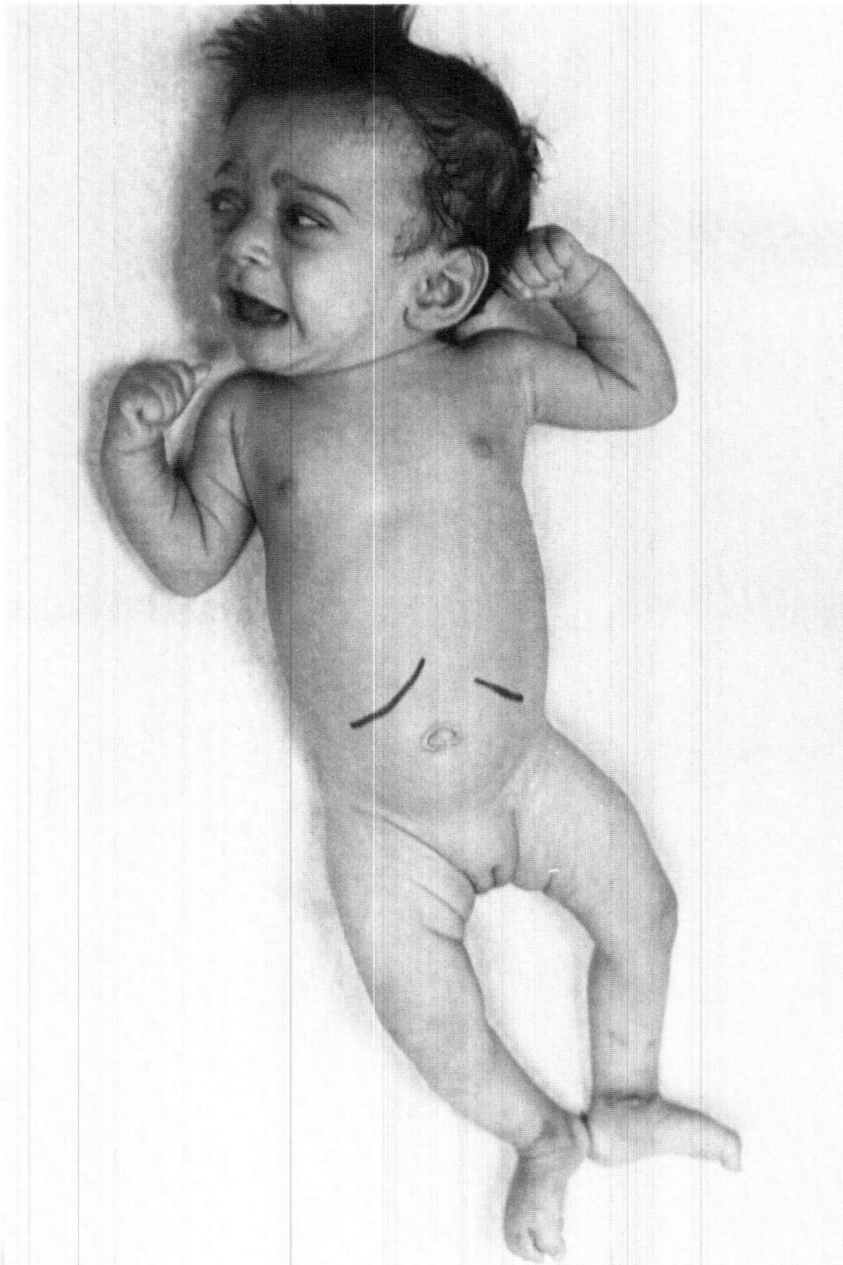

Figure 2 Supine view of patient at 4 months of age. Marked hepatosplenomegaly is noted.

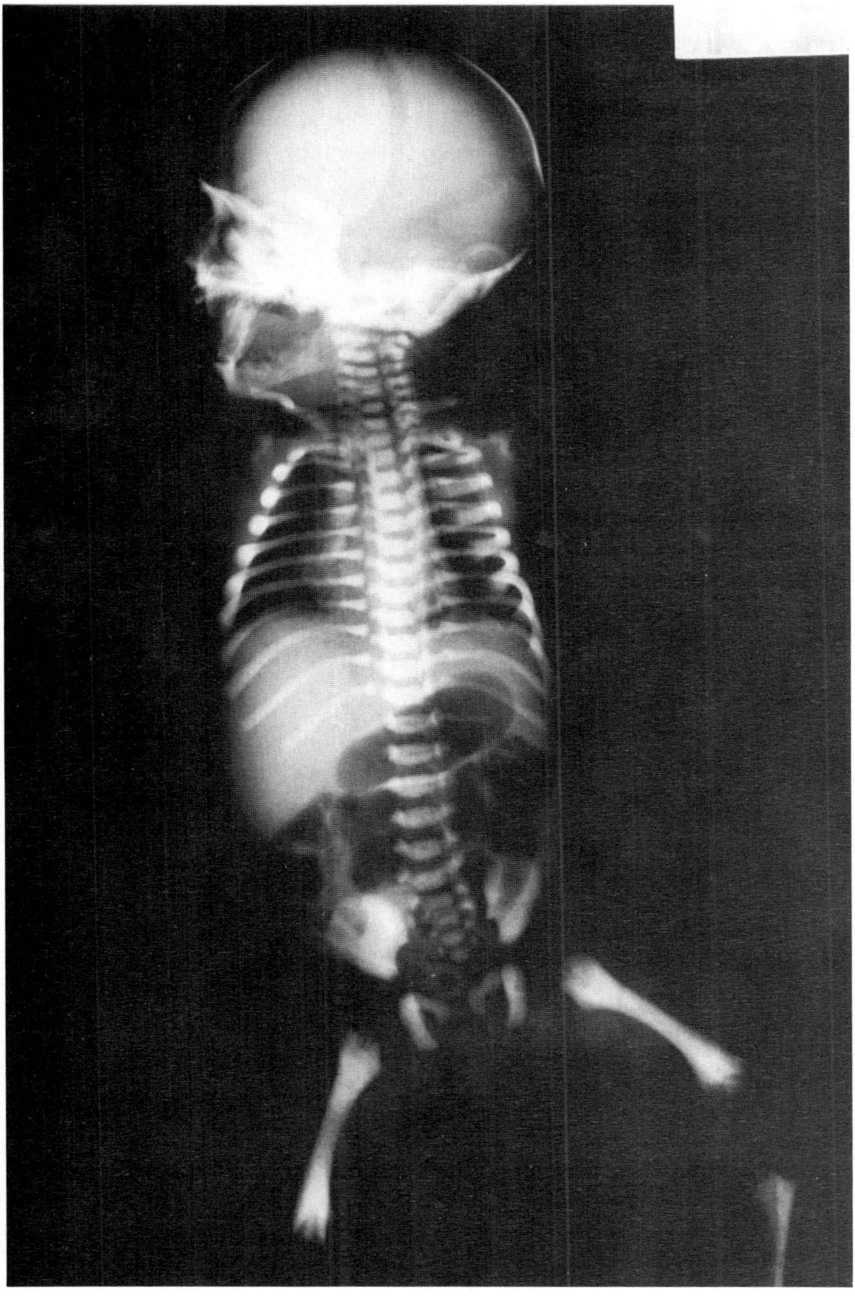

Figure 3 Radiographic findings at birth: increased density of the skull, spine, and long bones.

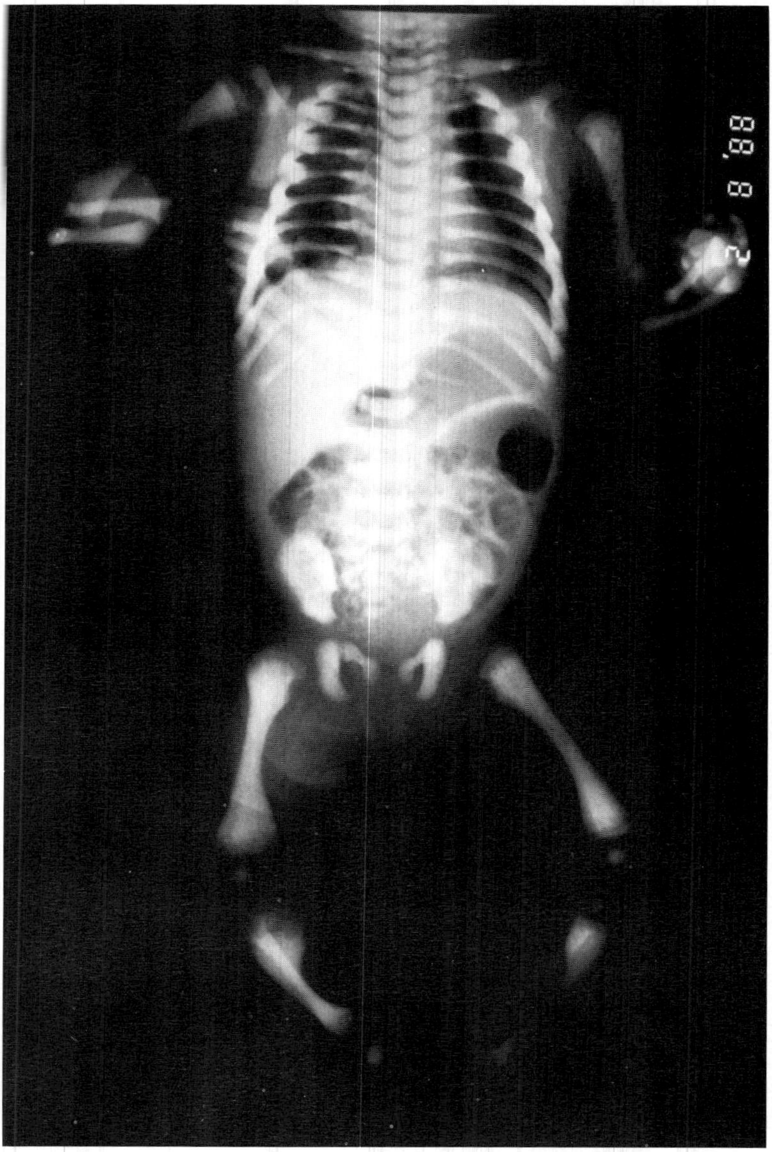

(A)

Figure 4 Radiographic findings at 4 months of age. A. Examination of the axial and appendicular skeleton shows diffuse sclerosis. B. Widening of the metaphyseal ends of the long bones. C. Marked sclerosis of the cranial base.

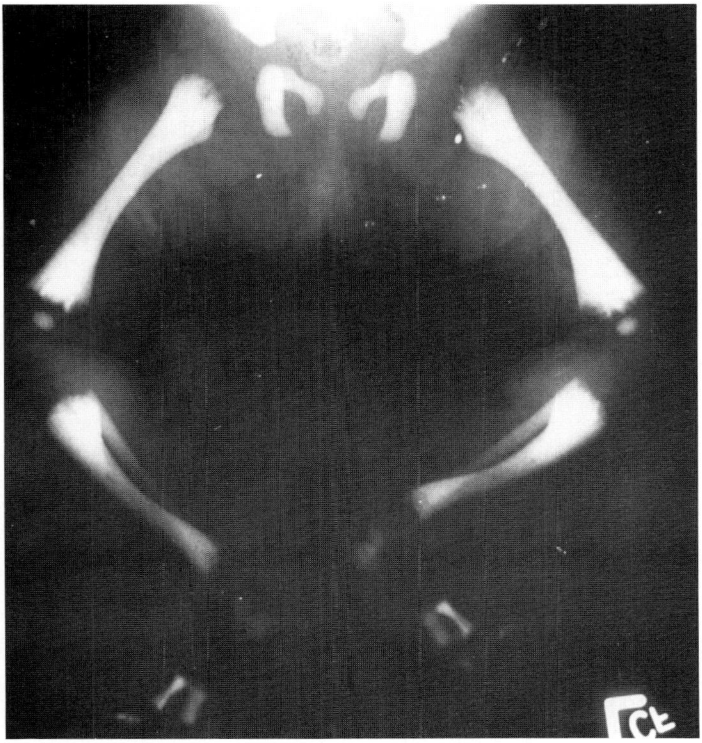

(B)

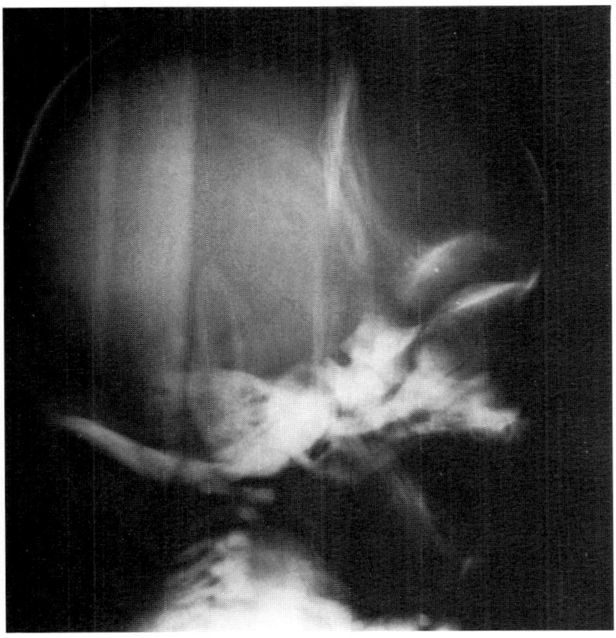

of renal tubular acidosis or metabolic acidosis. The hypocalcemia and hypophosphatemia were explained as resulting from massive uptake of these ions by bone.

The perinatal course was complicated by *Staphylococcus aureus* conjunctivitis, fever, and aseptic meningitis at 1 month of age. The parents were unwilling to consider bone marrow transplantation. The infant was discharged at 1-1/2 months of age. At 3-1/2 months of age the infant presented to a nearby hospital emergency room in hypocalcemic tetany. Platelet transfusion and packed red blood cell transfusions were given for treatment of thrombocytopenia and severe anemia. A course of antibiotics was given for possible sepsis.

At 4 months of age the patient was seen at our outpatient department. Physical examination showed a head circumference of 41.5 cm (75th percentile); weight, 9 lbs 15 ozs (below 5th percentile); length, 54-1/2 cm (below the 5th percentile). Bilateral proptosis, frontal bossing, and trapezoidal shape of the head were noted (Fig. 1). Funduscopic examination revealed bilateral pale discs. The pupils were unreactive to light. The infant was noted to react to sounds. The liver, palpable 5 cm below the right costal margin, was smooth. The spleen was enlarged and extended past the midline (Fig. 2).

Laboratory studies revealed a hematocrit of 26%, a hemoglobin level of 9.5 g/dl, and a reticulocyte count of 13.9%. The total white blood cell (WBC) count was 33,000/mm^3 (corrected WBC, 23,800). A differential count showed a leukoerythroblastic reaction with 60% lymphocytes, 9% monocytes, 2% eosinophils, 13% polymorphonuclear leukocytes, 16% band forms. Platelets were decreased in number. The serum calcium level was 7.5 mg/dl (range, 8.5–10.5 mg/dl). Total protein level was 5.3 g/dl (range, 6,0–8.5). Intact PTH level of 72 pg/ml (range, 10–65) was obtained with a simultaneous calcium level of 7.8 mg/dl.

Diffuse sclerosis (Figs. 3, 4) involving all bony structures including the thorax, abdomen, upper and lower extremities, and base of the skull was noted on the radiographs. Computed tomographic (CT) scan of the head excluded hydrocephalus. Bilateral optic atrophy and blindness were confirmed by visual-evoked response. Chronic rhinorrhea, the result of choanal atresia due to bony overgrowth, was confirmed by CT. Cultures of a purulent eye discharge grew *Hemophilus influenzae* and responded to antibiotic therapy. Oral prednisone (1 mg/kg per day) in conjunction with low-dose calcitriol (0.25 μg/day) was instituted with some improvement in the peripheral blood picture, and decrease in the hepatosplenomegaly. At 6 months of age, after 6 weeks of therapy, laboratory studies revealed a hematocrit of 31%, a hemoglobin level of 3.1 g/dl, and a reticulocyte count of 12.3%; the total white cell count was 28,000/mm^3 (corrected WBC, 22,400); platelets, 116,000. Serum calcium level was 9.8 mg/dl; phosphorus, 3.6 mg/dl; total protein, 5.5 g/dl; alkaline phosphatase, 512 g/dl.

B. Benign Osteopetrosis

The benign form of osteopetrosis is transmitted as an autosomal dominant trait. Incomplete penetrance and heterogeneity in the clinical expression are seen even among siblings within the same family (22,23). In almost of half of the cases, the patients are asymptomatic and the disorder is discovered incidentally by increased density found in bone. A normal life span can be expected. Hematological complications are rare. Symptoms, when present, include fractures (40%), bone pain (20-25%), cranial nerve palsy (10-20%), and early hip osteoarthritis. Gradual enlargement of the cranial vault and mandible, tall stature, genu valgum, clubbing of the long bones, and proptosis have been described. Osteomyelitis of the mandible (24,25) and, to a lesser extent of the maxilla (26) can also occur.

C. Intermediate Osteopetrosis

Both autosomal dominant and autosomal recessive inheritance have been found in cases associated with intermediate symptoms (27). An autosomal recessive form of osteopetrosis differs from the malignant autosomal recessive form by the relative mildness of clinical symptoms during infancy and childhood. Children with the disorder present with recurrent fractures, cranial nerve compression, and osteomyelitis (28).

Mild to moderate anemia may be present; however, marked hepatomegaly and severe anemia are absent. Survival into adult life is the rule. Radiographic evidence of disease is present. In many cases, parental consanguinity is ascertained and in all cases only one generation is affected. It may be clinically indistinguishable from the "benign" autosomal dominant form. Family evaluation and pedigree analysis are the only reliable methods of determining the pattern of gene transmission (4).

D. Osteopetrosis Associated with Renal Tubular Acidosis and Cerebral Calcification

This variant of osteopetrosis has been described in 21 patients from 12 unrelated families (29-34). It is inherited in an autosomal recessive manner. The biochemical hallmark is an almost complete deficiency of the enzyme carbonic anhydrase type II (CAII) in the erythrocytes of homozygote patients and decreased levels of the enzyme in obligate heterozygotes. The course is milder than that found in malignant osteopetrosis. Failure to thrive, hypotonia, and short stature may appear in infancy and midchildhood as the result of chronic systemic acidosis. Inability to acidify the urine (renal tubular acidosis [RTA] type I) and urinary wasting of bicarbonate (RTA type II) in the absence of phosphaturia and glycosuria are usually present. Blood urea nitrogen levels (BUN), serum creatinine levels, glomerular filtration rate (GFR), and intravenous pyelography (IVP) are normal. Skeletal roentgenograms and bone biopsies show evidence of osteopetrosis, but the incidence of bone fractures and cranial nerve palsies is less than in malignant osteopetrosis. Hematological complications are absent. Calcification of the basal ganglia and periventricular white matter can be demonstrated by CT scans of the head in patients older than 5 years (32). Psychomotor delay, mental retardation, and learning disabilities were present in 10 of the 12 pedigrees studied.

The deficiency of CAII in erythrocytes may be related to the skeletal, renal, and neurological abnormalities observed since the enzyme may also be deficient in these tissues. PTH can activate CAII in osteoclasts to secrete hydrogen ions (H+) and release calcium from the bone. A defect in this mechanism may be responsible for the bone sclerosis. In the kidney, CAII activity at the distal renal tubule is necessary for normal bicarbonate reabsorption. Cerebral calcifications and mental retardation may be the direct result of a deficiency of CAII in the brain or the indirect effect of chronic systemic acidosis.

There is variability of clinical expression among different pedigrees. Mental retardation and metabolic acidosis are prominent in some families (Saudi Arabia, Kuwait) (32,33), while repeated bone fractures with mild or absent mental retardation are seen in other families (Belgium, United States) (34).

E. Osteopetrosis in Association with Other Disorders

There have been reports of osteopetrosis associated with non-Hodgkins' lymphoma (35), Crohn's disease (36), bronchogenic carcinoma (37), icthyosis (38), and neuronal storage disease (39). The importance of these associations in the pathogenesis of the disease is unknown.

III. OSTEOCLAST BIOLOGY

The study of osteoclast biology has helped further our understanding of osteopetrosis and the bone resorptive process. The current concepts indicate that osteoclasts derive from progenitor lymphoidlike mononuclear elements that come from a hematopoietic milieu and are carried by the bloodstream into the bone surface, where they fuse with one another or with pre-existing osteoclasts and eventually differentiate (40–43).

The ultrastructural studies of the osteoclasts have helped to characterize the organelles involved in the resorptive process (42,44). The ruffled border represents a complex system of folds in the cell membrane resulting in fingerlike cytoplasmic projections linked to the disaggregating bone matrix in the outer side of the cell and to cytoplasmic vacuoles in the inner side. This is the site of active uptake and secretion, and its size is proportional to the degree of osteoclasts resorption.

The clear zone is an area along the osteoclast's membrane adjoining the bone where the cell membrane is smooth instead of ruffled. The cytoplasmic organelles are scarce and actinlike filaments are found in a finely granular amorphous substance. The clear zone is involved in the attachment of the osteoclasts to the bone and in maintaining a microenvironment for the resorptive activity.

There are other organelles that participate directly or indirectly in the resorptive process. The vesicles are important for endocytosis and exocytosis. The lysosomes are necessary for enzymatic digestion of intracellular and extracellular material. The microtubules may be involved in the secretory process of lysosomal enzymes and in the formation of ruffled borders. The mitochondria may serve as a storage site for calcium transported from the bone surface to the extracellular fluid.

A possible mechanism by which the osteoclasts disaggregate the bone matrix involves the release of lysosomal enzymes and proteinase-activatable procollagenase to dissolve partially the ground substance and collagen fibers and to release the mineral crystals (43). In this way all the material is phagocytosed through the channels of the ruffled border and is collected in the cytoplasmic vacuoles, where complete solubilization occurs.

The activation of osteoclastic bone resorption is mediated by factors of systemic and local origin. To maintain the plasma Ca^{2+} homeostasis, the osteoclastic resorption is regulated by calcitonin (CT), parathyroid hormone (PTH), and $1,25\text{-}(OH)_2D_3$. Calcitonin suppresses osteoclastic bone resorption by a cAMP-mediated mechanism that also inhibits the mobility of osteoclasts seen in time-lapse video experiment (45–47). The inhibition of cytoplasmic mobility can alter the processes of enzyme exocytosis and endocytosis required for bone resorption.

PTH and $1,25\text{-}(OH)_2D_3$ may activate osteoclastic bone resorption by inducing the osteoblast to secrete collagenase and tissue plasminogen activator (45). In this way the osteoid layer is removed, the mineral is exposed, and the bone becomes more susceptible to osteoclastic resorption. The activated osteoblasts may also transmit a signal to the osteoclasts by direct contact or by a short-range, unstable transmitter.

The effects of osteoclastic resorption in the morphogenesis of bone are regulated by local hormones such as prostaglandin E and osteoclast-activating factor (OAF) secreted by the osteoblasts in response to the shape of the bone and the mechanical stress on it (45). The PTH-like effects of these hormones may also be indirect and mediated by their actions on osteoblasts.

The normal function of osteoclast requires cellular and extracellular components. The cellular defects should be cured by transplantation of stem cells, while defects in the local microenvironment should not respond to transplantation. Defects in the stem cells should produce a small population of osteoclasts, while defects in the osteoclast should produce a large population of osteoclasts by compensatory hyperplasia. The validity of these speculations waits to be tested (43).

IV. CAUSES

The animal studies and clinical reports on osteopetrosis together with the recent studies on the biology of the osteoclasts seem to corroborate the notion that the osteopetrotic phenotype is the end result of multiple genetic defects (43). The osteoclast originates by differentiation from a stem cell described as a lymphoid-like mononuclear precursor. Local and systemic factors are necessary to activate the resorptive apparatus of the osteoclasts. In this sequence of events there are many potential sites of dysfunction, for which clinical examples have already been reported (49–58).

The transplantation studies in osteopetrosis have been helpful in clarifying the origin of the osteoclasts and have established the stem cell dysfunction as one of the causative factors in osteopetrosis. Walker et al. (40,41) demonstrated that the skeletal sclerosis of osteopetrotic microphthalmic mice can be removed within a few months after a brief period of parabiotic union to a normal littermate or after irradiation and transplantation of spleen or bone marrow cells from a normal littermate. They proposed that the transplanted cells supplied a local humoral factor for osteoclast function or provide stem cells for a new population of competent osteoclasts. In similar experiments with the osteopetrotic rat, Milhaud and Labot (48) proposed that the injected bone marrow cells potentiate the thymic epithelium to secrete hormones that may directly activate the osteoclasts or may promote the differentiation of thymic cells into osteoclast progenitors. The human counterpart of these experiments came when Coccia et al. (49) reported the case of a 5-month-old girl with malignant osteopetrosis who, after preparation with cyclophosphamide and modified total body irradiation, received a bone marrow transplantation from her human leukocyte antigen–major histocompatibility complex-HLA-MHC identical brother and started forming new osteoclasts of donor type, with significant clinical improvement.

Studying patients with malignant osteopetrosis, various authors have been able to detect defects at other levels of the osteoclast life cycle. Resistance of the stem cells to differentiation into osteoclasts and to osteoclast activation was described by Key et al. (50) in a patient whose condition improved with high doses of calcitriol. Defects intrinsic to the osteoclast have been proposed.

Ambler et al. (39) postulate that a lysosomal enzyme deficiency may explain the association of neuronal cytoplasmic storage disease with osteopetrosis. A defective osteoclast activation by local and systemic factors is also suggested by some of the clinical examples. Glorieux et al. (51) postulate the existance of physiologically defective PTH in a patient whose condition improved when treated with PTH extract. Shapiro et al. (52) described a defect in the resorptive function of the osteoclasts stimulated by PTH. Reeves et al. (53) described insensitivity of the osteoclasts to high levels of PTH, 1-25$(OH)_2D_3$, and OAF. A malfunction of the stem cell recruiting mechanism has been invoked by Teitelbaum et al. (54) to explain the osteoclast proliferation in malignant osteopetrosis. A neoplastic process of the osteoclast (54) and an abnormality of the matrix that renders it less susceptible to resorption (52) are also possible.

Like the studies of malignant osteopetrosis, the studies with the other clinical forms of osteopetrosis also suggest multiple etiologies. Horton et al. (55) also proposed a malfunction of the stem cell recruiting mechanism to explain the paucity of osteoclasts in a case of recessively inherited osteopetrosis with mild clinical course. Sly et al. (29,30) emphasize that the deficiency of carbonic anhydrase type II may have important clinical consequences in the syndrome of osteopetrosis, renal tubular acidosis, and cerebral calcifications. The enzyme is involved in the bicarbonate reclamation by the renal tubules and may be involved in the bone resorptive process by secreting H^+ ions that induce calcium release from the bone.

Although the actual model of the osteoclast biology has provided a theoretical framework of possible sites of dysfunction, many of the multisystemic manifestations of the disease still do not have an adequate explanation. Further studies are needed to clarify their pathophysiology.

V. HISTOLOGICAL FINDINGS

Bone histological examination in patients with osteopetrosis has shown abnormalities in the cortex, marrow, matrix, and osteoclasts (Table 2). The separation between the cortex and the marrow becomes indistinct due to an excess of wide bony trabeculae with a core of cartilage. Osteoid seams may be present. Decreased hematopoiesis is frequent and myelofibrosis is occasionally observed. The collagen fibers in the matrix are usually normal, but Bonucci et al. (56) have reported a patient in whom they detected anomalous collagen fibers and a decreased number of the round vesicles associated with mineralization. Studies of the cellular components of the bone revealed normal osteoblasts. The osteoclasts showed different types of abnormalities (Tables 2 and 3). Their number can be decreased, normal, or increased. Most of the time the osteoclasts are properly juxtaposed to bone but do not seem active in resorption. Howship's lacunae, ruffled borders, clear zones, and enzymatic secretion are frequently

Table 2 Histologic Findings in the Biopsies of Osteopetrotic Bone

Suggestive Cause	Onset	Severity	Inheritance	Cortex
Defective regulation of OS (55)	J	M	AR	Wide, bony trabeculae with a core of cartilage
Neoplastic proc. of OS (54)	J	S	AR	Bony trabeculae with a core of cartilage
Hyperplastic proc. of OS (54)	J	S		Bony trabeculae with a core of cartilage
Alteration of the matrix, chondrocytes, and OS (55)	J	S		
Carbonic anhydrase II deficiency (29)	J	I	AR	Bony trabecular with a core of cartilage
Defective PTH (51)	J	S		Excess of bone trabeculae with a core of cartilage
OS insensitivity to resorptive stimuli (53)	J	S		Wide osteoid seams over the bony trabeculae

Marrow	Cells	Matrix
Slightly reduced marrow space	Slightly reduced number of OS	
Abundant marrow space; focally abundant marrow fibrosis	Numerous OS juxtaposed to bone (huge, irregular, and with many nuclei) No ruffled borders No Howship's lacunae	
Reduced marrow space filled with spongiosa and small islands of hematopoietic tissue	Numerous OS juxtaposed to bone with ruffled borders, without Howship's lacunae	
	Normal osteoblasts Numerous OS juxtaposed to bone Prominent or absent ruffled border; Large vacuoles with amorphous material and electrondense granules (possibly abnormal lysosomes) Anomalous clusters of inorganic needle-shaped crystals in the mitochondria. Hypertrophic and degenerating chondrocytes with numerous vacuoles of mitochondrial origin.	Occasional anomalous collagen Less round vesicles associated with mineralization
	Normal osteoblast Normal OS number OS with clear zones Many mitochondria and well-developed rough endoplasmic reticulum No ruffled borders	Collagen fibers normal
Reduced marrow space	Numerous OS with large vacuoles and many dark-stained mitochondria No ruffled borders or clear zones	
Absent narrow space replaced by chondro-osseous tissue Decreased hematopoietic tissue Myelofibrosis	Normal osteoblast number Numerous OS	

Table 2 (Continued)

Suggested Cause	Onset	Severity	Inheritance	Cortex
OS defective resorptive function (52)	J	S		Irregular pattern of subperiosteal bone formation Moderate vascularity Increased amount of fibrous tissue Wide amount of collagen over the bony trabeculae Prominent lamina limitans
Cellular resistance to calcitriol-induced differentiation and OS activation (50)	J	S		Bony trabeculae with core of cartilage Many osteons Osteoid seams over the trabeculae
Poorly formed bone structure (3)	A	M	AD	

OS, osteoclast; J, juvenile; M, mild; S, severe; I, intermediate; A, adult; AR, autosomal recessive AD, autosomal dominant.

absent. In some of the osteoclasts, increased number of nuclei, large vacuoles (which may be abnormal lysosomes), and abnormal mitochondria may be seen.

VI. BONE METABOLISM

Several abnormalities have been detected in bone metabolism of osteopetrotic patients. No consistent pattern has emerged. Serological, histological, and radiographic evidence of rickets has been documented. Abnormalities in the PTH molecule, secondary hyperparathyroidism, cellular resistance to the action of PTH and $1{,}25(OH)_2D_3$, and decreased resorptive function of osteoclasts have been proposed to explain the findings in some patients.

Johnston et al. (3) studied five patients with the dominantly inherited benign osteopetrosis and they found normal serum levels of calcium, phosphorus, and alkaline phosphatase but increased levels of acid phosphatase. Urinary hydroxy-

Marrow	Cells	Matrix
Reduced marrow space filled with chondro-osseous tissue Virtually no marrow tissue	Numerous OS juxtaposed to bone No ruffled borders or clear zones Many nuclei Normal mitochondria, lysosomes, Golgi apparatus, and endoplasmic reticulum	
Absent marrow space Cellular marrow in enlarged osteons	Abundant OS juxtaposed to bone No ruffled borders or clear zones	
	Many osteoblasts and OS in foci	Few fibrils that seldom cross from one osteon to another

proline levels were normal. Chemical analysis of bone showed a normal calcium: phosphorus ratio and the calcium balance studies showed high-normal calcium accretion rates with modestly positive calcium balances. PTH infusion increased the serum calcium and the urinary calcium, phosphorus, and hydroxyproline. There was no derangement of calcium metabolism in these patients.

Reeves et al. (53) studied five patients with malignant osteopetrosis and reported low serum calcium and phosphorus, with high levels of PTH, alkaline, and acid phosphatase. X-rays showed rachitic changes in the metaphysis. In the urine the levels of cAMP were high and the levels of hydroxyproline were low. Calcium balances were positive. Bone biopsies showed abundant osteoid, myelofibrosis and numerous osteoclasts with decreased number of Howship's lacunae. The in vitro bone resorptive activity due to osteoclast activating factor (OAF) from cultured stimulated leukocytes was normal. There was evidence of rickets and decreased bone resorption in spite of increased humoral stimuli and increased osteoclast numbers

Table 3 Ultrastructural Findings of Osteoclasts and Parameters of Bone Metabolism in Osteopetrosis

				Ultrastructural findings					Serum values							Urine values		
Suggested cause	Onset	Severity	Inheritance	OS #	RB	CZ	HL	Enz. Rel	Ca	P	Alk P	Ac P	PTH	$1,25(OH)_2D_3$	CT	UcAMP	UOH PRO	Ca
Defective regulation of OS number (55)	J	M	AR	N or <					N	N		>	N					
Neoplastic OS (54)	J	S		>	-	+	-		<	<	>							
Hyperplastic OS (54)	J	S		>	+	+	-	+Ac.P	<		>	>						
Alteration in the matrix, chondrocytes, and OS (56)	J	S		>	±				<									
Carbonic anhydrase II deficiency (29)	J	I	AR	N	-	+	+	+Ac.P	N or <	N	N	N	N		N		N	N

Defective PTH (51)	J	S		>	–	–			<	<	>	>	N	>	N	>	>	<
OS insensitivity to resorptive stimulation (53)	J	S		>			+		<	<	>	>	>	>	N	>	<	
OS defective resorptive function (52)	J	S		>	–	–	–	colla-genase	<	<	>		N		N			
Cellular resistance to calcitriol-induced cell differentiation, and OS activation (50)	J	S		>	–	–			N	N	N		>	>			>	<
Not mentioned (49)	J	S		>			–		<	<	>	>	>	N	N			
Poorly formed bone structure (3)	A	M	AD	>					N	N	N	>						N

HL, Howship's lacunae; OS #, osteoclast number; RB, ruffled border; CZ, clear zone; Enz, rel., enzyme release; J, juvenile; A, adult, M, mild; S, severe; I, intermediate; N, normal, AR, autosomal recessive; AD, autosomal dominant; AcP, acid phosphate; >, increased; <, decreased, +, present, –absent.

Glorieux et al. (51) described a case of malignant osteopetrosis with low serum levels of calcium and phosphorus, high alkaline and acid phosphatases, normal 25-hydroxy-vitamin D levels and rachitic-like changes in the metaphysis of long bones. Serum PTH levels were low when urinary cAMP was high. PTH infusion increased the serum calcium and the urinary hydroxyproline and calcium levels. An abnormal PTH molecule with altered binding sites for antisera and osteoclast receptors but not for receptors on the renal tubules might explain this data.

Shapiro et al. (52) described a case of malignant osteopetrosis with low serum calcium and phosphorus, high alkaline phosphatase and normal PTH and calcitonin levels. Bone biopsy showed fibrosis, reduced marrow space filled with chondro-osseous tissue, osteoid seams, and prominent lamina limitans. In culture media, the osteopetrotic bone was able to release cAMP in response to PTH and calcitonin but did not release bone collagenase in response to PTH. There was evidence of rickets and decreased resorptive function inspite of an increased number of osteoclasts.

Aarskog et al. (57,58) described three children with severe osteopetrosis and low levels of plasma calcium, 25, hydroxyvitamin D and alkaline phosphatase. The serum levels of PTH and $1{,}25(OH)_2D$ were elevated. PTH infusion produced a blunted phosphaturic response and did not increase the serum levels of $1{,}25(OH)_2D$. In these patients, the levels of 25,hydroxy vitamin D were not as low as seen in vitamin D deficiency, the alkailine phosphatase levels were low and there were no radiological signs of rickets. They conclude that the increased levels of both PTH and $1{,}25(OH)_2D$ in their patients was probably due to lack or unresponsiveness of target cells in the bone.

Key et al. (50) described an 8-week-old female with malignant osteopetrosis in whom the serum levels of calcium, phosphorus, and alkaline phosphatase were normal but the levels of iPTH and $1{,}25(OH)_2D$ were elevated. In the urine, the calcium:creatinine ratio was low, the levels of hydroxylysine were high and gamma carboxyglutamic acid levels were normal. Treatment with a low-calcium diet and increasingly high doses of calcitriol for 3 months resulted in increased bone mineral and matrix turnover. Serum levels of osteocalcin, alkaline phosphatase, and iPTH rose, but the high levels of $1{,}25(OH)_2D$ were not altered by the low calcium diet. The patient's monocytes increased their in vitro bone resorptive capacity to 3.3 times control levels. In the bone biopsy, numerous osteoclasts with ruffled borders were associated with bony disruption. The lack of osteoclasts with ruffled borders at elevated basal levels of calcitriol and the high doses of calcitriol required for increasing bone resorption suggested a cellular resistance to calcitriol.

VII. TREATMENT

Allogenic bone marrow transplantation from HLA-matched sibling donors offers the greatest hope for long-term survival in infants with malignant disease (49,59–62). In a series of 14 marrow transplantations for infantile osteopetrosis, 6 of the patients achieved significant reversal of osseous abnormalities, with improvement in hematological status and immune function. By fluorescent Y-body analysis, osteoblasts and osteoclasts in the recipient have been demonstrated to be of host and donor origin, respectively. Preparatory immunosuppressive therapy to combat graft-versus-host reaction increases the likelihood of marrow engraftment. The failure of bone marrow transplantation therapy in some infants may reflect the heterogeneity of causes of the disorder. There are non-stem-cell causes for osteopetrosis, which would not respond to bone marrow transplantation (see Table 2). Hormonal therapy is an alternative for those patients who are unwilling, or unable, for lack of an appropriate donor, to undergo bone marrow transplantation. Potent stimulators of bone resorption, such as high-dose calcitriol (1,25-dihydroxyvitamin D_3) (50,63) and bovine PTH, have been used to induce osteoclast function.

Studies suggest a dual role for calcitriol in inducing bone resorption in patients with osteopetrosis. In vitro exposure to 1,25-dihydroxyvitamin D_3 stimulates cellular differentiation of the monocyte (and human myeloid leukemic cell) to cells capable of bone resorption (64,65).

Further, administration of 1-alpha hydroxylated vitamin D_3 stimulates functional osteoclasts to resorb bone at a higher rate than normal (66). Thus, the action of calcitriol is mediated both by its ability to increase the differentiation of precursors into competent bone resorbing cells and by directly stimulating cells to resorb bone more effectively. Cellular resistance to calcitriol is suggested by the need for very high dose therapy in these patients (16–32 μg/day) despite high basal levels of circulating 1,25-dihydroxyvitamin D.

A 3 month regimen of high-dose calcitriol (16–32 μg/day) and low calcium intake (4 mg/kg per day) given to a 2-month-old infant with malignant osteopetrosis induced an increase in bone turnover (50). Posttreatment bone marrow biopsy showed, for the first time, the presence of numerous osteoclasts with ruffled borders and associated bony disruption. In vitro monocytic resorptive capacity was increased to 3.3 times the pretreatment levels. Little clinical improvement was noted during this brief clinical trial. In contrast, in two infants with moderate to severe bone marrow fibrosis, no improvement in clinical symptoms or bone biopsy was found after 1 month of calcitriol therapy (63).

Brief clinical trials using intravenous infusion of parathyroid extract or bovine PTH for patients with severe disease have been unable to provide conclusive evidence of therapeutic efficacy (50). In two patients with plasma immunoreactive PTH (iPTH) levels at the upper normal range, resistance to the action of

PTH infusion was noted. In contrast, Glorieux et al. (51) studied a patient with malignant osteopetrosis with hypocalcemia and relative hypoparathyroidism in whom a 3 week infusion of PTH resulted in normalization of hypocalcemia and significant improvement in marrow space (23%). A dramatic increase in the number (93%) of osteoclasts, as well as significant improvement in the morphology and functional capacity of the osteoclast, was found. In this patient, physiologically "defective" PTH was suggested as the cause of osteopetrosis. Chronic steroid therapy (prednisone 1 mg/kg per day) (67) in combination with a low-calcium, high-phosphate diet resulted in improvement of hematological and skeletal complications in four patients with juvenile osteopetrosis. Short-term (1–6 months) therapy with high-dose intravenous methylprednisone (68) has been shown to induce regression of hepatosplenomegaly, increase the peripheral leukocyte and platelet count, normalize the hemoglobin concentration, and improve bone marrow cellularity. Potential side effects of high-dose steroid therapy include severe growth retardation, increased susceptibility to infection, and lowering of serum calcium levels. Long-term therapeutic trials with assessment of their impact on osteoclast morphology, biochemical parameters, degree of marrow fibrosis, and severity of clinical disease may help to delineate further the various disorders of osteoclast function and define those patients most likely to benefit from medical intervention (43,69–72).

REFERENCES

1. Albers-Schonberg, H. Roengenbilder ciner seltenen Knochenerkrankung. *Munch. Med. Wochenschr 51*:365 (1904).
2. Klintworth, G. K. The neurologic manifestations of osteopetrosis (Albers-Schonberg's disease). *Neurology 13*:512–519 (1963).
3. Johnston, C. C., Jr., Lavy, N., Lord, T., Vellios, F., Merritt, A. D., and Deiss, W. P. Osteopetrosis: A clinical, genetic, metabolic, and morphologic study of the dominantly inherited, benign form. *Medicine 47*:149–167 (1968).
4. Bollerslev, J. Osteopetrosis: A genetic and epidemiological study. *Clin. Genet. 31*:86–90 (1987).
5. El Khazen, N., Tanerly, D., Vamos, E., Van Regemorter, N., Flament-Durand, J., Carton, B., and Cremer-Perlmutter, N. Lethal osteopetrosis with multiple fractures in utero. *Am. J. Med. Genet. 23*(3):811–9 (1986).
6. Mathur, B. P., and Karan, S. Non-immune hydrops fetalis due to osteopetrosis congenita. *Indian Pediatr. 21*(8):651–653 (1984).
7. Chudhuri, J. N., Banerjee, S., Koshnia, B. R., Chatterji, P., and Soni, N. K. Marble bone disease in a child. *J. Laryngol. Otol. 100*(8):935–938 (1986).
8. Marula, A. A., and Ambegaikar, A. G. Choanal atresia: Early management and an association with marble bone disease. *J. Laryngol. Otol. 100*(8):959–963 (1986).

9. Oliveira, G., Boechat, M. I., Amaral, S. M., and Young, L. W. Osteopetrosis and rickets: An intriguing association. *Am. J. Dis. Child.* *140*(4):337–338 (1986).
10. McClearly, L., Rovit, R. L., and Murali, R. Case report: Myelopathy secondary to congenital osteopetrosis of the cervical spine. *Neurosurgery* *20*(3): 487–489 (1987).
11. Suzuki, S., and Awaya, G. Stress fracture of the vertebral arch in osteopetrosis. *Clin. Orthop.* *213*:232–236 (1986).
12. Greene, W. B., and Torre, B. A. Femoral neck fracture in a child with autosomal dominant osteopetrosis. *J. Pediatr. Orthop.* *5*(4):483–485 (1985).
13. Voisin, M. C., Kemeny, A., Pinaudeau, Y., Villiaumey, J., and Hioco, D. D. Variation of surface density and other parameters in remodeling of trabecular bone in various conditions. *Anal. Quant. Cytol. Histol.* *8*(4):333–337 (1986).
14. Kuo, T. T., and Davis, C. P. Osteopetrosis: A scanning electron microscopic study. *Human Pathol.* *12*:376–379 (1981).
15. Friede, H., Manaligod, J. R., Rosenthal, I. M., Craniofacial abnormalities in osteopetrosis with precocious manifestations: Report of a case with serial cephalometric roentgenograms. *J. Craniofac. Genet. Dev. Biol.* *5*(3): 247–257 (1985).
16. Smith, R. *Biochemical Disorders of the Skeleton*. Butterworth, Oxford, 1979, pp. 253-273.
17. Rao, V. M., Dalinka, M. K., Mitchell, D. G., Spritzer, C. E., Kaplan, F., August, C. S., Axel, L., and Kressel, H. Y. Osteopetrosis: MR characteristics at 1.5 T. *Radiology* *161*:217–220 (1986).
18. Nathan, D. G., and Oskie, F. A. *Hematology of Infancy and Childhood*, Vol. 1. W. B. Saunders, Philadelphia, 1987, pp. 214–215.
19. Beard, C. J., Key, L., Newburger, P. E., Ezekowitz, R. A., Arceci, R., Miller, B., Proto, P., Ryan, T., Arnast, C., and Simons, E. R. Neutrophil defect associated with malignant infantile osteopetrosis. *J. Lab. Clin. Med.* *108*(5): 498–505 (1986).
20. Miyamoto, R. T., House, W. F., and Brackman, D. E. Neurotologic manifestations of the osteopetroses, *Arch. Otolaryngol.* *106*:210–214 (1980).
21. Bajaj, S., Gupta, S. C., and Nigam, D. K. Osteopetrosis with bilateral facial nerve palsy. *J. Assoc. Physicians India* *34*(7):529–530 (1986).
22. Andersen, P. E., Jr., and Bollerslev, J. Heterogeneity of autosomal dominant osteopetrosis. *Radiology* *164*(1):223–225 (1987).
23. Silvestrini, G., Ferracciolli, G. F., Quaini, F., Palummeri, E., and Bonucci, E. Adult osteopetrosis: Study of two brothers. *Appl. Pathol.* *5*(3):184–189 (1987).
24. Gupta, D. S., Gupta, M. K., and Borle, R. M. Osteomyelitis of the mandible in marble bone disease. *Int. J. Oral Maxillofac. Surg.* *15*(2):201–205 (1986).
25. Steiner, M., Gould, A. R., and Means, W. R. Osteomyelitis of the mandible associated with osteopetrosis. *J. Oral Maxillofac. Surg.* *41*(6):395–405 (1983).

26. Crokett, D. M., Stanley, R. B., and Lubka, R. Osteomyelitis of the maxilla in a patient with osteopetrosis (Albers-Schonberg's disease). *Otolaryngol. Head Neck Surg. 95*(1):117–121 (1986).
27. Adeloye, A. The syndrome of osteopetrosis in siblings: Its occurrence in two sisters in Nigeria. *Childs. Nerv. Syst. 3*(2):128–131 (1987).
28. Osborn, R., Boland, T., DeLuchi, S., and Beirne, O. R. Osteomyelitis of the mandible in a patient with malignant osteopetrosis. *J. Oral Med. 40*(2): 76–80 (1985).
29. Sly, W. S., Hewett-Emmett, D., Whyte, M. P., Yu, Y. L., and Tashian, R. E. Carbonic anhydrase II deficiency identified as the primary defect in autosomal recessive syndrome of osteopetrosis with renal tubular acidosis and cerebral calcification. *Proc. Natl. Acad. Sci. USA 80* 2752–2756 (1983).
30. Sly, W. S., Whyte, M. P., Sundaram, V., Tashian, R. E., Hewett-Emmett, D., Guibaud, P., Vainsel, M., Baluarte, J., Gruskin, A., Al-Mosawi, M., Sakoti, N., and Ohlsson, A. Carbonic anhydrase II deficiency in 12 families with the autosomal recessive syndrome of osteopetrosis with renal tubular acidosis and cerebral calcification. *N. Engl. J. Med. 313*:139–145 (1985).
31. Ohlsson, A., Cumming, W. A., Paul, A., and Sly, W. S. Carbonic anhydrase II deficiency syndrome: Recessive osteopetrosis with renal tubular acidosis and cerebral calcification. *Pediatrics 77*(3):371–381 (1986).
32. Cumming, W. A., Ohlsson, A., Intracranial calcification in chidren with osteopetrosis caused by carbonic anhydrase II deficiency. *Radiology 157*: 325–327 (1985).
33. Ohlsson, A., Stark, G., and Sakati, N. Marble bone disease: Recessive osteopetrosis, renal tubular acidosis and cerebral calcification in three Saudi Arabian families. *Dev. Med. Child. Neurol. 22*:72–84 (1980).
34. Whyte, M. P., Murphy, W. A., Fallon, M. D., Sly, W. S., Teitelbaum, S. L., Mc. Alister, W. H., and Avioli, L. V. Osteopetrosis, renal tubular acidosis and basal ganglia calcification in three sisters. *Am. J. Med. 69*:64–74 (1980).
35. Shibuya, H., Suzuki, T., Matsubara, S., and Suzuki, S. Non-Hodgkin's lymphoma in a patient with osteopetrosis. *Lymphology 19*(2):90–92 (1986).
36. Henderson, R. G., Long, P. J., Al-Nafussi, A. I., Coombs, R. R., and Gibson, R. N. Paget's disease with benign osteopetrosis and Crohn's disease. *J. R. Soc. Med. 78*(9):766–768 (1985).
37. Sand, J. J., Biller, J., and Aschenbrener, C. A. Nonbacterial thrombotic endocarditis and nondisseminated malignancy associated with osteopetrosis. *Eur. Neurol. 27*(3):167–172 (1987).
38. Dowd, P. M., and Munro, D. D. Ichthyosis and osteopetrosis. *J. R. Soc. Med. 76*(5):423–426 (1983).
39. Ambler, M. W., Trice, J., Grauerholz, J., and O'Shea, P. A. Infantile osteopetrosis and neuronal storage disease. *Neurology 33*:437–441 (1983).
40. Walker, D. G. Osteopetrosis cured by temporary parabiosis. *Science 180*: 875 (1973).
41. Walker, D. G. Bone resorption restored in osteopetrotic mice by transplants of normal bone marrow and spleen cells. *Science 190*:784–787 (1975).

42. Bonucci, E. New knowledge on the origin, function and fate of osteoclasts. *Clin. Orthop. Rel. Res. 158*:252–269 (1981).
43. Mark, S. C. Osteopetrosis–multiple pathways for the interception of osteoclast function. *Bone Pathol. Appl. Pathol. 5*:172–183 (1987).
44. Holtrop, M. E., and King, G. J. The ultrastructure of the osteoclast and its functional implications. *Clin. Orthop. Rel. Res. 123*:177–196 (1977).
45. Chambers, T. J. The pathobiology of the osteoclast (review article). *J. Clin. Pathol. 38*:241–252 (1985).
46. Chambers, T. J., Revell, P. A., Fuller, K., and Athanasou, N. A. Resorption of bone by isolated rabbit osteoclasts. *J. Cell Sci. 66*:383–399 (1984).
47. Chambers, T. J., and Ali, N. N. Inhibition of osteoclastic motility by prostaglandin I_2, E_1, E_2 and 6-oxo E_1. *J. Pathol. 139*:383–397 (1983).
48. Milhaud, G., and Labat, M. L. Thymus and osteopetrosis. *Clin. Orthop. Rel. Res. 135*:260–271 (1978).
49. Coccia, P. F., Krivit, W., Cervenka, J., Clawson, C., Kersey, J. H., Kim, T. H., Nesbit, M. E., Ramsay, N. K., Warkentin, P. I., Teitelbaum, S. L., Kahn, A. J., and Brown, D. M. Successful bone-marrow transplantation for infantile malignant osteopetrosis. *N. Engl. J. Med. 302*:701–708 (1980).
50. Key, L., Carnes, D., Cole, S., Holtrop, M., Bar-Shavit, Z., Shapiro, F., Arceci, R., Steinberg, J., Gungdberg, C., Kahn, A., Teitelbaum, S., and Anast, C. Treatment of congenital osteopetrosis with high dose calcitriol. *N. Engl. J. Med. 310*:409–415 (1984).
51. Glorieux, F. H., Pettifor, J. M., Marie, P. J., Delvin, E. E., Travers, R., and Shepard, N. Induction of bone resorption by parathyroid hormone in congenital malignant osteopetrosis. *Metab. Bone Dis. Rel. Res. 3*:143–150 (1981).
52. Shapiro, F., Glimcher, M. J., Haltrop, M. E., Tashjian, A. H., Brickley-Parsons, D., and Kenzora, J. E. Human osteopetrosis. *J. Bone Joint Surg. 62A*:384–399 (1980).
53. Reeves, J., Arnaud, S., Gordon, S., Subryan, B., Block, M., Huffer, W., Arnaud, C., Mundy, G., and Haussler, M. The pathogenesis of infantile malignant osteopetrosis: Bone mineral metabolism and complications in five infants. *Metab. Bone Dis. Rel. Res. 3*:135–142 (1981).
54. Teitelbaum, S. L., Coccia, P. F., Brown, D. M., and Kahn, A. J. Malignant osteopetrosis: A disease of abnormal osteoclast proliferation. *Metab. Bone Dis. Rel. Res. 3*:99–105 (1981).
55. Horton, W. A., Schimke, R. N., and Iyama, T. Osteopetrosis: Further heterogeneity. *J. Pediatr. 97*:580–585 (1980).
56. Bonucci, E., Sartori, E., and Spina, M. Osteopetrosis fetalis: Report of a case with special reference to ultrastructure. *Virchows Arch.* [A] *368*: 109–121 (1975).
57. Aarskog, D., Aksnes, L., and Markestad, T. Acute response of parathyroid hormone in congenital osteopetrosis. *Acta Paediatr. Scand. Suppl. 277*: 75–80 (1979).
58. Aarskog, D., Aksnes, L., Markestad, T. Effect of parathyroid hormone on vitamin D metabolism in osteopetrosis. *Pediatrics 68*:108–112 (1981).

59. Sieff, C. A., Chessells, J. M., Levinsky, R. J., Pritchard, J., Rogers, D. W., Casey, A., Muller, K., and Hall, C. M. Allogenic bone-marrow transplantation in infantile malignant osteopetrosis. *Lancet 1*(8322):437–441 (1983).
60. Nisbet, N. W. Bone marrow transplantation in precocious osteopetrosis (editorial). *Br. Med. J. 294*(6570):463–464 (1987).
61. Fischer, A., Griscelli, C., Friedrich, W., Kubanek, B., Levinsky, R., Morgan, G., Vossen, J., Wagemaker, G., and Landais, P. Bone-marrow transplantation for immuno-deficiencies and osteopetrosis: European survey, 1968–1985. *Lancet 2*(8515):1080–1084 (1986).
62. Sorell, M., Kapoor, N., Kirkpatrick, D., Rosen, et al. Marrow transplantation for juvenile osteopetrosis. *Am. J. Med. 70*:1280–1287 (1987).
63. Blazar, B. R., Fallon, M. D., Teitelbaum, S. L., Ramsay, N. K., and Brown, D. M. Calcitriol for congenital osteopetrosis (letter). *N. Engl. J. Med. 311*(1):55 (1984).
64. Miyaura, C., Abe, E., Kuribayashi, T., et al. 1a,25 Dihydroxyvitamin D_3 induces differentiation of human myeloid leukemia cells. *Biochem. Biophys. Res. Commun. 102*:937–943 (1981).
65. Bar-Shavit, Z., Teitelbaum, S. L., Reitsma, P., et al. Induction of monocyte differentiation and bone resorption of 1,25-dihydroxyvitamin D_3. *Proc. Natl. Acad. Sci. USA 80*:5907–5911 (1983).
66. Tinkler, S. M. B., Williams, D. M., and Johnson, N. W. Osteoclast formation in response to intraperitoneal injection of 1a-hydroxycholecalciferol in mice. *J. Anat. 133*:91–97 (1981).
67. Dorantes, L. M., Mejia, A. M., and Dorantes, S. Juvenile osteopetrosis: Effects on blood and bone of prednisone and a low calcium, high phosphate diet. *Arch. Dis. Child. 61*(7):666–670 (1986).
68. Ozsoylu, S. High dose intravenous methylprednisolone in treatment of recessive osteopetrosis [letter]. *Arch. Dis. Child. 62*:214–215 (1987).
69. Van Tran, P., Dryll, A., Lansaman, J., Naveau, B., Treve, R., Miravet, L., and Ryckewaert, A. Osteoclast abnormalities in idiopathic osteopetrosis. Reference to the ultrastructural histochemistry study. *Virchows Arch* [A] *408*(2–3):269–280 (1985).
70. Pojda, Z. Pathogenesis and treatment of infantile osteopetrosis. *Mater. Med. Pol. 18*(1):40–42 (1986).
71. Conroy, C. W., and Maren, T. H. The determination of osteopetrotic phenotypes by selective inactivation of red cell carbonic anhydrase isoenzymes. *Clin. Chim. Acta 152*(3):347–354 (1985).
72. Marks, S. C., Jr. Congenital osteopetrotic mutations as probes of the origin, structure, and function of osteoclasts. *Clin. Orthop. 189*:239–263 (1984).

12

Osteoporosis

Salvador Castells

SUNY Health Science Center at Brooklyn,
Brooklyn, New York

I. INTRODUCTION

Osteoporosis in children is a heterogeneous group of metabolic bone diseases that have in common a loss of bone mass manifested by skeletal brittleness and rarefaction of bone with normal mineral metabolism.

Pommer (1,2) first described osteoporosis in 1885 and differentiated it from rickets and osteomalacia. He observed in osteoporosis the diminution of bone tissue, and the normal calcification of the remaining bone. One hundred years after Pommer's initial observation, osteoporosis in humans is still considered not to be a primary disease of mineral metabolism. It is the loss of bone tissue that secondarily affects bone mineral by increasing the liberalization of calcium and phosphorus into blood and urine. In some cases of osteoporosis, secondary hypercalcemia, hyperphosphatemia, and hypercalciuria may be found. In contrast, the term osteomalacia is used when uncalcified bone tissue is present and causes avidity for calcium and phosphorus. In patients with osteomalacia, blood calcium and phosphorus concentrations may be low.

Bone is a dynamic tissue, with the process of bone formation and resorption occurring at the same time. In children the rate of bone remodeling is very active. Age influences the turnover of bone, with two periods of very rapid bone gain: from birth to 2 years and during adolescence. Puberty is a period of increased bone mineral content (3). In boys at puberty, serum testosterone, alone or in combination with other factors such as growth hormone and somatomedin, increases bone formation (4). The significant difference in bone mass at different ages reflects a greater net formation relative to net resorption with the result of a larger skeleton mass than at previous ages. This may explain why in some types of childhood osteoporosis, such as osteogenesis imperfecta, and Down's syndrome, there is a significant clinical and radiological improvement during adolescence (5). In osteoporosis, accelerated bone resorption undertakes bone formation and the result is a loss of bone mass. Osteoporosis in children is characterized by a reduction in bone mass below normal for age, sex, and race of an individual.

By histological definition, osteoporosis is characterized by a reduction in trabecular bone mass with a ratio of mineral to organic matrix similar to normal bone. In osteomalacia, the ratio of mineral to organic matrix is low. In most instances, the distinction between osteoporosis and osteomalacia is only possible by bone biopsy when appropriately stained histological sections reveal undermineralization, a finding of osteomalacia.

II. CLASSIFICATION

Table 1 gives a classification of osteoporosis in children representing a heterogeneous group of disorders; some due to primary metabolic bone disease, others secondary to other metabolic disorders.

III. CLINICAL MANIFESTATIONS

Most children with osteoporosis are asymptomatic, and the clinician will only be able to suspect the diagnosis indirectly.

The general appearance of the child may give a clue to the diagnosis. Blue sclerae and easy bruisability may lead the astute clinician to the correct diagnosis of osteogenesis imperfecta. Progressive obesity with "buffalo hump" is characteristic of Cushing's syndrome.

A. Bone Pain

Generalized bone pain is not characteristic of any type of childhood osteoporosis. Acute localized pain and tenderness are usually found at the site of new fractures. Back pain is localized to the area of the deformed vertebrae. It is aggravated by vigorous movements and is relieved by rest, in contrast to the pain of bone tumors, which is persistent and more generalized.

B. Multiple Fractures

Children with osteoporosis have fragile bones. The bone fractures without any relation to the intensity of the trauma. Most metabolic bone diseases in children

Table 1 Classification of Osteoporosis

Congenital
Osteogenesis imperfecta
Osteolysis
Juvenile
Osteoporosis associated with accelerated bone formation: juvenile Paget's disease of bone
Immobilization
Endocrine disorders
Hypogonadism
Hyperthyroidism
Juvenile diabetes
Acromegaly
Hyperadrenocorticism
Progeria
Growth hormone deficiency
Arthritic disorders
Juvenile arthritis
Rheumatoid arthritis
Genetic disorders
Turner's syndrome (ovarian agenesis)
Down's syndrome
Metabolic disorders
Hemocystinuria
Marfan's syndrome
Ehlers-Danlos syndrome
Menkes syndrome
Riley-Day syndrome
Cystic fibrosis
Blood disorders
Wallerstrom's macroglobulinemia
Lymphoma
Leukemia
Multiple myeloma
Heparin therapy
Malnutrition
Anorexia nervosa
Scurvy
Protein deficiency

are diagnosed as a result of single or multiple fractures, frequently years after the bone disorder has been causing bone loss. The localization of the fractures may determine a characteristic gait. Hip fractures or aseptic necrosis may produce a waddling gait. The fractures occur most frequently in the long bones of the limbs, vertebral bodies, and the ribs, with the feet, sternum, and skull rarely affected.

C. Skeletal Deformities

Typical skeletal deformities are characteristic of some types of osteoporosis. In epiphyseal osteolysis, the clinical features of foreshortened, clawlike hands and feet with joint stiffness and contractures allow the clinician to suspect the syndrome. In osteogenesis imperfecta congenita, the presence of "wormian bones" in the skull is very characteristic. Marked kyphosis known as Scheuermann's kyphosis is considered a manifestation of juvenile osteoporosis (6).

D. Growth Retardation

Growth retardation is found in children with osteoporosis. It appears to be due to two factors: the disruption of the growth plate due to the osteoporotic process, and skeletal deformities and fractures. Compression fractures of the vertebrae and kyphosis determine loss of stature, with the trunk becoming shortened. Measurement of the arm span may be of value in estimating height loss. Growth retardation is marked in the most severe cases of osteoporosis.

IV. LABORATORY EXAMINATIONS

A. Serum Concentrations of Calcium, Phosphorus, and Alkaline Phosphatase

Serum concentrations of calcium, phosphorus, and alkaline phosphatase are normal in most children with osteoporosis. An exception has been the hypercalcemia found in the acute osteoporosis of disuse in children. Some diseases that occur secondary to osteoporosis may show characteristic changes in serum levels of phosphorus. In Cushing's disease, for example, the serum phosphate level is low due to the effect of corticoids in the renal tubule lowering tubular reabsorption of phosphate.

Urine calcium measurements are also of little value in the diagnosis of osteoporosis. Hypercalciuria is found in osteoporosis of immobilized children (7). Normal urine calcium excretion in children has been reported to be less than 4 mg/kg body weight per 24 hr (8,9). The urinary calcium–creatinine concentration ratio is a good index for screening the hypercalciuria. The normal values varies between ambulatory children (10) and hospitalized and partially immobilized children (11).

There is increased fecal calcium excretion in osteoporosis. It has been observed in patients with idiopathic juvenile osteoporosis (12) and osteoporosis of immobilization (13). The increase in fecal calcium in osteoporosis appears to be due to a diminution in dietary calcium absorption and not to an increase in calcium secreted into the intestine (14,15). The difficulty in measuring fecal calcium and in doing calcium balance studies makes this measurement useless for the clinician.

Serum alkaline phosphatase levels are normal or slightly above the norm for age, with a temporary elevation occurring following fractures.

B. Serum Concentrations of Osteocalcin

Human osteocalcin is a calcium-2^+-binding protein of bone matrix (16–18), which contains three carboxyglutamic acid (Gla) residues among its 49 amino acids at positions 17, 21, and 24 (17). The amino acid Gla side chain is directly involved in Ca^{2+} binding and the absorption of osteocalcin to hydroxylapatide surfaces in vivo and in vitro (18). Osteocalcin is present in developing bone at the onset of mineralization and may participate in bone formation (19). It may come from the proteolytic processing of a higher-molecular-weight "prohormone" (20). Osteocalcin can be detected in serum by radioimmunoassay (21) and its concentration may correlate with metabolic bone diseases (21); high plasma levels are observed in growing children (22). The synthesis of osteocalcin appears to be modulated by vitamin D. The bones of vitamin-D_3-deficient chicks contain 50% less osteocalcin than normal bones (23). The renal metabolite of vitamin D_3, 1,25$(OH)_2$-D_3, stimulates osteocalcin synthesis and secretion in osteosarcoma cells in culture (24). The administration of 1,25$(OHO)_2$-D_3 to experimental animals results in an elevation in serum osteocalcin levels (25). Children with X-linked hypophosphatemia and autosomal recessive vitamin-D-dependent rickets have elevated plasma osteocalcin levels during treatment with 1,25$(OH)_2$-D_3 (26). However, osteocalcin is elevated in renal failure patients receiving hemodialysis (27) when 1,25$(OH)_2$-D_3 levels are presumably low or absent.

Osteocalcin plays an important role in the regulation of mineral deposition and remodeling of bone. Studies of plasma levels of this peptide are helpful to our understanding of some of the underlying changes observed in metabolic bone diseases and provide a biochemical marker to monitor the effects of therapy with agents such as calcitonin, vitamin D_3, and calcitriol. We have found plasma osteocalcin levels to be elevated in patients with osteogenesis imperfecta (28) and to return to normal levels during treatment with calcitonin (29). In all types of rickets we have found decreased plasma osteocalcin levels (30), and a rapid increase in plasma osteocalcin concentrations (20,31) during treatment with vitamin D_3 or calcitriol. Thus, plasma osteocalcin concentrations can differentiate between osteoporosis of osteogenesis imperfecta and osteomalacia

Table 2 Plasma Osteocalcin Concentrations in Bone Disease

Bone Disease	Decrease	Elevated	Treatment
Osteoporosis			
Osteogenesis imperfecta		X	Calcitonin
hGH deficiency	X (or normal)		hGH
Juvenile idiopathic		X or normal	?
Osteomalacia			
Rickets	X		Vitamin D_3 Calcitriol

secondary to rickets, and allow the clinician to follow up the response to treatment with calcitonin or vitamin D_3 (Table 2). In some other types of osteoporosis, due to growth hormone deficiency, for example, serum plasma levels of osteocalcin have been reported to be lower compared to those of normal children and to increase towards normal with treatment with human growth hormone (32). In juvenile idiopathic osteoporosis, plasma osteocalcin concentrations have been reported to be normal or elevated (33).

V. RADIOLOGICAL EXAMINATION

A. Qualitative Radiography

Visual radiography is a poor technique for the early diagnosis of osteoporosis. On radiologic examination, osteoporosis shows increased radiolucency of bones. For a radiologist to be able to diagnose osteoporosis visually, loss of over 30% of bone mass is needed to detect the abnormality (34). In children, a constant increase in bone density as the child grows (35) is another cause of difficulty in diagnosing osteoporosis visually. Also, the skeletal mass is greater in males than females and greater in blacks than whites (36), creating another variable that is difficult to evaluate visually. In generalized osteoporosis, different bones may reflect the osteoporotic process with different intensity (37).

B. Quantitative Measurements

There are different methods for quantitating bone density (38). We have been using the radiographic method of photodensitometry (absorptiometry) of Colbert et al. (39,40). By using the left hand and wrist, one can simultaneously measure bone age and bone density. This method automatically compares the minimal value of the patient's middle phalanges with that of age- and sex-matched peer norms. A computer-controlled microdensitometer scans 1 mm "slices" of the image of each phalanx on a conventional nonscreen radiograph of the hand and wrist. For the baseline study and each subsequent determination, a pair of radiographs (exposed at 50–60 kvp) is obtained with an aluminum alloy reference wedge included in the field to permit correction for day-to-day variation in radiographic exposure and energy spectrum. The ratio of bone image area is the mineral concentration, expressed in computer units. The diagnosis of osteoporosis requires radiological evidence of bone loss greater than the normal skeletal mass for the age, race, and sex of the individual.

The mineral content of long bones may also be estimated by photon absorptiometry (41), computer tomography (42–43), and Compton photon-scattering technique (44). Other methods requiring bone biopsy are of limited use in children with osteoporosis. Qualitative methods are available (45). A morphometric quantitative method for measuring bone structure has been developed (46). This method measures only the portion of bone removed by biopsy. To follow the progress of the disease and response to treatment, repeat biopsies are needed. The difficulties in doing bone biopsies on children with osteoporotic bones considerably limit its use for research.

VI. OSTEOGENESIS IMPERFECTA

Osteogenesis imperfecta is an inherited disorder of connective tissue that primarily affects the skeletomuscular system. The genetic disorder causes generalized osteoporosis. The generalized osteoporosis determines bone fragility, multiple fractures, and deformities of the skeleton.

The other main clinical features are dwarfism, blue sclerae, dentinogenesis imperfecta, deafness, hypermobility of extremities, bruisability, excessive sweating, and muscle weakness.

The disease varies considerably in severity. Mildly affected individuals may only be detected when they see a physician because of short stature or sustain a fracture as a result of surprisingly mild trauma.

A. Classification

Two clinical varieties have been identified: the congenital and the tarda forms (Table 3). In osteogenesis imperfecta congenita, the osteoporosis is already present in utero and is so severe that minor trauma to the fetus produces numerous intrauterine fractures. The infant is born with multiple fractures at different stages of callus formation. The cranium is soft and membraneous. There are multiple wormian bones in the caput membranaceum. The extremities are short and clumsy. The affected infant has a characteristic appearance with striking micromelia and disproportionately large head (Fig. 1).

In osteogenesis imperfecta tarda, the disease is not apparent at birth, but fractures and deformities appear during or after the first year of life (Figs. 2 and 3). Falvo et al. (47) propose that the tarda group be subdivided according to the

Table 3 Classification of Osteogenesis Imperfecta

Clinical type[a] Congenita Tarda type I Tarda type II	Inheritance	Clinical findings
Genetic[b]		
Type I	Autosomal dominant	Bone fragility and blue sclerae. Scoliosis and growth retardation. Hearing loss. Walking independently.
Type II	Autosomal dominant or recessive	Marked bone fragility in utero. Blue sclerae Perinatal death
Type III	Autosomal dominant or recessive	Bone fragility and growth retardation. Mild blue sclerae
Type IV	Autosomal dominant	Osteoporosis, bone fragility, and fractures with variable deformity of long bones. Normal sclerae

[a]From Ref. 47.
[b]Modified from Ref. 48.

existence of bowing of the long bones. Patients with osteogenesis imperfecta tarda associated with bowing are classified as having tarda type I (OIT I), the patients without bowing have tarda type II (OIT II).

Silence et al. (48) classify osteogenesis imperfecta into four groups, taking into consideration the tarda or congenita type, mode of inheritance, and presence of blue sclerae. More recently, as clinical studies have progressed, both type I and type IV have been expanded to include varieties in which dentinogenesis imperfecta is either present or absent; autosomal dominant and autosomal recessive varieties have been included in type III; type II is now thought to be heterogeneous (49).

The attempts to classify osteogenesis imperfecta clinically are important. Most of the genetic diseases have at first appeared to be simple homogeneous entities, but as more biochemical and genetic knowledge about the disorder is obtained, several fundamentally distinct disorders are differentiated. An example has been the mucopolysaccharidoses. These were previously called Hurler's syndrome and considered a single entity. The clinical classification helps the clinician to predict the natural history of an infant with osteogenesis imper-

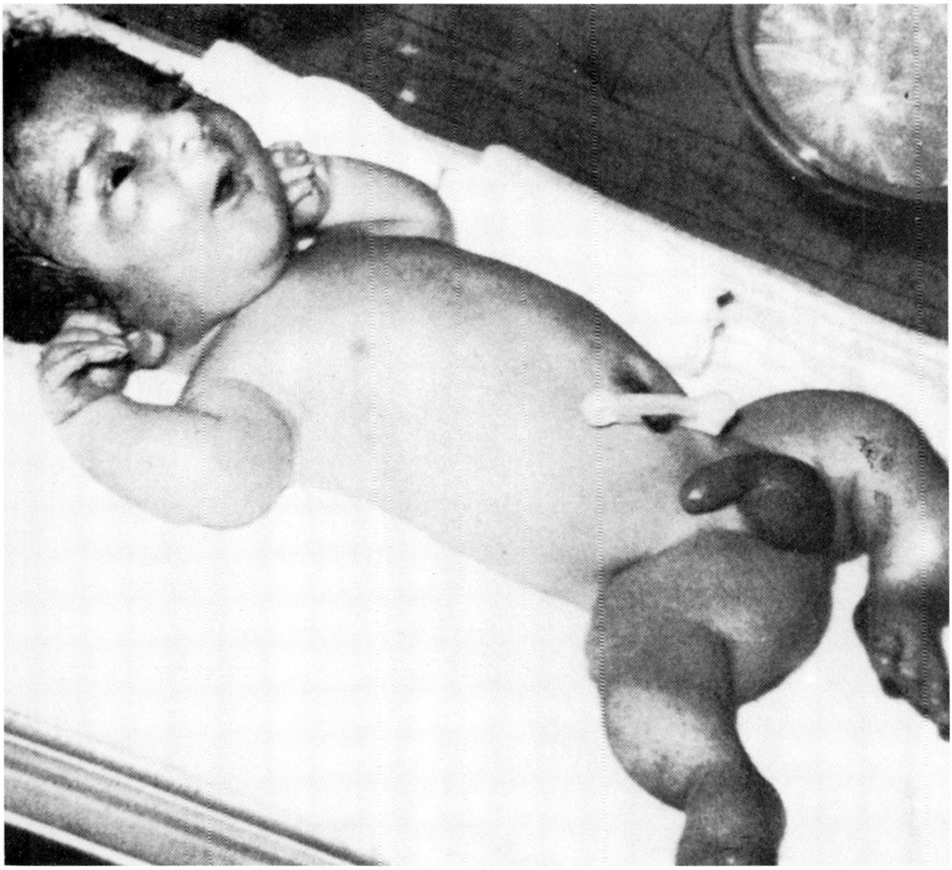

Figure 1 A typical case of osteogenesis imperfecta congenital. Numerous fractures were present at birth, at different stages of healing. There was no family history of osteogenesis imperfecta. The patient was treated at age 7 months with sodium fluoride for 6 months. There was no evidence of clinical or radiological improvement.

fecta, although it is still difficult to determine which infants with the congenital form may survive for a few days, weeks, or years. The clinical classification does not yet provide a basis to determine the type of inheritance. We hope that the biochemical studies of collagen metabolism in osteogenesis imperfecta will finally provide a way to put together the clinical, genetic, and biochemical groups.

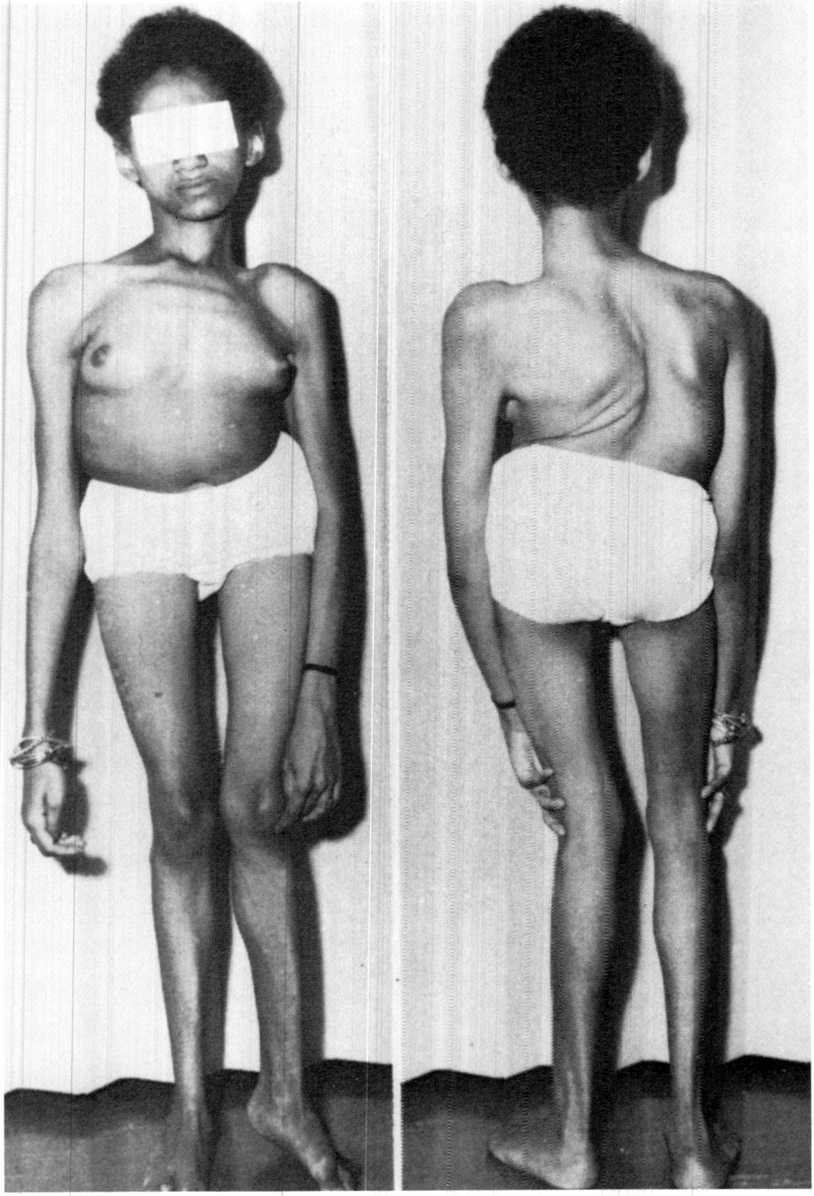

Figure 2 A 19-year-old woman with skeletal deformities seen in patients with osteogenesis imperfecta. She became pregnant and delivered an infant by cesarean section.

The frequency of osteogenesis imperfecta has been determined accurately for Edinburgh to be 5.77 × 10^{-5} (50), in Sweden to be 4.0 × 10^{-5} (51), and in Australia 3.5 × 10^{-5} (48). The overall frequency for osteogenesis imperfecta identifiable at birth is therefore around 1:20,000 total births.

B. Biochemical and Genetic Basis

Osteogenesis imperfecta is a disease of the connective tissue, with abnormalities in the structure or biosynthesis of the fibrillar collagens. The discovery in the last few years of heterogeneity of the collagens and the biosynthetic steps leading to fibrillogenesis (52,53) explains the variable degrees of expressivity and clinical complexity of the inherited connective tissue disorders. Osteogenesis imperfecta is considered at the present time to be, with Ehlers-Danlos syndrome, Marfan's syndrome, and possibly the chondrodystrophies, a genetic disorder of collagen structure and biosynthesis.

A number of osteogenesis imperfecta types have been extensively studied at the biochemical molecular levels of collagen structure and biosynthesis.

In type I osteogenesis imperfecta (Table 3), with blue sclerae and marked bone fragility, the structural collagen lesion appears to be due to quantitative defects in the production of type I procollagen (54,55). In this type of osteogenesis imperfecta, there is a decreased synthesis of the chain pro $\alpha 1$ (54), which results in decreased synthesis of mature triple helical type I collagen molecules. The mechanism for decreased synthesis appears to be to a decrease in RNA for pro $\alpha 1$ chain. In type II osteogenesis imperfecta, the lethal perinatal type (Table 3), there is decreased secretion of type I procollagen. A proportion of this procollagen has an abnormal structure. The cell strains studied from infants with type II osteogenesis imperfecta have revealed different disturbance in collagen structure (57–64).

There are several ways in which such abnormalities might arise at the genetic level. At the present time a collagen gene deletion appears to be the most likely (65–69) for pro $\alpha 1$ (I) and for pro α-2 (70). In type III osteogenesis imperfecta (Table 3), our knowledge of the molecular abnormalities is not well understood. Abnormal synthesis of type I procollagen (71) and a defect in assembling $\alpha 1$ (I) chains into type I procollagen molecules with secreted type I procollagen containing only pro α I chains have been described (71–74).

The type IV osteogenesis imperfecta (Table 3) is marked by a biochemical alteration in the type $\alpha 2$ (I) chain (75–76), suggesting a mutation in the pro α (I) collagen gene (77).

C. Biochemical Basis of the Osteoporotic Process in Osteogenesis Imperfecta

The osteoporotic process in osteogenesis imperfecta is due to increased bone resorption. Several studies (78–80) using tetracycline-based measurements of bone dynamics in patients with osteogenesis imperfecta have demonstrated an increased bone turnover at endosteal surfaces. We have undertaken the study of calcium kinetics in patients with osteogenesis imperfecta using ^{47}Ca. Our results also indicate that bone resorption in osteogenesis imperfecta is more generalized throughout the skeleton than has been demonstrated to date (81).

Radiocalcium turnover studies were performed on four patients, aged 4–13 years, with severe osteogenesis imperfecta, during a control period and during administration of calcitonin. A striking finding in these patients was a marked increase in the 24 hr exchangeable calcium pool, before calcitonin administration, compared to normal controls of the same age. The exchangeable calcium pool in mg/kg of body weight in the four patients with osteogenesis imperfecta was two to three times greater than in normal controls. Since an increase in exchangeable calcium pool often accompanies an increase in bone accretion rate, the osteoporotic process of osteogenesis imperfecta may result from a general increase in skeletal turnover, with resorption being more accelerated than bone accretion. Administration of salmon calcitonin reduced the exchangeable calcium pool size (81) (Fig. 4).

D. Natural History

The fractures in patient with osteogenesis imperfecta heal as fast as in normal individuals. In rare cases, osteosarcomas have appeared in patients with osteogenesis imperfecta (82).

Pregnancy has been reported in women severely deformed with osteogenesis imperfecta. We have had one such patient with severe skeletal deformities who delivered a normal infant by cesarean section (Fig. 4). The child returned to see us at age 12 years because of short stature. Densitometry studies revealed marked osteoporosis. She had only one fracture at age 12 years.

Patients with osteogenesis imperfecta improve considerably with pubertal development. There is a decrease in the incidence of fractures as puberty progresses, with a reappearance of fracturing after menopause. Serial measurements of bone density reveal an increase in bone density with puberty. The formation of bone matrix appears to be accelerated by sex hormones (83). The observation that the hormonal changes of puberty increase bone density and resistance to trauma should encourage researchers to find a therapeutic method to accomplish that before puberty in patients with osteogenesis imperfecta. Immobilization of a patient for treatment of fractures accentuates osteoporosis and contributes to fracturing.

Failure to grow is an important manifestation of the disease. It appears to correlate with the severity of the osteoporotic process. The marked shortness of the lower extremities is due in part to skeletal deformities, bowing, and multiple fractures of long bones. Also, multiple microfractures at the growth plate

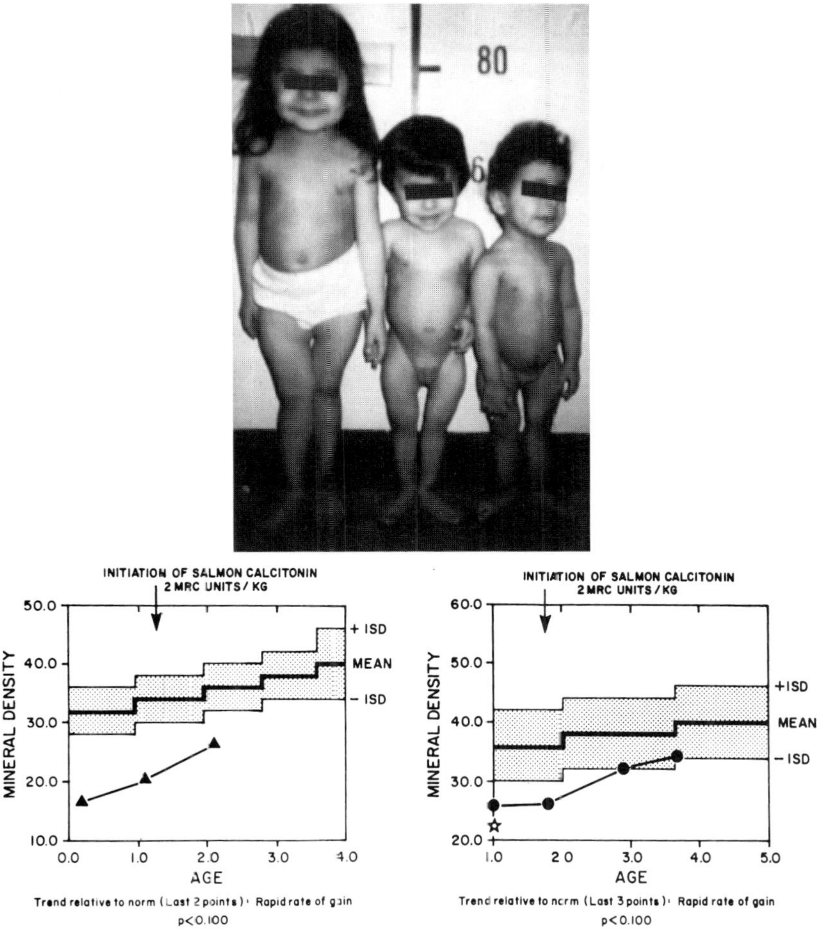

Figure 3 Three siblings with osteogenesis imperfecta tarda. Their father has osteogenesis imperfecta. The three siblings have blue sclerae, severe growth retardation, and skeletal deformities of the lower extremities. The oldest sibling, a 4-year-old-girl (left in photo), was started on salmon calcitonin at 2 MRC units/kg 3 days a week at age 22 months. Pins were placed on femurs to correct deformities on the right side; her bone density was markedly below normal for age and sex before treatment and increased to normal values after 2 years of therapy. The second sibling, a 2-year-old boy (center of photo), had markedly decreased bone density, which improved during 1 year of treatment with calcitonin. The third sibling, a 16-month-old girl with severe osteoporosis, has recently been started on calcitonin.

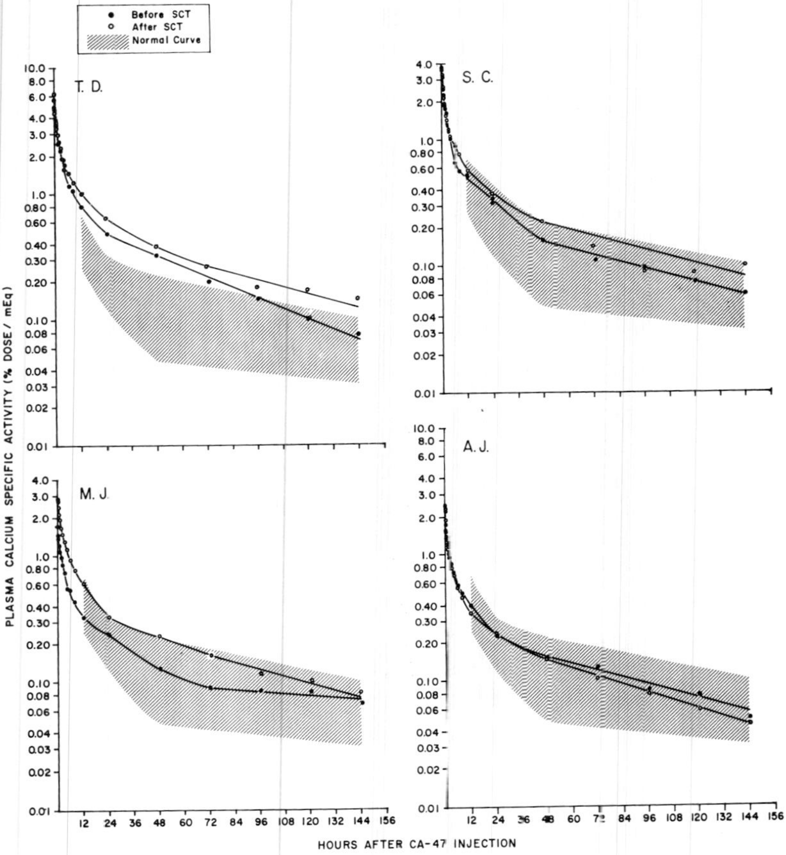

Figure 4 Plasma calcium specific activity curves in four patients with osteogenesis imperfecta (T. D., S. C., M. J., and A. J.). Closed circles represent data before calcitonin and open circles after 2–6 weeks of calcitonin. Cross-hatched area corresponds to values obtained in normal children by McPherson (McPherson, J. D. Estimation of the 24-hour exchangeable calcium pools in children using ^{48}Ca. *Acta Orthop. Scand. (Suppl.)* 78:189 [1985]) and Bronner (Bronner, F., Harris, R. S., Maletskos, C. J., and Benda, C. E. Studies of calcium metabolism: The fate of intravenously injected radiocalcium in human beings. *J. Clin. Invest.* 35:78 [1965]). The plasma calcium specific activity before calcitonin fell within the normal range in S. C., M. J., and A. J. In patient T. D., the plasma calcium-specific activity curve was above the normal range during the first 84 hr of the study. A decrease in radio calcium turnover during calcitonin was evident after at least 24 hr following radiocalcium injection in patients T. D., S. C., and M. J. The lack of significant response in radio calcium turnover in patient A. J. was probably due to the low dose of calcitonin administered.

may interfere with bone growth. Another important factor may be decreased responsiveness of the growth plate to growth factors. Plasma growth hormone and somatomedin levels have been reported to be normal in patients with osteogenesis imperfecta. We have seen several patients with no skeletal deformities, or history of fractures with marked short stature. The growth retardation in these patients can only be explained by an unresponsiveness of the growth plate to growth factors secondary to the osteoporotic process. Scoliosis and kyphoscoliosis may develop as a result of laxity of ligaments, as well as of vertebral osteoporosis. The vertebrae develop a characteristic "codfish" or "hourglass" deformity due to the pressure of the normally elastic nucleolus pulposus on the abnormally osteoporotic vertebrae. The scoliosis is often extreme and appears to progress during adolescence, when the number of fractures markedly decreases.

E. Prenatal Diagnosis

Prenatal osteogenesis imperfecta can be detected very early in the second trimester by sonographic studies (84-86). We have found the presence of osteocalcin in the amniotic fluid of normal fetuses during the first weeks of pregnancy (unpublished data). The fetus with osteogenesis imperfecta might have elevated amniotic fluid levels of osteocalcin compared to the normal fetus, similar to the elevated plasma osteocalcin levels found in osteogenesis imperfecta patients. If this theory is supported by present research, a biochemical index for prenatal osteogenesis imperfecta might be found.

F. Treatment

The management of patients with osteogenesis imperfecta includes medical and surgical treatment. The surgical treatment is discussed in a separate chapter.

Since the osseous manifestations greatly outweigh the other manifestations in clinical significance, all the attempts to treat the disease have been directed to correcting the generalized osteoporosis. It is expected that if mineralization of the bone can be increased, its resistance to trauma would improve. The primary difficulty is that the evaluation of therapeutic programs for children with osteogenesis imperfecta has been complicated by extreme differences in the clinical manifestations of bone fragility and variation in the natural course of the disease.

Other factors besides the disease itself affect the frequency of fractures: patient's activity, age, exposure to trauma, mobility, and degree of parental supervision.

Several forms of therapy have been used in the past and found to be of no beneficial value, such as treatment with thyroid hormone (87), parathyroid hormone (88), parathyroidectomy (89) and thymus extract (90,91).

1. Anabolic Steroids

The role of sex hormones in the treatment of osteogenesis imperfecta has been based on the clinical observation of a decrease in the incidence of fractures at puberty and an increase after the menopause. In osteogenesis imperfecta in cats, sex hormones have been reported to be beneficial (92). Since the effects of steroids on bone vary depending on the species studied (93), this observation may not be of value for humans. Cattell and Clayton (94) have studied the effects of different anabolic steroids in children with osteogenesis imperfecta. In their study there was no evidence that anabolic hormones produced increased retention of calcium by the skeleton. The drugs produced no dramatic alleviation of the disease, although a reduced incidence of fractures was observed in some patients. The use of anabolic steroids in their study produced severe side effects, such as masculinizing changes and short stature, by inducing early closure of the epiphysis.

Considering the severity of the side effects of anabolic steroids and their failure to produce increased deposition of calcium in the bone, it is our conclusion that they should not be administered either to children or adults with osteogenesis imperfecta.

2. Fluoride

The use of fluoride in the treatment of osteogenesis imperfecta is based on observations suggesting that sodium fluoride given over a prolonged period of time has beneficial effects in the treatment of osteoporosis (95-102), multiple myeloma (103,104), and Paget's disease (105-108).

Fluoride administration to osteoporotic patients at 0.4 mg/kg body weight per day or more frequently produced a decrease in urinary calcium excretion accompanied by an unaltered fecal and blood calcium level, suggesting an increase in skeletal deposition (109).

Purves (108) reported a decrease in ^{47}Ca deposition in osteoporotic bone after fluoride treatment, suggesting that fluoride induces new bone formation. Increased bone mass has been reported in adult osteoporotic patients treatment with fluoride (103).

Aeschlimann et al. (10) were the first to use sodium fluoride for the treatment of patients with osteogenesis imperfecta. They administered sodium fluoride to an infant from 1 month to 13 months of age in an attempt to modify the course of the disease. Sodium fluoride was given at a dosage of 0.3-0.7 mg/kg body weight daily. The calcium and phosphorus metabolic balances were not significantly altered by sodium fluoride therapy. Pierog et al. (111) administered 1 mg sodium fluoride/kg body weight daily to a 43-day-old baby with osteogenesis imperfecta congenita. The patient did well without evidence of new fractures during the period of treatment.

Bilginturan and Ozsolylu (112) gave sodium fluoride to several children with osteogenesis imperfecta. They reported radiological improvement of bone density during the treatment. Kuzemko (113) administered sodium fluoride at a dosage of 0.5–0.7 mg/kg body weight daily to a 20-month-old child with osteogenesis imperfecta.

Albright and Grunt (114) treated 13 patients with osteogenesis imperfecta of differing degrees of severity with sodium fluoride. The dosage ranged from 0.25 to 0.90 mg/kg of body weight per day. Results of calcium and phosphorus balance studies did not vary significantly during the period of sodium fluoride therapy. Although the incidence of fractures decreased in some patients during the period of fluoride therapy, the authors considered that the overall results did not warrant the general use of fluoride for the treatment of patients with osteogenesis imperfecta.

Our experience in the treatment of osteogenesis imperfecta with fluoride is limited to one case. This boy was born with multiple fractures of both upper and lower extremities and hydrocephalus. At age 7 months, he was placed on 0.5 mg/kg body weight per day of sodium fluoride. The therapy was continued for 6 months with no radiological or clinical improvement (Fig. 1).

Can fluoride be considered a therapeutic agent in osteogenesis imperfecta? Evidence at present is negative. Even if the reports of increased bone density during fluoride therapy are taken without question, the value of the new bone formed by fluoride stimulation is subject to debate. Histological examination shows that the new bone formed during fluoride administration is poorly organized and poorly mineralized, raising questions about its strength (115). There is also evidence that fluoride depresses collagen formation. Rats given fluorinated water to drink exhibited a decreased rate of collagen formation and a decreased total amount of collagen (116). Fluoride added to the media of bone cultures reduced the incorporation of [^{14}C]proline in protein (117). The decrease in the rate of collagen formation by fluoride administration could be a severe handicap in the therapeutic use of fluoride in children with osteogenesis imperfecta. Normal growth and maturation of the skeleton require an optimal mechanism of collagen formation. Furthermore, children with osteogenesis imperfecta may already have a genetic impairment in collagen formation, as previously discussed; further interference in collagen metabolism by fluoride may be detrimental to skeletal growth.

3. *Magnesium Oxide*

The use of magnesium oxide for the treatment of osteogenesis imperfecta is based on the work of Solomons and Styner (118). It was found that the bone collagen of patients with osteogenesis imperfecta is a potent inhibitor of calcification in vitro. This inhibition was removed by treatment of the collagen from patients with osteogenesis imperfecta with pyrophosphatase in the presence of magnesium ions. It was also found that serum and urinary levels of inorganic pyrophosphate were elevated in 281 patients with osteogenesis imperfecta. Oral administration of magnesium oxide to four of these patients reduced their serum and urinary levels of pyrophosphate.

It has been known for several years that both plasma and urine of normal individuals contain small quantities of inorganic pyrophosphate (119,120), a compound that strongly inhibits the precipitation of calcium phosphate in vitro. Fleish et al. (121,122) suggested that pyrophosphate might be one of the physiological regulators of calcification, with calcium phosphate deposition taking place only after the destruction of the pyrophosphate by pyrophosphatase, an enzyme present in large concentrations in calcifying tissues (123,124). The effect of magnesium in reducing pyrophosphate levels might be explained by the allosteric activation of pyrophosphatase (125).

Russell et al. (126) have reported normal levels of pyrophosphate in the serum and urine of patients with osteogenesis imperfecta. The results do not agree with those of Solomons and Styner (118), who claimed that patients with osteogenesis imperfecta had elevated serum and urine pyrophosphate concentrations.

Thus, the precise role of pyrophosphate metabolism in osteogenesis imperfecta is not clear. Nevertheless, Solomons (American Academy of Orthopedic Surgeons, 1961) has described in a preliminary report a decrease in fracture rate during the administration of magnesium oxide to patients with osteogenesis imperfecta. Magnesium oxide was administered orally at 10 mg/kg per day for 8 months, followed by an increase to 15 mg/kg per day for another 4 months.

4. *Calcitonin*

Calcitonin is a polypeptide hormone secreted in mammals by the parafollicular cells of the thyroid gland and in lower animals by the ultimobranchial body (127).

The major action of calcitonin is to inhibit bone resorption (128), which leads to a definite increase in total bone mass in experimental animals (129, 130). In adults, calcitonin seems to be more effective in treating diseases characterized by an abnormally high rate of bone resorption. Information on the prolonged effects of calcitonin in humans and its effectiveness as a therapeutic agent have recently been accumulated. Several investigators have reported favorable results of clinical trials of calcitonin in osteoporosis of adults (131,135), which is characterized by a low or normal bone formation but a high resorption rate. There is evidence that 50% or more of postmenopausal and idiopathic osteoporotic patients can expect sustained clinical improvement after treatment with calcitonin (136). In Paget's disease, which is characterized by high rate of bone turnover, the effects of calcitonin in clinical and biochemical parameters have been even more encouraging than in osteoporosis (137–140).

The possibility that calcitonin might also be beneficial in the treatment of osteogenesis imperfecta is based on the presence of increased bone resorption in osteogenesis imperfecta and the decrease in abnormally high bone absorption rates by calcitonin. Logic suggests that treatment directed at decreasing bone resorption may improve the osteopenia of osteogenesis imperfecta.

Our results indicating a reduction in the 24-hr exchangeable calcium pool during administration of salmon calcitonin in four patients with osteogenesis imperfecta seem to show that calcitonin decreased bone resorption in osteogenesis imperfecta (81) (Fig. 4).

Further evidence for inhibition in bone resorption by calcitonin is indicated by our findings (141–142) that administration of porcine calcitonin to patients with osteogenesis imperfecta tarda produced a retention of calcium and phosphorus and a decrease in urinary hydroxypyroline during treatment with calcitonin.

The absence of adverse reactions and the apparent improvement in the abnormal bone metabolism observed in patients with osteogenesis imperfecta treated with porcine and salmon calcitonin indicate that calcitonin administration in osteogenesis imperfecta may improve bone mineralization and decrease skeletal fragility.

Further evidence for increased bone resorption in osteogenesis imperfecta was given by our finding of increased bone collagenase before calcitonin administration in one patient and decreased collagenase during calcitonin therapy (143). Bone collagenase is considered an index of bone breakdown (144,145).

The pathophysiological events in osteogenesis imperfecta can be postulated to follow a certain order. Initially, there is a basic defect in the formation of the connective tissue of bone matrix. The defect in bone matrix accelerates the rate of bone turnover. The increased skeleton turnover results in bone of further poor architectural quality.

Synthetic salmon calcitonin, a peptide containing the same number and linear sequence of amino acids as calcitonin extracted from the ultimobranchial glands of salmon, has been found to have a more potent and longer-lasting effect than calcitonin obtained from porcine thryoid. Salmon calcitonin may provide a more convenient and more effective form for long-term therapy of osteogenesis imperfecta than porcine calcitonin.

We have treated 50 patients with osteogenesis imperfecta with synthetic salmon calcitonin for several years. The patients were classified as having osteogenesis imperfecta congenita or tarda (type 1 and 2) according to the clinical classifications of Falvo et al. (47). There was a significant improvement in fracture rate and bone density during treatment with salmon calcitonin (146). Figure 3 shows three siblings with osteogenesis imperfecta, two of whom have been treated over periods of 1 and 2 years, with marked clinical improvement and increase bone density.

VII. JUVENILE PAGET'S DISEASE OF BONE

Paget's disease usually is not detected before the age of 40 years. Although uncommon in children and adolescents, there have been several cases reported in children (147-149).

Initially there is excessive bone resorption followed by excessive and disorganized new bone formation. Paget's disease goes through various phases of activity and may become dormant. The first phase is characterized by increased osteoclastic activity, followed soon by overactive osteoblastic activity. Bone formation and bone destruction follow. In the second phase, hyperactive osteoclasts resorb bone at a very rapid rate. In the next phase (mixed), the osteoclasts and osteoblasts are hyperactive.

The cause of Paget's disease is unknown, but recent data support the belief that the disorder results from a slow viral infection that occurs years before the clinical manifestations appear. Intranuclear and cytoplasmic inclusions have been found in osteoclasts of patients with Paget's disease, suggesting such a viral cause (150).

Serum alkaline phosphatase concentrations are elevated and high rates of urinary hydroxyproline excretion occur. Radiological evidence for abundant bone formation, with thickening of the cortex, osteosclerosis, and osteoporosis, is characteristic. Bone biopsy in children reveals resorption and formation of bone, as described in adult patients with Paget's disease.

Calcitonin has been found to be effective in the treatment of adult patients with Paget's disease (151,152). Similar results have been reported in the juvenile form (147-153).

The differential diagnosis of juvenile Paget's disease is congenital hyperphosphatasia (hyperostosis corticolis deformans juvenilis). The disease is a rare disorder of children, characterized by high serum alkaline phosphatase concentration, and increased urinary hydroxypyroline excretion with lack of normal cortical remodeling and bone deformities. In juvenile Paget's disease, the classic mosaic pattern is characteristic and is not seen in cases of congenital hyperphosphatasia.

VIII. OSTEOLYTIC DISEASES

Osteolytic diseases are manifest by accelerated destruction of bone, which localize mainly in the extremities (Table 4).

In the advanced form of the disease there are characteristic deformities of the hands and feet, which appear foreshortened and clawlike. There is a progressive

Table 4 Types of Osteolytic Disease

Carpal and tarsal osteolysis
Cranioskeletal dysplasia with acro-osteolysis
Acro-osteolysis alone
Multicentric osteolysis
Hereditary
Nonfamilial with nephropathy
Massive osteolysis
Angiomatosis of bone (lymphangiomatosis, hemangiomastosis) with osteolysis
Skin lesions and corneal opacities with osteolysis (Winchester syndrome)
Selective muscle fiber hypoplasia and epiphyseal osteolysis

shortening of the limbs, which makes the term "vanishing limbs" appropriate. The joints are swollen, tender, and stiff. Fractures are frequently present and kyphoscoliosis is found in many patients. Growth retardation is marked.

Roentgenographic studies show osteoporosis with destruction of the distal portion of long bones.

A. Types

1. Carpal and Tarsal Osteolysis

One type, cranioskeletal dysplasia with acro-osteolysis maxillae, is inherited as an autosomal dominant trait with variable expressivity (154–159). The syndrome consists of dissolution of the terminal phalanges of the hands and feet, associated with specific skull deformities. The cranial deformities are dolichocephaly with multiple wormian bones, delayed closure of cranial sutures, absence of frontal sinuses, and small maxillae. A prominent occipital ridge, skeletal demineralization, vertebral and long bone fractures, joint laxity, and thick and coarse hair are also present. In another type, the acro-osteolysis presents with only the deformity of fingers and toes.

2. Multicentric Osteolysis

In this disorder the disease is manifest as an autosomal recessive trait (160–162). There is a second type in which the multicentric osteolysis is associated with nephropathy (163–166). The disease process can involve any skeletal site and is characterized by progressive shortening of the limbs with severe deformities of the joints.

3. Massive Osteolysis

This appears to be nonfamilial and in some cases trauma and fractures have preceded the osteolytic process (167).

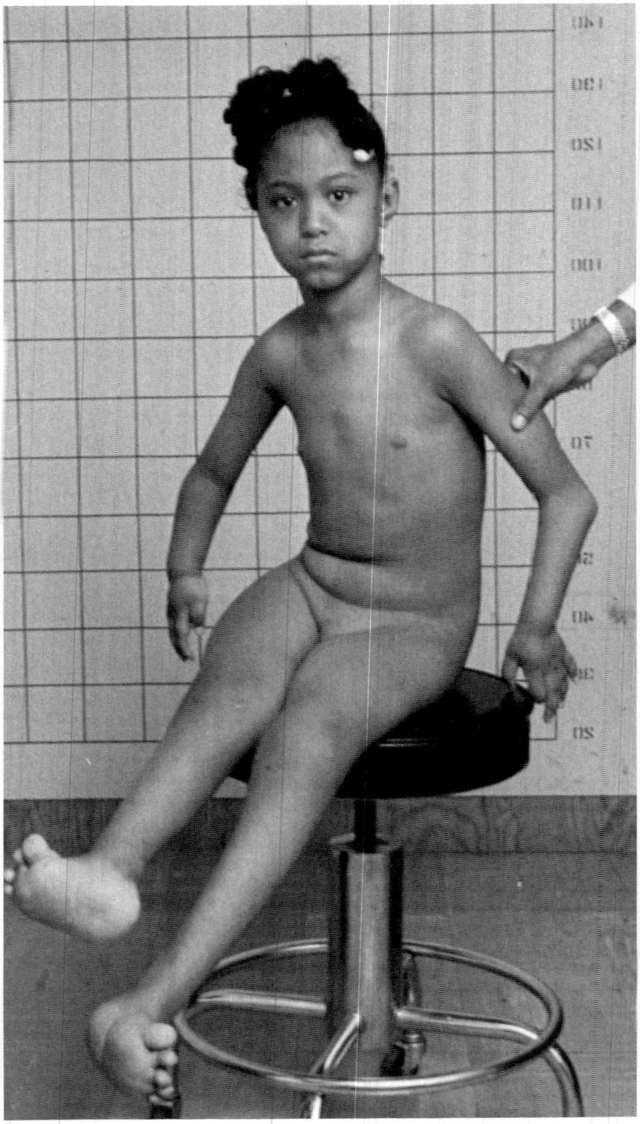

Figure 5 Patient with osteolytic disease and muscle hypoplasia. The foreshortened clawlike hands and feet are characteristic. There is also marked stiffness of lower and upper extremities and an inability to stand.

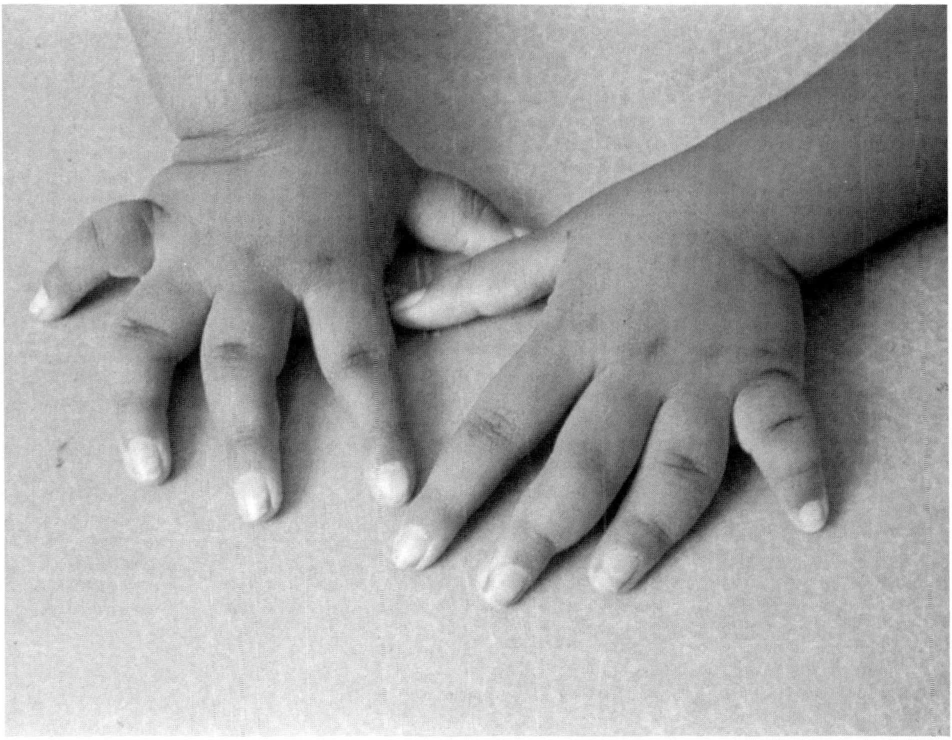

Figure 6 Small, foreshortened, clawlike hands.

4. Osteolysis Associated with Hemangiomatosis of Bone (168).

5. Winchester Syndrome

This is associated with dissolution of the carpal and tarsal bones, generalized osteoporosis, coarsened facial features, thickened and hypertrichotic skin, corneal opacities, and joing stiffness and contractures (169–171). Biopsy of the skin lesions in the Winchester syndrome reveals considerable diffuse proliferation of fibroblasts deep in the dermis, with highly vacuolated mitochondria (172).

6. Epiphyseal Osteolysis and Selective Muscle Fiber Hypoplasia (173)

One patient described by us was found to have clinical features of foreshortened, clawlike hands and feet, joint stiffness, and contractures with severe joint pain and muscle atrophy. A selective muscle fiber hypoplasia affecting types I

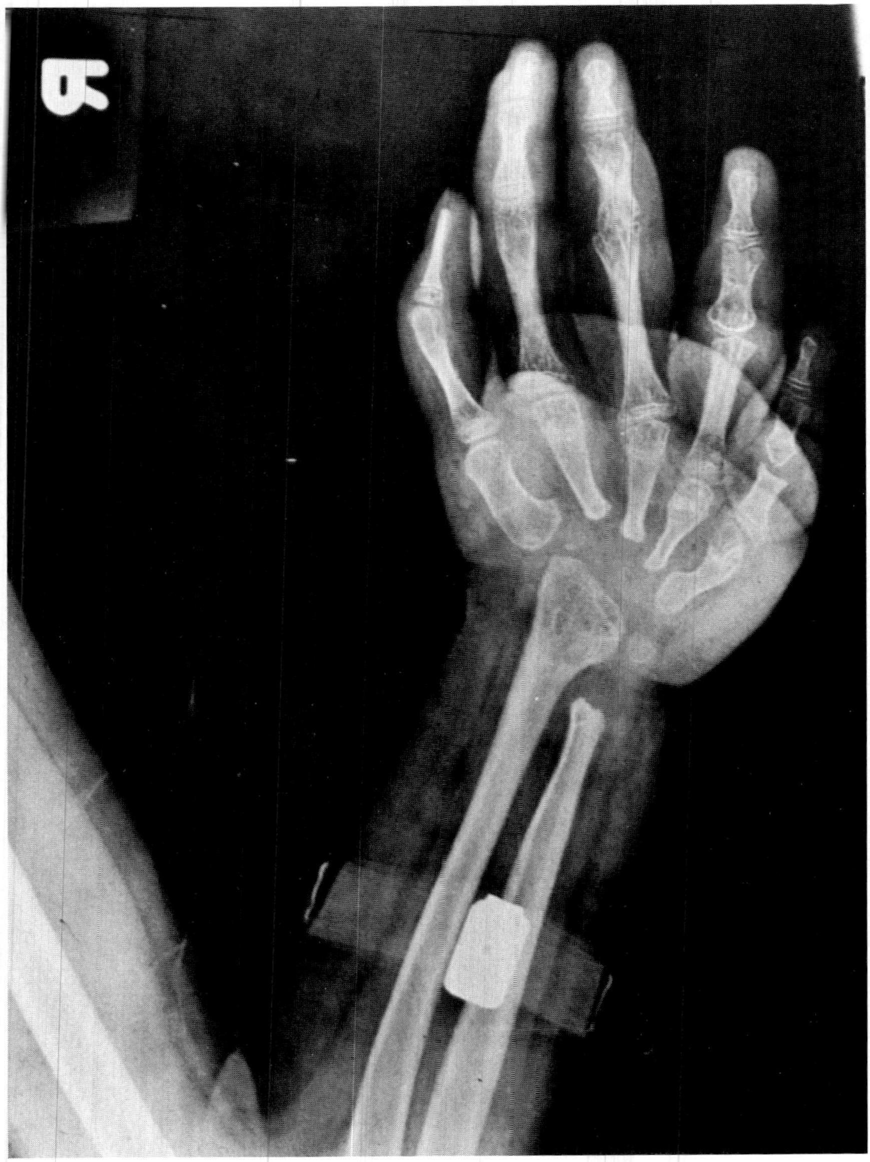

Figure 7 The carpals are almost totally destroyed, with erosion of the proximal metacarpals and the distal portion of the radius and ulna. Severe generalized osteoporosis is present in all bone.

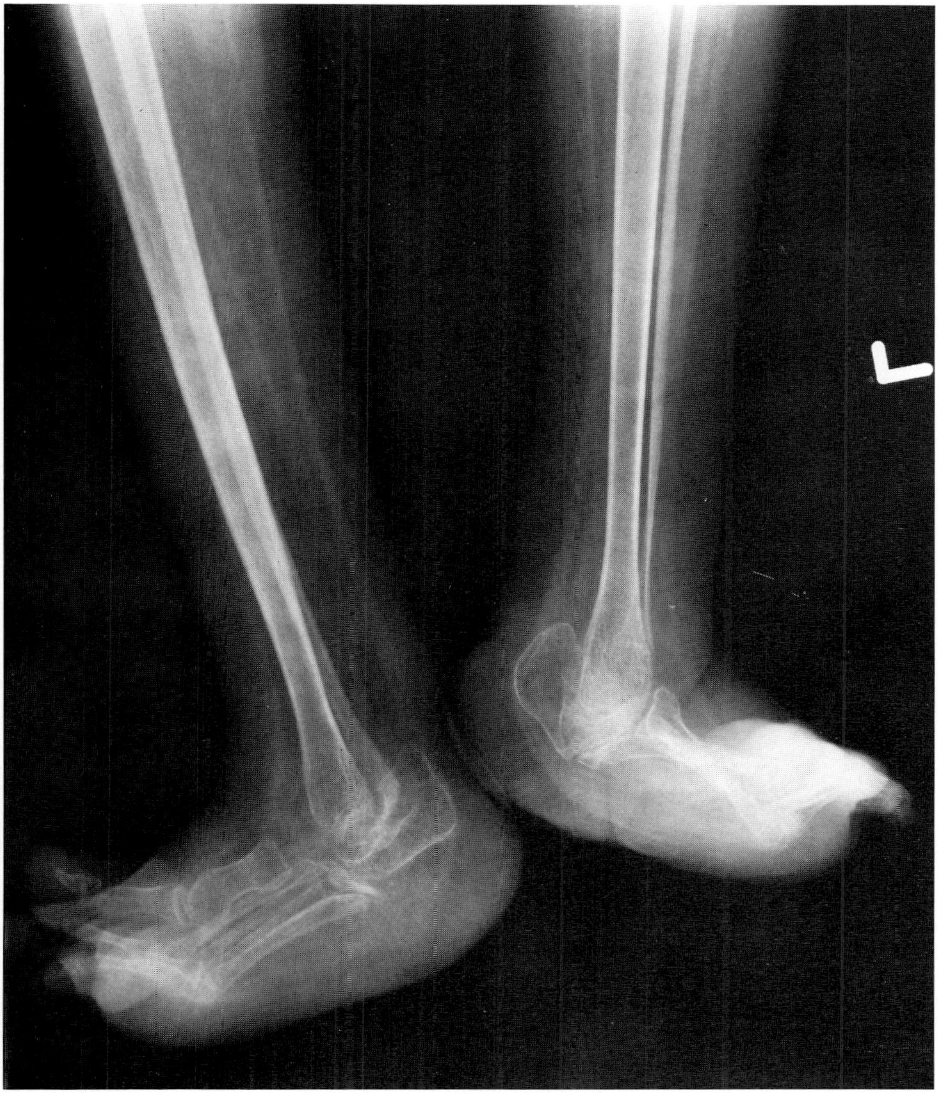

Figure 8 The tarsals and metatarsal bones are destroyed. Severe generalized osteoporosis is present.

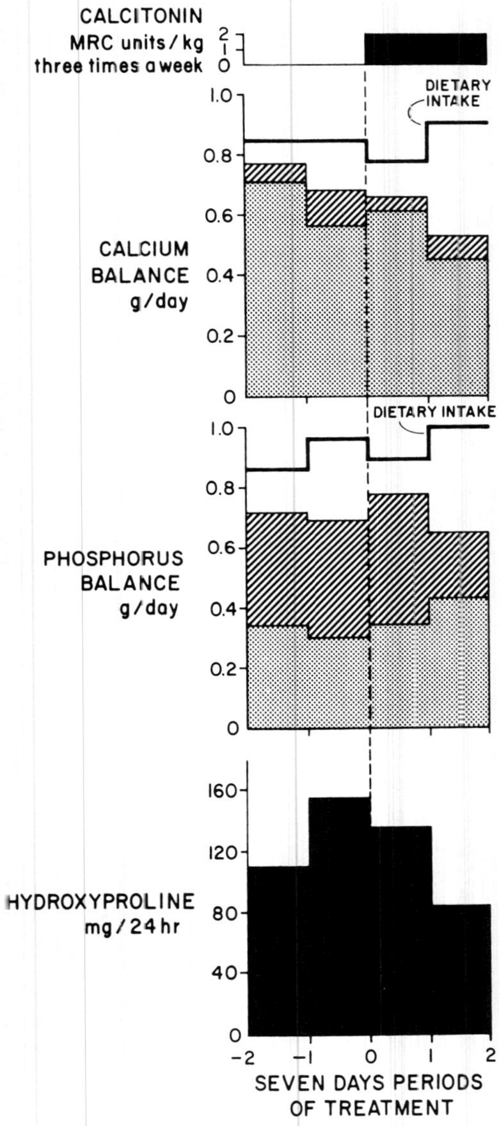

Figure 9 Calcium and phosphorus balance studies and 24 hr urinary hydroxyproline excretion rate two weeks before and two weeks during calcitonin treatment. Fecal excretion is represented by a stipped area and urinary excretion is represented by a cross-hatched area. The clear space below the dietary intake line in calcium balance became markedly increased by the second week of calcitonin therapy.

and IIA fibers was found to be associated with the marked osteolytic process (Fig. 5-8).

B. Etiopathology

There is increased bone resorption in patients with osteolysis. One patient studied by us had an increaed exchangeable calcium pool of 17.20 g (normal in control children, 9.70 ± 2.4) (173).

The cause of the accelerated osteolytic process is unknown. It may be due to multiple causes, including a genetic disorder, a biochemical abnormality of fibroblasts and muscle fibers, and renal and hemangiomatosis disorders.

C. Treatment

Physical therapy and orthopedic treatment of fractures and deformities have until now been the only available treatment modalities.

Calcitonin seems to be an effective medical treatment. We treated one patient with synthetic salmon calcitonin at 2 MRC units/kg for 3 days a week with oral supplementation of calcium. The patient had a marked improvement during calcitonin therapy, with marked amelioration of bone pain (173) (Fig. 9).

IX. IDIOPATHIC JUVENILE OSTEOPOROSIS

Idiopathic juvenile osteoporosis is a rare disorder of prepubertal children that manifest clinically between the ages of 8 and 14 years. Juvenile osteoporosis, compared with postmenopausal or senile osteoporosis, is uncommon. The disorder may be more common if kyphosis is taken as a manifestation of the disease (174). More boys than girls (3:1) seem to be affected (175). From evidence available at the present time, there is no suggestion of a hereditary factor.

A. Clinical Manifestations

The appearance of bone pain seems to be the main symptom. This can be localized in the lower extremities, which increases further with walking. It is described by patients as a constant dull ache, which makes walking difficult. Another frequent localization of the pain is the spine. The backache is generalized.

In other cases, the clinical onset of the disease is manifested by a fracture of one or more bones, usually due to minimal trauma. Metaphyseal impaction fractures cause the knee and ankle pains. The presence of swelling may make the differentiation of this disorder from arthritis difficult. Some patients manifest deformities of the long bones due to malalignment of poorly treated fractures.

Table 5 Differentiation Between Idiopathic Juvenile Osteoporosis (IJO) and Osteogenesis Imperfecta (OI)

	IJO	OI
Family history	Negative	May be positive
Onset	2–3 yrs before puberty	Birth or during 1–2 yr of life
Duration	1–4 yr, recovery after puberty	Lifelong
Clinical findings	Bone pain	Blue sclerae
	Fractures	Dentincgenesis imperfecta
	Kyphosis	Lax ligaments, deafness
Radiographic findings	Generalized osteoporosis	Generalized osteoporosis
	Normal length and width of long bones	Abnormally short, narrow, and deformed long bones
	Thin cortices	
	Metaphyseal fractures common	Metaphyseal fractures uncommon

Kyphosis appears to be present in all cases to a greater or lesser extent. In severe cases of lumbar-dorsal kyphosis, there is a protuberant stenum: a diminution of the separation between the lower ribs and the iliac crest. In most cases only temporary limitation of activity is present, but in a few cases patients have spent various periods of time in wheelchairs.

Growth impairment is found in some patients, but the ultimate height loss is small since the patients recover in a few years.

The differential diagnosis with osteogenesis imperfecta is important (Table 5). Scheuermann's kyphosis is considered to be a form of juvenile osteoporosis (174,175). Like idiopathic juvenile osteoporosis, it tends to be self-limiting and appears between the age of 8 and 15 years. The arcurate deformity of Scheuermann's juvenile kyphosis is caused by wedge-shaped deformities of the vertebrae (176).

B. Mechanism of the Osteoporotic Process

Roentgenographic and clinical studies seem to indicate that bone formation is normal and suggest a predominance of bone resorption over bone formation. Microradiographic studies indicate that there is an increase in resorption surface compared to that of age-matched controls (177). The clinical improvement coincides with a decrease in the abnormally increased bone resorption (178). However, other investigators using tetracycline labeling have reported reduction in bone formation rather than increased bone resorption (179).

Plasma calcium, phosphorus, and alkaline phosphatase levels have been reported normal in some patients, but some authors have found that plasma alkaline phosphatase and urinary total hydroxyproline levels were slightly increased in some patients compared with their age-matched controls (178).

During the active phase of the disease, calcium balance studies have been reported to be negative in the majority of patients (180–183), due to increased fecal calcium levels. Dent and Friedman (184) have also reported that the fecal calcium level was greater than the dietary calcium intake, suggesting a malabsorption of calcium from the bowel. Marder et al. (185) have reported low plasma calcitriol and normal serum calcitriol levels in one case of idiopathic juvenile osteoporosis. There was marked improvement with daily treatment with 1.0 μg calcitriol. Since calcitriol promotes calcium absorption from the intestine (186), a deficiency will produce a negative calcium balance with increased fecal calcium excretion, as has been found to occur in idiopathic juvenile osteoporosis.

C. Treatment

Dihydrotachisterol, vitamin D_2, or its active metabolites have been used to correct the calcium malabsorption in this disease (182–185). Since hypercalciuria has been reported in some cases, some clinicians have been reluctant to use vitamin D_2 or calcitriol in the treatment of idiopathic juvenile osteoporosis. Calcium supplements, to maintain a 1 g calcium intake, have been advocated. The use of sex hormones has been recommended based on the theoretical assumption that there is a temporary hormonal disturbance associated with the hormonal changes of puberty (9). No laboratory evidence for such an abnormality has been found. The main complication of administering sex hormones for this condition in children is dwarfism, and we do not advise the use of these agents at the present time. Calcitonin has been used in a few cases, with inconclusive results (7).

Because of the self-limited course of this disease and spontaneous recovery, we advise a conservative approach consisting of physical therapy, appropriate calcium intake, and vitamin D_2 supplementation in the diet.

X. OSTEOPOROSIS AND HYPERCALCEMIA FOLLOWING IMMOBILIZATION

Long-standing immobilization may produce bone demineralization, hypercalcemia, and occasionally diminished renal function (187–191). The symptoms of immobilization hypercalcemia may occur early or late during immobilization or may appear suddenly or insidiously. The symptoms include headaches (sometimes described as migraine attacks), anorexia, malaise, nausea and vomiting,

Table 6 Causes of Hypercalciuria in Children with Normal or Elevated Blood Calcium Levels

Normocalcemic	Hypercalcemic
Furosemide or ethacrynate sodium therapy	Immobilization
Corticosteroid therapy	Vitamin D intoxication
Distal renal tubular acidosis	Calcium gluconate therapy
Lead poisoning	Idiopathic hypercalcemia of infancy (Williams' syndrome)
Faconi's syndrome	
Wilson's disease	Subcutaneous fat necrosis in neonates
Syndrome of excess secretion of antidiuretic hormone	Hyperparathyroidism
Idiopathic hypercalciuria	Sarcoidosis
	Malignancy
	Tuberculosis

Source: Ref. 196.

abdominal pain, constipation, and weight loss. Polydipsia and polyuria may be found in some cases. If the patient is not treated, renal insufficiency, hypertension, seizures, and hearing loss may develop. Blood analysis shows elevated serum calcium concentrations with normal phosphorus levels, metabolic alkalosis, hypercalciuria, hyperphosphaturia, normal to elevated alkaline phosphatase levels, decreased glomerular filtration rates and creatinine clearance. Serum parathyroid hormone concentration has been found to be normal in all cases. The rise in serum calcium during immobilization is more clear when determinations of serum ionized calcium are made (192).

The osteoporosis and hypercalcemia of immobilization have been explained by an increase in bone resorption, with the rise in serum calcium coming from bone (193). There is also an increase in calcium excretion, which causes a negative calcium balance; more calcium is excreted than is taken in by diet (194).

Adolescence is a period of rapid bone growth during which accelerated bone formation and bone resorption occur. Root et al. (193) studied the kinetics of calcium metabolism utilizing nonradioactive strontium in an adolescent boy who fractured his femur and developed hypercalcemia secondary to immobilization. There was a decreased exchangeable pool of strontium and a decreased bone deposition rate. After he began walking there was a progressive increase in the exchangeable strontium pool and the serum calcium concentration returned to normal. The bone deposition rate increased after he became mobile again.

Bronner et al. (195) have reported similar results, with a decrease in bone deposition rate in subjects with scoliosis immobilized in a cast, while the rate of bone resorption increased. It appears that in immobilized children and adolescents the first response of the immobilized bone is increased bone resorption and decreased bone formation secondary to the loss of mechanical factors stimulating bone during ambulation. Hypercalcemia is a consequence of the increased rate of calcium resorption from bone. Following the loss of bone mineral, osteoporosis appears.

The diagnosis of this condition requires serial measurements of serum calcium, phosphorus, and alkaline phosphatase during immobilization. Urinary calcium excretion should also be evaluated. Normal urine calcium excretion in children is less than 4 mg/kg body weight/24 hr (196). The calcium-creatinine (Ca/Cr) concentration ratio (mg/mg), determined from a randomly collected urine sample, can be also used to screen for hypercalcuria.

Moore et al. (197) and Stapelton et al. (198) have shown that the normal Ca/Cr ratio in random urine samples of children from 3 months to 18 years of age is 0.66 ± 0.06 (mean ± SD). Ratios greater than 0.18 require a 24 hr urine collection to demonstrate urinary calcium excretion greater than 4 mg/kg body weight.

Calcium is filtered by the glomerulus and resorbed in the tubules. There is an increase in the filtered load of calcium in immobilized children, which is responsible for the hypercalciuria (191).

The differential diagnosis of hypercalcemia and hypercalciuria in children is given in Table 6.

The treatment of hypercalcemia and hypercalciuria is very important to prevent the severe complications of renal damage with hypertension and seizures. Osteoporosis and hypercalcemia of immobilization can be prevented by mobilization at the earliest possible time. Hypercalcemia responds quickly to weight-bearing mobilization. Recovery proceeds at a very rapid rate after walking is begun again (194), contrary to studies that question the reversibility of mineral loss due to immobilization (199). The use of oral phosphates to decrease serum calcium levels has been recommended in the treatment of hypercalcemia (200). Supplemental oral phosphate reduces urinary calcium excretion but does not prevent osteoporosis during immobilization (194), making oral phosphatase therapy of little value for the treatment of hypercalcemia of immobilization. Rapid diuresis induced by furosemide may be useful for short-term treatment of hypercalcemia (201). Furosemide, a potent natriuretic agent, also increases calcium excretion in direct proportion to sodium excretion (202). The careful replacement of water and electrolyte losses is essential. Steroid therapy, 25-40 mg/m^2 per 24 hr of prednisone for 1-2 weeks, is regarded as an effective treatment (191). Mithramycin also produces a decrease in serum calcium concentrations (203) by reducing bone resorption. We have found good results with the use of salmon calcitonin (Calcimar) at a dosage of 2-4 MRC units subcutaneously/kg body weight. The plasma calcium concentrations should be evaluated carefully and the administration of salmon calcitonin should be repeated if increases in plasma calcium concentrations occur to above the normal values.

REFERENCES

1. Pommer, G. *Rachitis and Osteomalacia*. Vogel, Leipzig (1885).
2. Pommer, G. *Arch. Klin. Chir.* 136:1 (1885).
3. Christiansen, C., Rodbro, P., and Nielsen, C. T. Bone mineral content and estimated total body calcium in normal children and adolescents. *Scand. J. Clin. Lab. Invest.* 35:501–510 (1977).
4. Riis, B. J., Krabbe, S., Christiansen, C., Catherwood, B. D., and Deftos, L. J. Bone turnover in male puberty: A longitudinal study. *Calcif. Tissue Int.* 37:213–217 (1985).
5. Garn, S. M., Gall, J. C., Jr., and Nagy, J. M. Preliminary radiogrammetric analysis of the bone recovery phase in adolescents with Down's syndrome. *Invest. Radiol.* 7:97–101 (1972).
6. Bradford, D. S., Brown, D. M., Moe, J. H., Winter, R. B., and Owsey, J. Scheuermann's kyphosis: a form of juvenile osteoporosis? *Clin. Orthop.* 118:10–15 (1976).
7. Langman, C. B., and Moore, E. S. Hypercalciuria in clinical pediatrics. *Clin. Pediatr.* 23:135–137 (1984).
8. Royer, P. Explorations biologiques due métabolisme calcique chez l'enfant. *Helv. Pediatr. Acta* 16:320 (1961).
9. Macy, I. *Nutrition and Chemical Growth in Childhood*. Charles C. Thomas, Springfield, IL, 1946, p. 138.
10. Moore, E. S., Coe, F. L., McMann, B. J., and Favus, M. J. Idiopathic hypercalciuria in children. Prevalence and metabolic characteristics. *J. Pediatr.* 92: 906–910 (1978).
11. Ghazali, S., and Barratt, T. M. Urinary excretion of calcium and magnesium in children. *Arch. Dis. Child.* 49:97 (1974).
12. Dent, C. E., and Friedman, M. Idiopathic juvenile osteoporosis. *Q. J. Med.* 34:177–210 (1965).
13. Heaney, R. P. Radiocalcium metabolism in diffuse osteoporosis in man. *Am. J. Med.* 33:188 (1962).
14. Rose, G. A. Immobilization osteoporosis: A study of the extent, severity and treatment with bendrofluazide. *Br. J. Surg.* 53:769 (1966).
15. Spencer, H., Menczel, J., Lewin, I., and Samachson, J. Absorption of calcium in osteoporosis. *Am. J. Med.* 37:223 (1964).
16. Price, P. A., Otsuka, A. A., Poser, J. W., Kristaponis, J., and Raman, N. Characterization of a γ-carboxyglutamic acid-containing protein from bone. *Proc. Natl. Acad. Sci. USA* 73:1447–1451 (1976).
17. Price, P. A., Otsuka, A., and Poser, J. W. Comparing γ-carboxyglutamic acid-containing proteins from bovine and swordfish bone: Primary structure

and Ca^{2-} binding. In *Calcium-Binding Proteins and Calcium Function.* (R. H. Wasserman, R. A. Corradino, E. Carafoli, R. H. Kretsinger, D. H. McLennan, and F. L. Siegel, eds.) North Holland, New York, 1977, pp. 333-337.

18. Hauschka, P. V., and Gallop, P. M. Purification and calcium-binding properties of osteocalcin, the γ-carboxyglutamate-containing protein of bone. In *Calcium-Binding Proteins and Calcium Function.* (R. H. Wasserman, R. A. Corradino, E. Carafoli, R. H. Kretsinger, D. H. McLenan, and F. L. Sieger, eds.). North Holland, New York, 1977, p. 338.
19. Hauschka, P. V., and Reid, M. L. Vitamin K dependence of a calcium-binding protein containing gamma carboxyglutamine acid in chicken bone. *J. Biol. Chem.* 253:9063-9068 (1978).
20. Nishimoto, S. K., and Price, P. A. Secretion of the vitamin K-dependent protein of bone by rate osteosarcoma cells. *J. Biol. Chem.* 255:6579-6583 (1980).
21. Price, P. A., Parthemore, J. G., and Deftos, L. J. New biochemical marker for bone metabolism: Measurement by radioimmunoassay of bone GLA protein in the plasma of normal subjects and patient with bone disease. *J. Clin. Invest.* 66:878-883 (1980).
22. Gundberg, C. M., Lian, J. B., and Gallop, P. M. Measurements of γ-carboxyglutamate and circulating osteocalcin in normal children and adults. *Clin. Chim. Acta* 128:1-8 (1983).
23. Lian, J. B., Glimcher, M. J., Roufosse, A. H., Hauschka, P. V., Gallop, P. M., Cohen-Solal, L., and Reit, B. Alteration of the carboxyglutamic acid and osteocalcin concentrations in the vitamin D-deficient chick bone. *J. Biol. Chem.* 257:4999-5003 (1982).
24. Price, P. A., and Baukol, S. A. 1,25-Dihydroxy-vitamin D_3 increases synthesis of the vitamin K-dependent bone protein by osteosarcoma cells. *J. Biol. Chem.* 255:11600-11603 (1980).
25. Price, P. A., and Baukol, S. A. 1,25-dihydroxy-vitamin D_3 increases serum levels of the vitamin K-dependent bone protein. *Biochem. Biophys. Res. Commun.* 99:928 (1981).
26. Gundberg, C. M., Cole, D. E. C., Lian, J. B., Reade, T. N., and Gallop, P. M. Serum osteocalcin in the treatment of inherited rickets with 1,25-dihydroxy-vitamin D. *J. Clin. Endocrinol. Metab.* 35:1063-1067 (1983).
27. Cole, D. E. C., Gundberg, C. M., Hanning, R. M., Hotkin, S. Y., Balfe, J. W., and Gallop, P. M. Clearance of osteocalcin by continuous ambulatory peritoneal dialysis in renal failure. *Am. Soc. Bone Mineral Res.* abstract (1983).
28. Castells, S., Yasumura, S., Fusi, M. A., Colbert, C., Bachtell, R. S., and Smith, S. Plasma osteocalcin levels in patients with osteogenesis imperfecta. *J. Pediatr.* 109:88-91 (1986).
29. Castells, S., Yasumura, S., Smith, S., and Casas, J. Calcitonin suppresses elevated plasma levels of osteocalcin in children with osteogenesis imperfecta. *Pediatric. Res.* 20:327A (1986).

30. Greig, F., Casas, J., and Castells, S. Changes in plasma osteocalcin concentrations during treatment of rickets. *J. Pediatr*. 114:820–823 (1989).
31. Castells, S., Greig, F., Fusi, M. A., Finberg, L., Yasumura, S., Lieberman, U. A., Eil, C., and Marx, S. J. Severely deficient binding of 1,25-dihydroxyvitamin D to its receptors in a patient responsive to high doses of this hormone. *Clin. Endocrinol. Metab*. 63:252–256 (1986).
32. Delmas, D. D., Chatelain, P., Malaval, L., and Bonne, G. Serum bone GLA-protein in growth hormone deficient children. *J. Bone Mineral Res*. 1:333–338 (1986).
33. Cole, D. E. C., Carperter, T. O., and Gundberg, C. M. Serum osteocalcin concentrations in children with metabolic bone disease. *J. Pediatr*. 106:770–776 (1985).
34. Wray, J. B., Sugarman, E. D., and Schneider, A. J. Bone composition in senile osteoporosis. *J.A.M.A*. 183:118–122 (1963).
35. Smith, D. A., Anderson, J. B., Shimmins, J., Speirs, C. E., and Barnett, E. Changes in metacarpal mineral content and density in normal male and female subjects with age. *Clin. Radiol*. 20:23–31 (1969).
36. Trotter, M., Broman, G. E., and Peterson, R. R. Densities of bones of white and negro skeletons. *J. Bone Joint Surg*. 42A:50–58 (1960).
37. Jowsey, J. Bone density measurement in metabolic diseases of bone. *Monogr. Clin. Orthop*. Vol. I, pages 96–114 (1977).
38. Steinbach, H. L. The roentgen appearance of osteoporosis. *Radiol. Clin. North Am*. 2:191 (1964).
39. Colbert, C., Spruit, J. J., and Davila, L. R. Biophysical properties of bone: Determining mineral concentration from the x-ray image. *Trans. NY Acad. Sci*. 30:271 (1967–1968).
40. Colbert, C., and Bachtell, R. S. Radiographic absorptiometry (photodensitometry). In *Non-Invasive Measurements of Bone Mass and Their Clinical Application*. (S. H. Cohn, ed.). CRC Press, Boca Raton, FL, 1981.
41. Cameron, J., and Sorensen, J. Measurement of bone mineral in vivo: An improved method. *Science* 142:230–232 (1963).
42. Revak, C. S. Mineral content of cortical bone measured by computed tomography. *J. Comput. Assist. Tomogr*. 4:342–350 (1980).
43. Wickman, G., and Wing, K. R. Bone mineralization control by CT scanning of the proximal tibia. *Calcif. Tissue Int*. 31:254 (1980).
44. Stein, H., Sabato, S., Leichter, I., Nir, D., and Weinreb, A. A new method of measuring bone density in the lower tibia of normal and post-injury limbs. *Clin. Ortho. Rel. Res*. 174:181–187 (1983).
45. Dempster, D. W., Shane, E., Horbert, W., and Lindsay, R. A simple method for correlative light and scanning electron microscopy of human iliac crest bone biopsies. Qualitative observations in normal and osteoporotic subjects. *J. Bone Mineral Res*. 1:15 (1986).
46. Teitelbaum, S. L. Pathological manifestations of osteomalacia and rickets. *Clin. Endocrinol. Metab*. 42:43–62 (1980).
47. Falvo, K. A., Root, L., and Bullough, P. G. Osteogenesis imperfecta: Clinical evaluation and management. *J. Bone Joint Surg*. 56A:783–793 (1974).

48. Silence, D. O., Senn, A., and Danks, D. M. Genetic heterogeneity in osteogenesis imperfecta. *J. Med. Genet.* 16:101–116 (1979).
49. Byers, P. H., Bonadio, J. F., and Steinman, B. Invited editorial comment: Osteogenesis imperfecta: Update and perspective. *Am. J. Med. Genet.* 17: 429—435 (1984).
50. Wynne-Davies, R., and Gormley, J. Clinical and genetic patterns in osteogenesis imperfecta. *Clin. Orthop. Rel. Res.* 159:26–35 (1981).
51. Gunnar, S. *Osteogenesis Imperfecta in Sweden.* University Books, Stockholm, 1961.
52. Miller, E. J. A review of biochemical studies on the genetically distinct collagens of the skeletal system. *Clin. Orthop.* 92:260 (1973).
53. Rowe, D. W., Poirier, M., and Shapiro, J. R. Osteogenesis imperfecta: A genetic probe to study Type I collagen biosynthesis. In Veis, A. (ed.). The chemistry and biology of mineralized connective tissues. Elsevier North-Holland, Inc., N.Y., pp. 155–162.
54. Bornstein, P. Structurally distinct collagen types. *Annu. Rev. Biochem.* 49:957–1003 (1980).
55. Sykes, B., Francis, M. J. O., and Smith, R. Altered relation of two collagen types in osteogenesis imperfecta. *N. Engl. J. Med.* 296:1200–1203 (1977).
56. Barsh, G. S., David, K. E., and Pyers, P. H. Type I osteogenesis imperfecta: A nonfunctional allele for pro $\alpha 1$ (I) chains of type I procollagen. *Proc. Natl. Acad. Sci. USA* 79:3838–3842 (1982).
57. Trelstad, R. L., Rubin, D., and Gross, J. Osteogenesis imperfecta congenita: Evidence for a generalized molecular disorder of collagen. *Lab. Invest.* 36: 501–508 (1977).
58. Barsh, G. S., and Byers, P. H. Reduced secretion of structurally abnormal Type I procollagen in a form of osteogenesis imperfecta. *Proc. Natl. Acad. Sci. USA* 78:5142–5146 (1981).
59. Williams, C., and Prockop, D. J. Synthesis and processing of a type I procollagen containing shortened pro $\alpha 1$ (I) chains by fibroblasts from a patient with osteogenesis imperfecta. *J. Biol. Chem.* 258:5915–5921 (1983).
60. Kirsch, E., Glanville, R. W., Krieg, T., and Muller, P. Analysis of cyanogen bromide peptides of type I collagen from a patient with lethal osteogenesis imperfecta. *Biochem. J.* 211:599–603 (1983).
61. DeWet, W. J., Philajaniemi, T., Myers, J., Kelly, T. E., and Prockop, D. J. Synthesis of a shortened pro $\alpha 2$ (I) chains and decreased synthesis of pro-$\alpha 2$ (I) chains in a proband with osteogenesis imperfecta. *J. Biol. Chem.* 258: 7721–7728 (1983).
62. Batman, J. F., Mascara, T., Chan, D., and Cole, W. G. Abnormal type I collagen metabolism by cultured fibroblasts in fetal perinatal osteogenesis imperfecta. *Biochem. J.* 217:103–115 (1984).
63. Steinmann, B., Rao, V. H., Vogel, A., Bruchner, P., Gitzelmann, R., and Byers, P. H. Cysteine in triple-helical domain of one allelic product of the $\alpha 1$ (I) gene of type I collagen produces a lethal form of osteogenesis imperfecta. *J. Biol. Chem.* 259:1129–1138 (1984).

64. Bonadio, J., Holbroook, K. A., Gelinas, R. E., Jacob, J., and Byers, P. H. Altered triple-helical structure of type I procollagen in lethal perinatal osteogenesis imperfecta. *J. Biol. Chem.* 260:1734–1742 (1985).
65. Pope, F. M., and Nicholls, A. C. Intra- or extragenic deletions are associated with Ehlers-Danlos syndrome type II and broad-boned lethal osteogenesis imperfecta. *J. Med. Genet.* 20:455–458 (1983).
66. Barsh, G. S., and Byers, P. H. Reduced secretion of structurally abnormal type I procollagen in a form of osteogenesis imperfecta. *Proc. Natl. Acad. Sci. USA* 78:5142–5146 (1981).
67. Pope, F. M., Cheah, K. S. E., Nicholls, A. C., Price, A. B., and Graveld, F. G. Lethal osteogenesis imperfecta congenita and a 300 base pair gene deletion for an α (1)-like collagen. *Br. Med. J.* 288:431–434 (1984).
68. Sykes, B. C., Ogilvie, D. J., and Wordsworth, B. P. Lethal osteogenesis imperfecta and a collagen gene deletion. Length polymorphism provides an alternative explanation. *Hum. Genet.* 70:35–37 (1985).
69. Chu, M-L., Williams, C. J., Pepe, G., Hirsch, J. L., Prockop, D. J., and Ramirez, F. Internal deletion in a collagen gene in a perinatal lethal form of osteogenesis imperfecta. *Nature* 304:78–80 (1983).
70. Ramirez, F., Sangiorgi, F. O., and Tsipouras, P. Human collagens. Biochemical molecular and genetic features in normal and diseases states. In *Human Genes and Diseases*. (F. Blasi, ed.). Johy Wiley, New York, pp. 341–375 (1986).
71. Peltonen, L., Palotie, A., and Prockop, D. J. A defect in the structure of type I procollagen in a patient who had osteogenesis imperfecta: Excess mannose in the COOH-terminal propeptide. *Proc. Natl. Acad. Sci. USA* 77: 6179–6183 (1980).
72. Pope, F. M., and Nicholls, A. C. Heterogeneity of osteogenesis imperfecta congenita. *Lancet* 1:820–821 (1980).
73. Deak, S., Chu, M-L., Myers, T. C., Nicholls, A. C., Pope, F. M., Rowe, D., and Prockop, D. J. A term of osteogenesis imperfecta in which the MRNA for pro $\alpha 2$ (I) is inefficiently translated in fibroblasts. *Fed. Proc.* 41:825A (1982).
74. Chu, M.-L., Rowe, D., Nicholls, A. C., Pope, F. M., Rowe, D., and Prockop, D. J. Presence of translatable in RNA for pro $\alpha 2$ (I) chains in fibroblasts from a patient with osteogenesis imperfecta where type I collagen does not contain $\alpha 2$ (I) chains. *Collagen Rel. Res.* 4:389 (1984).
75. Byers, P. H., Shapiro, J. R., Rowe, D. W., David, K. E., and Holbrook, K. A. Abnormal 2 chain in type I collagen from a patient with a form of osteogenesis imperfecta. *J. Clin. Invest.* 71:689–694 (1983).
76. Byers, P. H., Bonadio, J. F., and Steinmann, B. Osteogenesis imperfecta: Update and prospective. *Am. J. Med. Genet.* 17:429–435 (1984).
77. Tsipouras, P., Myers, J. C., Ramirez, F., and Prockop, D. J. Restriction fragment and length polymorphism associated with the pro alpha 2(1) gene of human type I procollagen. Application to a family with an autosomal dominant form of osteogenesis imperfecta. *J. Clin. Invest.* 72:1262–1267 (1983).

78. Jett, S., Ramser, J. R., Forst, H. M., and Villanueva, A. R. Bone turnover and osteogenesis imperfecta. *Arch. Pathol.* 81:112–116 (1966).
79. Lee, W. R., A quantitative microscopic study of bone formation in a normal child and 2 children suffering from osteogenesis imperfecta. In: *Proceedings of the Second Symposium of Calcified Tissues.* Liege, Belgium, 1965, p. 451.
80. Ramser, J. R., Villanueva, A. R., Pirok, D., and Frost, H. M. Tetracycline-based measurement of bone dynamics in 3 women with osteogenesis imperfecta. *Clin. Orthop.* 49:151–162 (1966).
81. Castells, S., Lu, C., Baker, R. K., and Wallach, S. Effects of synthetic salmon calcitonin in osteogenesis imperfecta. *Curr. Ther. Res.* 16:1–13 (1974).
82. Rutkowski, R., Resnick, P., and McMaster, J. H. Osteosarcoma occurring in osteogenesis imperfecta. *Br. J. Surg.* 61A:606–608 (1979).
83. Gardner, W.U., and Pfeffier, C. A. Influence of estrogen and androgens on the skeletal system. *Physiol. Rev.* 23:139–165 (1943).
84. Shapiro, J. E., Phillips, J. A., III, Byers, P. H., Saunders, R., Holbrook, K. A., Levin, L. S., Dorst, J., Barsh, G. S., Peterson, K. E., and Goldstein, P. Prenatal diagnosis of lethal perinatal osteogenesis imperfecta (OI Type II). *J. Pediatr.* 100:127–133 (1982).
85. Elejalde, B. R., and de Eljalde, M. D. Prenatal diagnosis of perinatally lethal osteogenesis imperfecta. *Am. J. Med. Genet.* 14:353–359 (1983).
86. Hobbins, J. C., Bracken, M. B., and Mahoney, M. J. Diagnosis of fetal skeletal dysplasia with ultrasound. *Am. J. Obstet. Gynecol.* 142:306–312 (1982).
87. Schabad, I. D. Der stoffwechsel bei angerborener Knochenbruchigkeit (osteogenesis imperfecta). *Z. Kinderheilk.* 11:230 (1914).
88. Hansen, A. E. Influence of Viosterol and parathyroid extract on mineral metabolism in osteogenesis imperfecta. *Am. J. Dis. Child.* 50:132 (1935).
89. LaFort, R. Osteopasatirose. *Bull. Soc. Belg. Orthop.* 10:129 (1938).
90. Ryan, W. J. Osteogenesis imperfecta. With a suggestion for treatment. *J. Bone Joint Surg.* 65:939 (1932).
91. Secord, E. W., Wilder, R. M., and Henderson, M. S. Osteogenesis imperfecta tarda treated with thymus extract. *Proc. Mayo Clin.* 11:1 (1936).
92. Coop, M. C. A treatment for osteoporosis imperfecta in kittens. *J. Am. Vet. Med. Assoc.* 132:299–300 (1958).
93. McLean, F. C., and Urist, M. R. *Bone*, 2nd ed. University of Chicago Press, Chicago, 1961, p. 104.
94. Cattell, H. S., and Clayton, B. Failure of anabolic steroids in the therapy of osteogenesis imperfecta. *J. Bone Joint Surg.* 50A:123–141 (1968).
95. Bernstein, D. S., and Cohen, P. Use of sodium fluoride in the treatment of osteoporosis. *J. Clin. Endocrinol. Metab.* 27:197–210 (1967).
96. Cass, R. M., Croft, J. D , Jr., Perkins, P., Nye, W., Waterhouse, C., and Terry, R. New bone formation in osteoporosis following treatment with sodium fluoride. *Arch. Intern. Med.* 118:111–116 (1966).
97. Cohen, M. B., and Rubini, M. E. The treatment of osteoporosis with sodium fluoride. *Clin. Orthop.* 40:147–152 (1965).

98. Geal, M. G., and Beilin, L. J. Sodium fluoride and optic neuritis. *Br. Med. J.* 2:355-356 (1964).
99. Rich, C., and Ensinck, J. Effect of sodium fluoride on calcium metabolism of human beings. *Nature* 191:184-195 (1961).
100. Slayton, R., Ensinck, J., and Ivanovich, P. The effects of sodium fluoride on calcium metabolism of subjects with metabolic bone disease. *J. Clin. Invest.* 43:545-556 (1964).
101. Rich, C., and Ivanovich, P. Response to sodium fluoride in severe primary osteoporosis. *Ann. Intern. Med.* 63:1069-1074 (1965).
102. Rose, G. A. A study of the treatment of osteoporosis with fluoride therapy and high calcium intake. *Proc. R. Soc. Med.* 58:436-440 (1965).
103. Cohen, P., and Gardner, F. H. Induction of skeletal fluorosis in two common dimineralizing disorders. *J.A.M.A.* 195:962-963 (1964).
104. Neer, R. M., Zipkin, I., Carbone, P. P., and Rosenberg, L. E. Effects of sodium fluoride therapy on calcium metabolism in multiple myeloma. *J. Clin. Endocrinol. Metab.* 26:1059-1068 (1966).
105. De Deuxchaisnes, C. N., and Krane, S. M. Paget's disease of bone: Clinical and metabolic observation. *Medicine* 43:233-266 (1964).
106. Faglia, G., and Norbiato, G. Effetti della sominstrazione de fluoruro di sodio in un caso di morbo di Paget. *Metabolismo* 1:399 (1965).
107. Higgens, B. A., Nassim, J. R., Alexander, R., and Hilb, A. Effect of sodium fluoride on calcitonin phosphorus, nitrogen balance in patient with Paget's disease. *Br. Med. J.* 1:1159-1161 (1965).
108. Hodge, H. C., and Smith, F. A. Fluorides and man. *Annu. Rev. Pharmacol.* 8:395-408 (1968).
110. Aeschlimann, M. I., Grunt, J. A., and Crigler, J. F., Jr. Effects of sodium fluoride on the clinical course and metabolic balance of an infant with osteogenesis imperfecta congenita. *Metabolism* 15:905-914 (1966).
111. Pierog, S. H., Fontana, V. J., and Ferrar, A. Osteogenesis imperfecta. Therapeutic challenge. *N.Y. State J. Med.* 69:310-313 (1969).
112. Bilginturan, N., and Ozsoylu, S. The results of sodium fluoride treatment in osteogenesis imperfecta. *Turk. J. Pediatr.* 8:129 (1966).
113. Kuzemko, J. A. Osteogenesis imperfecta tarda treated with sodium fluoride. *Arch. Dis. Child.* 45:481-482 (1970).
114. Albright, J. A., and Grunt, J. A. Studies of patients with osteogenesis imperfecta. *J. Bone Joint Surg.* 53A:1415-1425 (1971).
115. Baylink, D. J., and Bernstein, D. S. The effects of fluoride therapy on metabolic bone disease. *Clin. Orthop.* 55:51-85 (1967).
116. Peck, W. A., Ziplin, I., and Whedon, G. D. Fluoride inhibition of bone collagen synthesis. *Clin. Res.* 13:330-331 (1965).
117. Proffit, W. R., and Ackermann, J. Fluoride: Its effects on two parameters of bone growth in organ culture. *Science* 145:932-934 (1964).
118. Solomons, C. C., and Styner, J. Osteogenesis imperfecta. Effect of magnesium administration on pyrophosphate metabolism. *Calcif. Tissue Res.* 3:318-326 (1969).

119. Fleisch, H., and Bisaz, S. Isolation from urine of pyrophosphate, a calcification inhibitor. *Am. J. Physiol.* 203:671–675 (1962).
120. Fleisch, H., and Bisaz, S. Mechanism of calcification: Inhibitory role of pyrophosphate. *Nature* 195:911 (1962).
121. Fleisch, H. Role of nucleation and inhibition in calcification. *Clin. Orthop.* 32:170–180 (1964).
122. Fleisch, H., Russell, R. G. G., and Straumann, F. Effect of pyrophosphate on hydroxyapatite and its implication in calcium homeostasis. *Nature* 212: 901-903 (1966).
123. Cartier, P., and Picard, J. La mineralization du cartilage ossifiable. *Bull. Soc. Chem. Biol.* 37:1159 (1955).
124. Perkins, H. R., and Walker, P. G. The occurrence of pyrophosphate in bone. *J. Bone Joint Surg.* 40B:333–339 (1958).
125. Horn, A., Borning, H., and Theliele, G. Allosteric properties of the magnesium-dependent inorganic pyrophosphate in mouse liver cytoplasm. *Eur. J. Biochem.* 22:243 (1967).
126. Russell, R. G. G., Bisaz, S., Ddonath, A., Morgan, D. B., and Fleisch, H. Inorganic pyrophosphate in plasma in normal persons and in patients with hypophosphatasia, osteogenesis imperfecta, and other disorders of bone. *J. Clin. Invest.* 50:961-969 (1971).
127. Hirsch, P. F., and Munson, P. L. Thyrocalcitonin. *Physiol. Res.* 49:547 (1969).
128. Rasmussen, H., and Tenenhous, A. Thyrocalcitonin, osteoporosis, and osteolysis. *Am. J. Med.* 43:711–726 (1967).
129. Foster, G. V., Doyle, F. H., Bordier, P., and Matrajt, H. Effect of thyrocalcitonin on bone. *Lancet* 2:1428–1431 (1966).
130. Wase, A. W., Peterson, A., Rickets, E., and Solewski, J. Some effects of thyrocalcitonin on the calcium metabolism of the rat. *Endocrinology* 79: 687–691 (1966).
131. Baude, C. A., de Siebenthal, J., Langer, B., Tuplin, M. R., and Mach, R. S. The effects of prolonged administration of thyrocalcitonin in human senile osteoporosis. *Proceedings of the Second International Symposium on Calcitonin.* Springer-Verlag, New York, 1970, p. 531.
132. Brown, P., Thin, C. G., Malone, D. N. S., Roscoe, P., and Strong, J. A. Metabolic studies with porcine calcitonin in osteoporosis. *Scot. Med. J.* 15: 206 (1970).
133. Caniggia, A., Gennari, C., Bencini, M., Cesari, L., and Borrello, G. Calcium metabolism and ^{47}Ca kinetics before and after long term thyrocalcitonin treatment in senile osteoporosis. *Clin. Soc.* 38:397–407 (1975).
134. Cohn, S. H., Dombrowski, C. S., Hauser, W., Klopper, J., and Atkins, H. L. Effects of porcine calcitonin on calcium metabolism in osteoporosis. *J. Clin. Endocrinol. Metab.* 33:719–729 (1971).
135. Jowsey, J., Riggs, B. L. Goldsmith, R. S., Kelly, P. J., and Arnaud, C. D. Effects of prolonged administration of porcine calcitonin in postmenopausal osteoporosis. *J. Clin. Endocrinol. Metab.* 33:752–758 (1971).

136. Wallach, S., Aloia, J., and Cohn, S. Treatment of osteoporosis with calcitonin. *Semin. Drug Treat.* 2:21 (1972).
137. DeRose, J., Avramides, A., Baker, R. K., and Wallach, S. Treatment of Paget's disease with calcitonin. *Semin. Drug Treat.* 2:51 (1972).
138. Haddad, J. G., Birge, S. J., and Avioli, L. V. Effects of prolonged thyrocalcitonin administration on Paget's diseases of bone. *N. Engl. J. Med.* 283:549–555 (1970).
139. Shai, F., Baker, R. K., and Wallach, S. The clinical and metabolic effects of porcine calcitonin on Paget's disease of bone. *J. Clin. Invest.* 50:1927–1940 (1971).
140. Woodhouse, N. J. Y., Bordier, P. H., Fisher, M., Joplic, G. F., Reiner, M., Kalu, D. N., Foster, G. V., and MacIntyre, I. Human calcitonin in the treatment of Paget's bone disease. *Lancet* 1:1139–1143 (1971).
141. Castells, S., Inamdar, S., Baker, R., and Wallach, S. Effect of porcine calcitonin on calcium and phosphorus in patients with osteogenesis imperfecta tarda. In *Proceedings of the XII International Congress of Pediatrics*, Wien, Austria, 1971.
142. Castells, S., Inadmar, S., Baker, R. K., and Wallach, S. Effects of porcine calcitonin in osteogenesis imperfecta tarda. *J. Pediatr.* 80:757–762 (1972).
143. Castells, S. New approaches to treatment of osteogenesis imperfecta. *Clin. Orthop.* 93:239–249 (1973).
144. Gardner, B., Gray, H., and Hedayati, H. Bone collagenase as a test of osteolysis. *Curr. Top. Surg. Res.* 2:175 (1970).
145. Gardner, B., Gray, H., and Hetayata, H. Bone collagenase in osteolytic stress of rats and humans. *Surg. Forum* 21:467 (1970).
146. Castells, S., Colbert, C., Chakrabarti, C., Bachtell, R. S., Kassner, E. G., and Yasumura, S. Therapy of osteogenesis imperfecta with synthetic salmon calcitonin. *J. Pediatr.* 95:807–811 (1979).
147. Woodhouse, N. J. Y., Fisher, M. T., Sigurdsson, G., Joplin, G. F., and McIntyre, I. Paget's disease in a 5-year-old: Acute response to human calcitonin. *Br. Med. J.* 4:267–269 (1972).
148. Choremis, C., Yannakos, D., Papadatos, C., and Baroutsou, E. Osteitis deformans (Paget's disease) in an 11 year old boy. *Helv. Pediatr. Acta* 13: 185–188 (1958).
149. Irving, R. E. Familial Paget's disease with early onset. *J. Bone Joint Surg.* 35B:106–111 (1953).
150. Mills, B., and Singer, F. Nuclear inclusions in Paget's disease of bone. Science 194:201–202 (1976).
151. DeRose, J., Singer, F. R., Avramides, A., Flores, A., Dziadin, W. R., Baker, R. K., and Wallach, S. Response of Paget's disease to porcine and salmon calcitonins: Effects of long-term treatment. *Am. J. Med.* 56:858–866 (1974).
152. Goldfield, E. B., Braiker, B. M., Prendergast, J. J., and Kolb, F. O. Synthetic salmon calcitonin: Treatment of Paget's disease and osteogenesis imperfecta. *J.A.M.A.* 22:1127–1129 (1972).

153. Doyle, F. H., Woodhouse, N. J. Y., Glen, A. C. A., Joplin, G. F., and McIntyre, I. Healing of the bones in juvenile Paget's disease treated with human calcitonin. *Br. J. Radiol.* 47:9–15 (1974).
154. Chawla, S. Cranio-skeletal dysplasia with acro-osteolysis. *Br. J. Radiol.* 37:702–705 (1964).
155. Cheney, W. D. Acro-osteolysis. *A.J.R.* 94:595–607 (1985).
156. Kohler, E., Babbitt, D., Huizenga, B., and Good, T. A. Hereditary osteolysis. *Pediatr. Radiol.* 108:99–105 (1973).
157. Beals, K., and Bird, C. B. Carpal and tarsal osteolysis. *J. Bone Joint Surg.* 57A:681–686 (1975).
158. Gluck, J., and Miller, J. J. III, Familial osteolysis of the carpal and tarsal bones. *J. Pediatr.* 81:506–510 (1972).
159. Brown, D. M., Bradford, D. S., Gorlin, R. J., Desnick, R. J., Langer, L. O., Jr., Jowsey, J., and Sauk, J. J., Jr. The acro-osteolysis syndrome: Morphologic and biochemical studies. *J. Pediatr.* 88:573–580 (1976).
160. Torg, J. S., DiGeorge, A. M., Kirkpatrick, J. A., and Trujill, M. D. Heredity of multicentric osteolysis with recessive transmission. A new syndrome. *J. Pediatr.* 75:243–252 (1969).
161. Tyler, T., and Rosenbaum, H. D. Idiopathic multicentric osteolysis. *Am. J. Roentgenol.* 126:23–31 (1976).
162. Hemingway, A. P., Leung, A., and Lavender, J. P. Familial vanishing limbs: Four generations of idiopathic multicentric osteolysis. *Clin. Radiol.* 34: 585–588 (1983).
163. Mahoudeau, D., Durbisay, J., Elissalde, B., and Sraer, C. Osteolyse éssentielle et néphrite. *Bull. Mem. Soc Med.Hop.* 77:229–234 (1961).
164. Marie, J., Leveque, B., Lyon, G., Bebe, M., and Watchi, T. M. Acro-osteolyse essentielle compliquée d'insuffisance renale d'évaluation fétale. *Presse Med.* 71:249–252 (1963).
165. Torg, J. S., and Steel, H. H. Essential osteolysis with nephropathy. A review of the literature and case report of an unusual syndrome. *J. Bone Joint Surg.* 50A:1629–1638 (1968).
166. Shurtleff, D. B., Sparkes, R. S., Clawson, K., Guntheroth, W. G., and Mottet, N. K. Hereditary osteclysis with hypertension and nephropathy. J.A.M.A. 188:133–118 (1964).
167. Gorham, L. W., Wright, A. W., Schultz, H. H., and Maxon, F. C., Jr. Disappearing bone: A rare form of massive osteolysis. *Am. J. Med.* 17:674–682 (1954).
168. Halliday, D. R., Dahlin, D. C., Pugh, D. G., and Young, H. H. Massive osteolysis and angiomatosis. *Radiology* 82:637–644 (1964).
169. Winchester, P., Grossman, H., Lim, W. N., and Danes, B. S. A new acid mucopolysaccharidosis with skeletal deformities stimulating rheumatoid arthritis. *Am. J. Roentogenol.* 106:121–128 (1969).
170. Brown, S. I., and Kuwabara, T. Peripheral corneal opacification and skeletal deformities. *Arch. Ophthalmol.* 83:667–677 (1970).

171. Holister, D. W., Rimoin, D. L., Lachman, R. S., Cohen, A. H., Reed, W. B., and Westin, G. W. The Winchester syndrome: A nonlysosomal connective tissue disease. *J. Pediatr.* 84:701–709 (1974).
172. Cohen, A. H., Hollister, D. W., and Reed, W. B. The skin in Winchester syndrome: Histological and ultrastructural studies. *Arch. Dermatol.* 111: 230–236 (1975).
173. Castells, S., Sher, J. H., Rose, J., Anderson, H. C., Shafig, S., and Hashemi, S. E. Selective muscle fiber hyoplasia and epiphyseal osteolysis. *Pediatr. Res.* 2:920–928 (1977).
174. Bradford, D. S., Brown, D. M., Moe, J. H., Winter, R. B., and Towsey, J. Scheuermann's kyphosis: A form of juvenile osteoporosis? *Clin. Orthop.* 118:10–15 (1976).
175. Jones, E. T., and Hesinger, R. N. Spinal deformity in idiopathic juvenile osteoporosis. *Spine* 6:1–4 (1981).
176. Bradford, D. S., and Moe, J. H. Scheuermann's juvenile kyphosis. *Clin. Orthop.* 110:45 (1975).
177. Jowsey, J., and Johnson, K. A. Juvenile osteoporosis: Bone findings in seven patients. *J. Pediatr.* 81:511–517 (1972).
178. Cloutier, M. D., Hayles, A. B., Riggs, B. L., Jowsey, J., and Bickel, W. H. Juvenile osteoporosis: Report of a case including a description of some metabolic and microradiographic studies. *Pediatrics* 40:649–655 (1967).
179. Evans, R. A., Dunstan, C. R., and Hills, E. Bone metabolism in idiopathic juvenile osteoporosis: A case report. *Calcif. Tissue Int.* 35:5–8 (1983).
180. Brenton, D. P., and Dent, C. E. Idiopathic juvenile osteoporosis: In: *Inborn Errors of Calcium and Bone Metabolism*. 1976, pp. 223–255. Edited by H. Bickel and J. Stern, University Park Press, Baltimore.
181. Gooding, C. A., and Ball, J. H. Idiopathic juvenile osteoporosis. *Radiology* 93:1349–1350 (1969).
182. Teotia, M., Teotia, S. P. S., and Singh, R. K. Idiopathic juvenile osteoporosis. *Am. J. Dis. Child.* 133:894–900 (1979).
183. Lapatsanis, P., Kavadias, A., and Uretos, K. Juvenile osteoporosis. *Arch. Dis. Child.* 46:66–71 (1971).
184. Dent, C. E., and Friedman, M. Idiopathic juvenile osteoporosis. *Q. J. Med.* 34:177–210 (1965).
185. Marder, H. K., Tsang, R. C., Hug, G., and Crawford, A. C. Calcitriol deficiency in idiopathic juvenile osteoporosis. *Am. J. Dis. Child.* 136:914–917 (1982).
186. Ribovich, M. L., and DeLuca, H. F. The influence of dietary calcium and phosphorus on intestinal calcium transport in rats given vitamin D metabolites. *Arch. Biochem. Biophys.* 170:529–535 (1975).
187. Dodd, K., Grawbarth, H., and Rapoport, S. Hypercalcemia, nephropathy and encephalopathy following immobilization. *Pediatrics* 6:124–130 (1952).
188. Halvorsen, L. Osteoporosis, hypercalcemia and nephropathy following immobilization in children. *Acta Med. Scand.* 149:401–408 (1954).

189. Mason, A. S. Acute osteoporosis with hypercalcemia. *Lancet* 1:911–913 (1957).
190. Winters, J. L., Kleinschmidt, A. G., Jr., Frensilli, J. J., and Sutton, M. Hypercalcemia complicating immobilization in the treatment of fractures. *J. Bone Joint Surg.* 48A:1182–1184 (1966).
191. Hyman, L. R., Boner, G., Thomas, J. C., and Segar, W. E. Immobilization hypercalcemia. *Am. J. Dis. Child.* 124:723–727 (1972).
192. Heath, H., Earll, J. M., Schaaf, M., Piechocki, J. T., and Li, T-K, Serum ionized calcium during bed rest in fracture patients and normal men. *Metabolism* 21:633–640 (1972).
193. Root, A. W., Bongiovanni, A. M., and Eberlein, W. R. Measurement of the kinetics of calcium metabolism in children and adolescents utilizing non-radioactive strontium. *J. Clin. Endocrinol. Metab.* 26:537–544 (1966).
194. Hulley, S. B., Vogel, J. M., Donaldson, C. L., Bayer, J. H., Friedman, R. J., and Rosen, S. N. The effect of supplemental oral phosphate on the bone mineral changes during prolonged bed rest. *J. Clin. Invest.* 50:2506–2518 (1971).
195. Bronner, F., Richelle, L. J., Saville, P. D., Nicholas, J. S., and Cobb, J. R. Quantitation of calcium-metabolism in postmenopausal osteoporosis and in scoliosis. *J. Clin. Invest.* 42:898–905 (1963).
196. Langman, C. B., and Moore, E. S. Hypercalcemia in clinical pediatrics. *Clin. Pediatr.* 23:135–137 (1984).
197. Moore, E. S., Coe, F. L., McMann, B. J., and Favus, M. J. Idiopathic hypercalcemia in children: Prevalence and metabolic characteristics. *J. Pediatr.* 92:906–910 (1978).
198. Stapleton, F. B., Noe, H. N., and Jerkins, G. Urinary excretion of calcium following an oral calcium loading test in healthy children. *Pediatrics* 69: 594–597 (1982).
199. Rose, A. Immobilization osteoporosis. A study of the extent, severity and treatment with bendrofluazide. *Br. J. Surg.* 53:769–777 (1966).
200. Goldsmith, R. S., and Ingbar, S. H. Inorganic phosphate treatment of diverse etiologies. *N. Engl. J. Med.* 274:1–7 (1966).
201. Suki, W. N., Yium, J. J., Von Minden, M., Saller-Hebert, C., Eknoyan, G., and Martinez-Maldonado, M. Acute treatment of hypercalcemia with furosemide. *N. Engl. J. Med.* 283:836–840 (1970).
202. Eknoyan, G., Suki, W. N., and Martinez-Maldonado, M. Effect of diuretics on urinary excretion of phosphate, calcium, and magnesium in thyroparathyroidectomized dogs. *J. Lab. Clin. Med.* 76:257–268 (1970).
203. Singer, F. R., Neer, R. M., Murray, T. M., Keutmann, H. T., Deftos, L. J., and Potts, J. T., Jr. Mithramycin treatment of intractable hypercalcemia due to parathyroid carcinoma. *N. Engl. J. Med.* 282:634–636 (1970).

13

Orthopedic Management of Osteogenesis Imperfecta

Charles R. Spero
Kings County Hospital Center, Brooklyn, New York
Carl Barbera
SUNY Health Science Center at Brooklyn, Brooklyn, New York

Since the recognition of the syndrome that is today known as osteogenesis imperfecta, and its description by Ekman (1) in 1788, comparatively little change has taken place in its treatment. The patients themselves, as well as their families and members of the medical community who care for them, often become frustrated at the apparent lack of improvement either medically or in their adaptation in the social sphere.

Despite some modest progress in the medical treatment of the metabolic disorder of this disease, and some insight into its basic histochemical and biochemical derangement, physicians remain confined to providing "symptomatic" treatment.

Though challenging, however, the picture is not dismal. Appropriate care has greatly lengthened the life expectancy of these patients, and the variability of the disease's severity allows all but a few to become productive members of society.

The role of the orthopedic surgeon in the treatment of osteogenesis imperfecta has expanded, due to advances in surgical as well as nonoperative and preventive modes of therapy. An understanding of the characteristics and natural history of the disease permits educated selection and timing of the treatments available.

The clinical manifestations of increased bony fragility, excessive ligamentous laxity, and scoliosis can be controlled by proper and timely orthopedic intervention so as greatly to enhance self-image, productivity, and the ability to carry out activities of daily living. Treatment concerns itself with more than acute fracture care, since this falls short of long-term goals. Such goals may not have been realistic in the past; however, they are certainly attainable now. Advances in bioengineering, orthotic construction, physical and occupational therapy, rehabilitative medicine, and surgical management have changed the previously dismal outlook for patients with osteogenesis imperfecta (OI).

It is important to appreciate that many patients with OI experience a spontaneous increase in their level of function with maturity. This may be due to abatement of the clinical severity of their disease, increased confidence in their ability to function, or both (2). Children who have been very limited ambulators may significantly increase their activity level during adolescence. It is therefore appropriate to maintain an aggressive attitude toward treatment of these patients.

With these things kept in mind, the urgency and intensity of therapy should reflect several factors, most important among them being the age of the patient and the severity of the disease. In the past, medical providers have been timid in recommending physical therapy for these patients. Today, however, it is assuming a larger and larger role in their care (3,4).

Whereas immobilization, particularly that required after a fracture, will compound the brittleness of the patient's bone by superimposing disuse osteoporosis upon the metabolic disease, a well thought-out and applied program of physical therapy will reduce the incidence of fracture, increase bone density, and promote a more rapid return to function after an acute fracture. Even patients with more severe forms of osteogenesis imperfecta can be placed on a program of light resistance exercises, or can participate in swimming or water therapy. Weight bearing is encouraged whenever possible (3). Adjunctive to this philosophy of maximizing function, and a part of it, is the practice of functional bracing.

Relatively newer techniques and lightweight materials have made it practical to provide orthotics that will be neither too cumbersome nor too heavy for these small, injury-prone patients to use effectively. Patients with osteogenesis imperfecta have a normal healing response to fractures. Although the bone's final strength will never exceed its premorbid state, the time to healing is no different than in any other patient (2). This permits the use of functional bracing to shorten the time of immobilization after a fracture, and permit an earlier return to weight bearing. Furthermore, the routine use of orthotics can permit a higher level of function than a patient with osteogenesis imperfecta would otherwise have. Not only can bracing increase function and protect against fracture, but the greater use of muscle forces and the stress of weight bearing will also improve the baseline quality of the patient's bones. There comes a point, however, when it becomes impractical or impossible to provide a patient with adequate bracing.

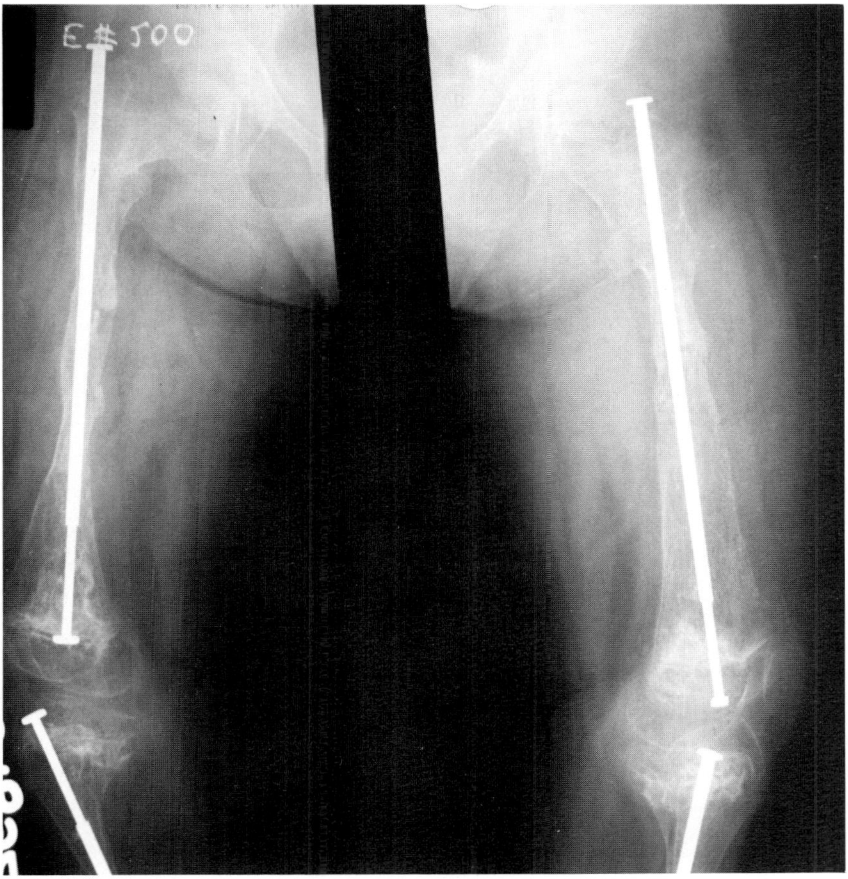

Figure 1 Patient with severe osteogenesis imperfecta had nails placed in both femurs and tibias, resulting in a remarkable improvement in mobility and ability to participate in physical therapy.

Severely deformed extremities, aside from being technically difficult to brace, present a biomechanical situation that limits an orthotic device's effectiveness. As a bone becomes more and more bowed, the compressive forces of weight bearing are transformed into bending forces. Rather than being constructively stressed to increase its mass and strength, therefore, the bone is at greater risk of fracture. As deformity increases, it also becomes increasingly more difficult to protect such a limb from injury. In such a case, corrective surgery is indicated. If a limb shows progressive deformity or recurrent fractures despite

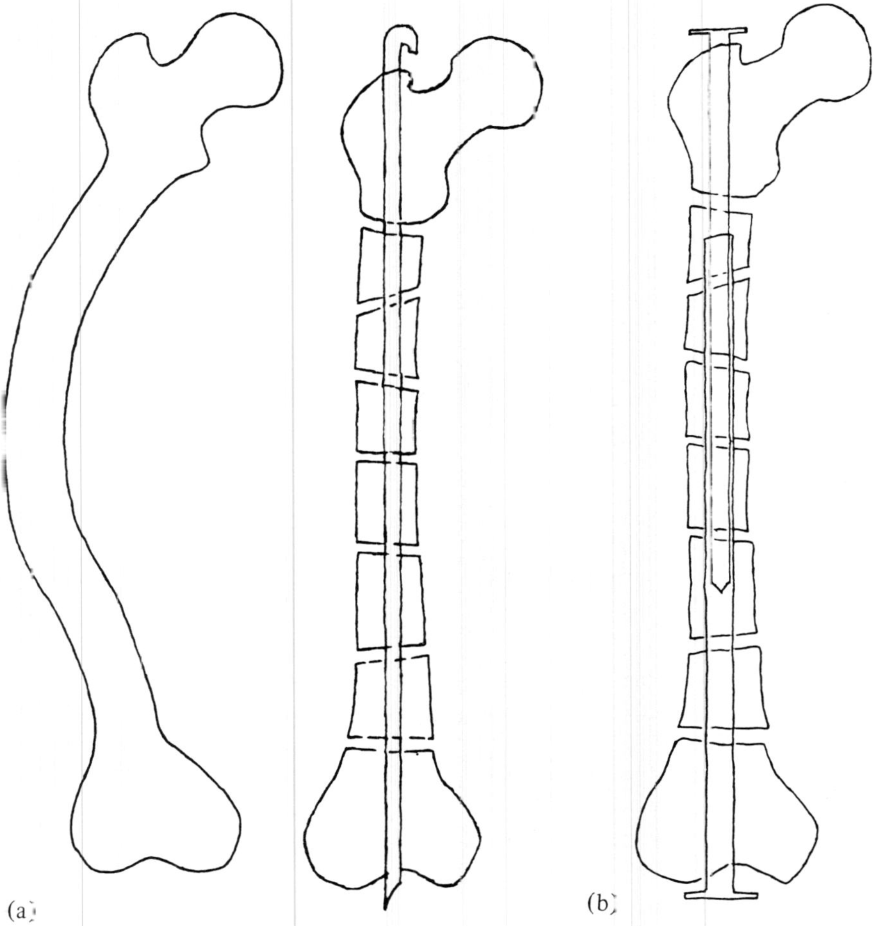

(a) (b)

Figure 2

adequate conservative treatment, or if a child demonstrates a lag in development or functional capability to fear of fracture, surgery can be undertaken (5).

The procedure most commonly performed is that described by Sofield and Millar (Fig. 2a) in 1959 (6). The entire length of the involved bone is exposed, and the periosteum is longitudinally split and separated from the underlying bone. The bone is transected in multiple places, to separate it into multiple cylindrical segments. The medullary canal of each segment is then individually and extracorporeally reamed wide enough to accept an intramedullary rod.

Each segment is threaded onto the rod and laid back into its periosteal sheath. A periosteum and overlying soft tissue is closed and the patient immobilized. A long-leg toe-to-groin cast is used for tibial osteotomies while femoral osteotomies require a hip spica cast. As originally described, the osteotomized bone was threaded onto a straight solid rod. It is introduced through the greater trochanter in the case of the femur, or the proximal metaphysis in the case of the tibia, and extends to the metaphyseal portion of the distal end of either bone (7,8).

The incidence of nonunion or infection with this procedure is surprisingly low, but several complications do occur.

There is a tendency for the nail to migrate, gradually backing out of the bone and becoming symptomatic. This would necessitate its removal. Another, perhaps more frustrating, problem was the fact that although the rod was of fixed length, the child continued to grow. The bone would therefore overgrow the rod, and either be again prone to fracture, or begin to angulate as it had done before the operation.

These problems were addressed by Bailey and Dubow, who described in 1969 (Fig. 2b) their experiences tih an extensible intramedullary rod (9). This is a two-piece device; one is a straight rod and the other is a hollow outer sleeve that slips over the rod. The opposite end of each half of the rod is "T"-shaped, which allows it to be well secured in the bone.

The surgical technique is similar to that used with the solid rod, except that the extensible rod is inserted transarticularly through the epiphysis, crossing the growth plate. One half of the rod is passed from distal to proximal while the other is passed from proximal to distal, and the two halves are fitted together.

As the child grows and the bone increases in length, the sleeve slips over the inner rod and the device elongates. This obviates the previously mentioned problems of migration and overgrowth. Even though the rod crosses the physis, if it is inserted with care there is no interference with the child's normal growth (9,10).

These same principles can be applied to the upper extremities. The need for operative correction is less common, however, since the limbs are typically subjected to less stress, and greater deformity can be accepted without disabling impairment of function (11).

Another area of orthopedic treatment for the patient with osteogenesis imperfecta involves spinal deformity. There is an increased incidence of progressive scoliosis with the disorder; reported incidence ranges from 44 to 96%. Curvatures tend to be mild in young children and become more severe with advancing age. In general, the more advanced the osteoporosis, the greater the risk of serious spinal deformity (12). The inherent malleability of OI bone contributes to the progression of scoliosis and kyphosis. Compounding this material tendency to deform is the added effect of gravity and body weight (13).

The consequences of progressive spinal deformity are cosmetic deformity; decreased pulmonary function with advanced curvature; neurological compromise with advanced deformity, especially kyphosis, pain, loss of function, and loss of the ability to sit. In these patients, it is difficult to apply the standard methods of treatment used in patients with idiopathic scoliosis.

Bracing is often impractical. A standard brace corrects spinal curvature through indirect forces applied through the pelvis and ribs. The soft bones of the patient with osteogenesis imperfecta will themselves deform under these forces (14). The standard Milwaukee brace treatment protocol for this disorder therefore does not correct the spinal deformity and may lead to secondary thoracic cage deformity. The use of custom-molded plastic total contact body jacket type orthoses may be better tolerated by the patient and lessen the chance of secondary thoracic deformity (3); however, they do not correct spinal deformity or halt curve progression. Under the best of circumstances these devices may slow down, but not halt or reverse, a deforming spine in OI.

Operative spinal stabilization may be indicated and is challenging. Standard instrumentation for spinal fusion in the treatment of scoliosis included posterior spinal rods. These rods apply their corrective forces to the spine via metal hooks that engage the spinal laminae. The high forces concentrated upon the laminae through these hooks themselves deform the laminae, sometimes fracture them, and lead to instrument failure (13). Furthermore, the eventual success of any scoliosis surgery hinges upon the solidity of the resulting fusion mass. It is difficult to obtain fusion in these patients, due to the scant amount of donor bone available. When fusion is obtained, it tends to be no stronger than the patient's inherent metabolic disease will permit.

Several advances have been made in this area. Primary among them is the use of autologous banked bone to induce fusion. Attempts are also being made to reinforce the strength of the hook sites, either by the use of polymethyl methacrylate cement, or by staging the fusion procedure. In the latter technique, the hooks are inserted, and bone graft applied to the hook sites in one procedure. In a second operation, the rods are inserted and the spine fused.

Several surgeons are attempting to increase the success of the operative treatment of scoliosis in the patient with osteogenesis imperfecta by instrumenting and fusing the spine anteriorly (13). Not enough is known at present, however, to indicate an advantage of any one of these techniques over the others.

Advances in bioengineering have made available functional custom transportation and seating devices. Patients are no longer prisoners of nonfunctional, cumbersome wheelchair devices. No longer must the nonambulator remain captive in his or her own home. Modular wheelchair units, hydraulic and mechanical lifts, custom vans, and computer-assisted environments now provide for and assist the patient in transportation for both recreational and vocational purposes.

In summary, with the provision of physical and occupational therapy, functional bracing and wheelchair design, vocational training, aggressive and physiological fracture management and prevention, along with prophylactic surgery and spinal stabilization, the quality of life for the OI patient can be and should be greatly improved.

REFERENCES

1. Ekman, O. J. *Descriptionem et Casus Aliquot Osteomalaciae sistems*. Dissertatio Medica Upsaline (1788).
2. Albright, J. A. Management overview of osteogenesis imperfecta. *Clin. Orthop.* 159:80 (1981).
3. Bleck, E. E. Non-operative treatment of osteogenesis imperfecta. *Clin. Orthop.* 159:111 (1981).
4. Salvo, J. A., Root, L., and Bullough, P. G. Osteogenesis imperfecta: clinical evaluation and management. *J. Bone Joint Surg.* 56A:783 (1974).
5. Millar, E. A. Observations in the surgical management of osteogenesis imperfecta. *Clin. Orthop.* 159:154 (1981).
6. Sofield, H. A., and Millar, E. A. Fragmentation, realignment, and intramedullary rod fixation of deformities of long bones in children. A ten year appraisal. *J. Bone Joint Surg.* 41A:1371 (1959).
7. Neimann, K. M. Surgical treatment of the tibia in osteogenesis imperfecta. *Clin. Orthop.* 159:134 (1981).
8. Rodriguez, R. P., and Bailey, R. W. Internal fixation of the femur in patients with osteogenesis imperfecta. *Clin. Orthop.* 159:126 (1981).
9. Bailey, R. W., Rodriguez, R. P., and Dubow, H. I. Clinical experiences with the use of an intermedullary extensible rod in children with brittle bones. *J. Bone Joint Surg.* 58A:725 (1976).
10. Bailey, R. W. Further clinical experience with the extensible nail. *Clin. Orthop.* 159:171 (1981).
11. Root, L., Upper limb surgery in osteogenesis imperfecta. *Clin. Orthop.* 159: 141 (1981).
12. Benson, D. R., Donaldson, D., and Millar, E. A. The spine in osteogenesis imperfecta. *J. Bone Joint Surg.* 60A:925 (1978).
13. Benson, D. R., and Newman, D. C. The spine and surgical treatment in osteogenesis imperfecta. *Clin. Orthop.* 159:147 (1981).
14. Hoek, K. J. Scoliosis in osteogenesis imperfecta: Proceedings of the Western Orthopaedics Association. *J. Bone Joint Surg.* 57A(1):136 (1975).

14

Skeletal Dysplasias with Primary Abnormalities in Carbohydrate, Lipid, and Amino Acid Metabolism

Cecilia D. Cervantes and Fima Lifshitz

North Shore University Hospital, Manhasset, and
Cornell University Medical College, New York, New York

Over 80 entities presently make up the skeletal dysplasias (1). These conditions may involve multiple organ systems of which the skeletal system is primarily affected. The skull, spine, and limbs show various degrees and forms of abnormalities, and disproportionate short stature frequently results. These conditions are congenital, some of which are identifiable at birth, but many only become evident in later life. The classification of this heterogeneous group of skeletal dysplasias has been revised because new entities become identified, more conditions become well defined, and the primary defects of some of the conditions became better understood (2).

This chapter will mainly discuss those skeletal dysplasias that already have an identified specific abnormality in carbohydrate, lipid, or amino acid metabolism (3-6). This, therefore, excludes all the other conditions that are not yet completely understood (7-9).

I. MUCOPOLYSACCHARIDE STORAGE DISORDERS

The mucopolysaccharide storage disorders (MPS) result from defective lysosomal hydrolase activities involved in the degradation of three major glycosaminoglycans: heparan sulfate, dermatan sulfate, and keratan sulfate (4). These substances, which are a major component of bone organic matrix, are normally degraded in a stepwise fashion, each reaction being catalyzed by a glycosidase sul-

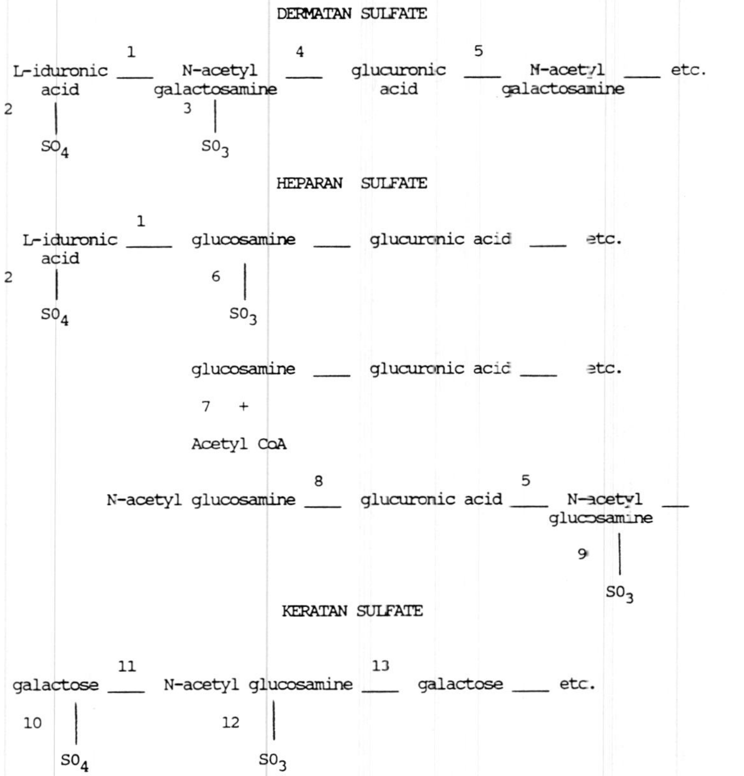

Cleavage Site	Enzyme	Deficiency Disorder
1	alpha-L-iduronidase	Hurler's, Scheie, Hurler-Scheie
2	iduronate sulfatase	Hunter
3	N-acetyl galactosamine sulfatase	Maroteaux-Lamy
4	N-acetyl-β-galactosaminidase	?
5	β-glucuronidase	Sly
6	heparan-N-sulfatase	Sanfilippo A
7 *	acetyl transferase	Sanfilippo C
8	N-acetyl glucosaminidase	Sanfilippo B
9	N-acetyl alpha-D-glucosamine-6-sulfatase	Sanfilippo D
10	galactosamine-6-sulfate sulfatase	Morquio A
11	β-galactosidase	Morquio B
12	N-acetyl glucosamine-6-sulfatase	?
13	β-hexosaminidase	?

Figure 1 Structure of the three major glycosaminoglycans that accumulate in mucopolysaccharide storage diseases and the site of cleavage by various lysosomal enzymes. *, Not a bond cleavage but a transfer reaction. ?, Uncertain.

Table 1 Dysostosis Multiplex

Head
Enlarged calvaria with thickened cranial vault
Scaphocephaly, brachycephaly, or dolichocephaly
Shallow orbits
Enlarged, J-shaped sella turcica
Hypoplastic sinuses
Thorax
Widened medial end of clavicles
Hypoplastic lateral end of clavicles
Oar-shaped ribs
Spine
Rounded vertebral bodies
Odontoid hypoplasia
Atlantoaxial subluxation
Thoracolumbar gibbus
Anterior and inferior beaking of thoracolumbar vertebrae
Pelvis
Iliac flaring
Hypoplastic ilium
Shallow acetabulum
Coxa valga
Extremities
Widened diaphyses of long bones
Varus deformity of humeral neck
Claw-hand deformity
Tapering of proximal ends of metacarpals
Demineralization of long bones

fatase or deacetylase (4). In the mucopolysaccharide storage diseases, there is a deficiency of one of these enzymes resulting in incomplete breakdown and generalized accumulation of these glycosaminoglycans, most markedly in the tissues where they predominate. The different enzymes involved in the degradation of the three important bone mucopolysaccharides and the resulting diseases are shown in Figure 1.

The clinical syndrome of mucopolysaccharidosis includes a variety of manifestations with different degrees of skeletal involvement called "dysostoses multiplex" (Table 1). This pattern of dysplastic lesions shows that the developing skeleton reacts stereotypically to various disturbances of a single metabolic pathway (10). There are about 15 types of mucopolysaccharidosis and 8 distinct enzymatic defects of which all except the Morquio syndrome or type IV are characterized by dysostosis multiplex (Table 2). Flattened vertebral bodies and

Table 2 The Mucopolysaccharide Storage Disorders

Type	Enzyme deficiency	Urinary MPS	Dysostosis multiplex	Mental retardation	Short stature	Corneal clouding
I H (Hurler's)	Alpha-L-iduronidase	HS, DS	+++	+++	+++	+
I S (Scheie)	Alpha-L-iduronidase	HS, DS	+	–	–	+
I H/S (Hurler-Scheie's)	Alpha-L-iduronidase	HS, DS	+++	++	++	+
II (Hunter's)	Iduronate sulfatase	HS, DS	+++	++	+++	–
III A (Sanfilippo's A)	Heparan-N-sulfatase	HS	+	+++	+	–
III B (Sanfilippo's B)	N-acetyl-alpha glucosaminidase	HS	+	+++	+	–
III C (Sanfilippo's C)	Acetyl CoA-alpha glucosaminide-N-acetyltransferase	HS	+	+++	+	–
III D (Sanfilippo's D)	N-acetyl-alpha D-glucosaminide-6-sulfatase	HS	+	+++	+	–
IV A (Morquio A)	Galactosamine-6-sulfate sulfatase	KS	+++	+/–	+++	+
IV B (Morquio B)	Beta-galactosidase	KS	++	+	+++	+
V (Now I S)						
VI (Maroteaux-Lamy)	N-acetylgalactosamine-4-sulfatase	DS	+++	–	+++	+
VII (Sly's)	Beta-glucuronides	DS, HS	+	+/–	+/–	+

Deafness	Coarse facies	Hepato-splenomegaly	Cardiac disease	Life span	Others
+	+	+++	Coronary artery disease	<10 yrs	Umbilical and inguinal hernia
+/-	+	+	Aortic stenosis	3rd decade	Stiff joints, myelopathy
+	+	+	Valvular disease	3rd decade	Micrognathia
+	+	+	Valvular disease	Normal	Papilledema, pachymeningitis
+/-	+	+	Valvular disease	<20 yrs	Hirsutism
+/-	+	+	Valvular disease	>20 yrs	Hirsutism
+/-	+	+	Valvular disease	>20 yrs	Hirsutism
+/-	+	+	Valvular disease	<20 yrs	Hirsutism
+++	+	-	Aortic insufficiency	Normal	Short trunk loose joints, thin enamel
+	+/-	-	Valvular disease	Normal	Short trunk, loose joints
+/-	+	+/-	Aortic stenosis	3rd decade	Hydrocephalus, odontoid hypoplasia
+/-	+	+	Aortic insufficiency	<2nd decade	Metatarsus, adductus, diastasis recti

genu valgum are unique to Morquio syndrome. All these conditions are recessively inherited. Hunter's syndrome or type II is X-linked while the others are autosomal (11). There is a wide interfamilial variability in clinical severity among the various types of mucopolysaccharidosis even when the same enzyme deficiency is involved. This illustrates the concept of genetic heterogeneity and allelic variation (12).

The various types of mucopolysaccharidosis can be differentiated by the clinical picture and by the type of glycosaminoglycan excreted in the urine (Table 2). The latter can be determined by a simple paper spot test combined with monodimensional electrophoresis (13), or by spectroscopy (14). A more definite diagnosis can be obtained by demonstrating the enzyme deficiency as suggested by the above screening tests in cell cultures.

A. MPS I H (Hurler's Syndrome)

Hurler's syndrome is the prototype for all the mucopolysaccharidoses (15). However, it is the most severely progressive of all the lysosomal storage disorders, characterized by early death (usually before age 10 years) and corneal clouding. Although affected patients appear normal at birth, they subsequently deteriorate in both mental and physical development. This disorder is caused by absence of alpha-L-iduronidase activity, which is necessary in the cleavage of L-iduronic acid residues present in both heparan sulfate and dermatan sulfate (11). Other clinical characteristics may include head enlargement, which is often scaphocephalic, with thickened nostrils and ears, coarse hair, harsh voice, hepatosplenomegaly, hydrocephalus, inguinal and umbilical hernia, neurosensory and conductive hearing loss, cardiomegaly, cardiac murmurs, psychomotor retardation, severe dwarfing, and dysostosis multiplex (4,11,16).

The dysostoses multiplex are best characterized radiographically and include widening of the medial end of the clavicle and anterior portion of the ribs, and hypoplastic or absent lateral portions. Due to the early closure of the sagittal sutures, the head is scaphocephalic and enlarged. The sella is J-shaped and the orbits are shallow, causing proptosis. There is mild gibbus resulting from smaller upper and lower thoracic vertebral bodies that are ovoid (4,11). The iliac wing is flared, the iliac body small, and the acetabulum is shallow. There is absence of diaphyseal constriction of the metacarpals, and the shafts of long bones may be wider than the metaphyses. The femoral neck has a varus deformity. Atlanto-axial subluxation due to hypoplastic odontoids is less often seen than in the other mucopolysaccharidoses.

On microscopic examination, there is accumulation of mucopolysaccharides, mainly dermatan and heparan sulfate, in the lysosomes of parenchymal and mesenchymal cells. The coronary arteries are lined with MPS deposits, resulting in pseudoatheromatosis with massive proliferation of collagen and elastic fibers (17). The liver may have diffuse fibrosis with extensive hepatocyte and Kupffer's cell vacuolization (18). The cause of the hepatic fibrosis is not well defined, but it is believed to be due to the abnormal accumulation of a hepatotoxic metabolite.

Diagnosis is based on excessive dermatan sulfaturia and heparan sulfaturia usually at a 7:3 ratio, but definite diagnosis is made by assay of alpha-L-iduronidase activity in the leukocytes or cultured fibroblasts. Prenatal diagnosis can be made by assaying the enzymatic activity of amniotic fluid cells (11).

B. MPS I S (Scheie's Syndrome)

Scheie's syndrome, formerly classified as MPS V, is caused by the same enzyme deficiency as Hurler's syndrome, alpha-L-iduronidase (19). However, the clinical findings are similar to those seen in Hurler's syndrome except for normal stature and intelligence and a longer life span. Deafness and corneal clouding may be present. In addition to the dysostosis multiplex, bone cysts of the femoral head have also been reported (20). The aortic and mitral valves may be stenotic or insufficient, or both (11).

Histological findings are similar to those in MPS I H, except that cortical neurons appear normal. There is also much less glycosaminoglycan content in the brain in contrast to MPS I H.

It is difficult to differentiate MPS I S from MPS I H biochemically. The distinction can be made clinically on the basis of height, which is normal or near normal in MPS I S and reduced significantly in the other mild MPS syndromes (11). There have been reports of residual alpha-L-iduronidase activity in MPS I S, which might explain the mild clinical picture, but these findings have been inconsistent. Some studies have shown no correlation between the clinical severity of these disorders and the amount of alpha-L-iduronidase activity of fibroblasts (21). Moreover, some investigators point out that low activity of alpha-L-iduronidase in both plasma and leukocytes is never found in normal individuals and should identify Scheie's syndrome (22).

C. MPS I H/S (Hurler-Scheie's Syndrome)

MPS I H/S is also caused by a deficiency of alpha-L-iduronidase activity, as in MPS I H and MPS I S. The clinical characteristics of these patients are intermediate between the Hurler and Scheie's syndromes. They are short and mentally retarded and have severe dysostoses multiplex but have a longer life span than patients with Hurler's syndrome. An almost consistent feature is the presence of micrognathia (23).

Microscopically, there are mucopolysaccharide cytoplasmic inclusions in all connective tissues, liver, and brain. Inclusions are also prominent in the anterior horn motor neurons of the spinal cord and less frequent in the cerebral cortex, cerebellum, and brain stem (24).

Diagnosis is based on the demonstration of deficient alpha-L-iduronidase activity in cultured leukocytes or fibroblasts in addition to the presence of clinical characteristics including micrognathia, which is usually not seen in the other two types of MPS I syndromes.

D. MPS II (Hunter's Syndrome)

In contrast to the other forms of MPS, which are inherited as autosomal recessive, Hunter's syndrome is an X-linked recessive deficiency of iduronate sulfatase, which is needed in the degradation of heparan sulfate and dermatan sulfate. It is, therefore, limited to the male sex, although there have been reports of an autosomal recessive transmission (11). Skeletal manifestations are similar to those of MPS I. However, lumbar gibbus does not occur and nodular skin lesions may be present on the posterior thorax or arms (25). Instead of corneal clouding, eye changes include chronic papilledema or retinitis pigmentosa. Affected patients are also characterized by a longer life span, milder mental retardation, and better auditory acuity than the MPS type I. Just like in Hurler's syndrome, the conductive hearing loss relates to chronic eustachian tube obstruction and thickened middle ear secretions (26). The excessive and thickened secretions in the respiratory tract also explain the obstructive apnea observed in both conditions. The radiographic features, however, are similar to or less marked than those of MPS I (27).

Other long-term complications that have been reported in Hunter's syndrome include myelopathy, which has resulted from impingement upon the cervical spinal cord (28), and papilledema, which may result from premature fusion of cranial sutures (29).

Microscopically, there are metachromatic cytoplasmic materials and vacuoles in the fibrocytes and ganglion and satellite cells of the rectal intramural plexi (30).

Diagnosis is made by demonstrating high levels of dermatan sulfate and heparan sulfate in the urine and, specifically, by deficient activity of the enzyme iduronate sulfatase in leukocytes, fibroblasts, or amniotic fluid cells (11,31). An abnormal level of [^{35}S] sulfate-labelled mucopolysaccharide characteristic of Hunter's syndrome has been detected in amniotic fluid cell cultures of a female fetus at risk for the condition (32).

E. MPS III (Sanfilippo's Syndrome)

The Sanfilippo's syndrome involves a deficiency of one of four enzymatic steps necessary for the removal of N-sulfated or N-acetylated alpha-linked glucosamine residues from the heparan sulfate chain (11). There are four types of Sanfilippo's syndrome: type A is due to a deficiency of heparan-N-sulfatase (33), type B is due to a deficiency of alpha-N acetyl glucosaminidase (34), type C is due to a deficiency of N-acetyl transferase (35), and type D is due to alpha-N-acetyl glucosamine-6-sulfatase (36).

The four types of Sanfilippo's syndrome are clinically indistinguishable. Moreover, this is the most frequently undiagnosed form of MPS because of its very mild somatic manifestations (37). The most prominent feature of MPS III, however, is progressive and severe psychomotor retardation (11). The dysostoses multiplex, short stature, hepatosplenomegaly, and joint stiffness are of mild degree. There may also be hirsutism, corneal clouding, and mitral valve disorders.

On microscopic examination, water-soluble metachromatic granules are seen in the viscera, which consist of finely granular, floccular, or filamentous material that is bound in cytoplasmic vacuoles. This material is believed to be glycosaminoglycans (38). The heart valves and arterial walls are infiltrated by foam cells. Zebra bodies are seen in both viscera and nervous system; these are lipid soluble and represent stored gangliosides (39).

The diagnosis of Sanfilippo's syndrome is suspected when there is a marked increase in the urinary excretion of heparan sulfate. Definite diagnosis of the enzyme deficiency can be made by assay of the enzymatic activity in fibroblasts and leukocytes and, prenatally, in amniotic fluid cells (11,40).

F. MPS IV (Morquio's Syndrome)

Two types of Morquio's syndrome are known. Classic Morquio syndrome, or MPS type IV A, is caused by a deficiency of N-acetylgalactosamine-6-sulfatase, while type IV B is due to a deficiency of beta-galactosidase. The two types of Morquio's syndrome are differentiated clinically by a milder degree of involvement in type B. Patients with Morquio's syndrome have skeletal changes that differ from the dysostosis multiplex of the other types of MPS. The most prominent skeletal features include severe short trunk dwarfism, genu valgum, pectus carinatum, platyspondyly, and short neck (4,11). There is also severe hypoplasia of the odontoid process of the second cervical vertebra resulting in atlantoaxial subluxation. The 2nd to 5th metacarpal bones have cone-shaped bases. The proximal capital epiphyses are irregular and the superior aspect of the acetabula is poorly ossified. Patients usually stop growing at the age of 7 or 8 years. Intelligence is usually normal or only minimally diminished.

Other findings include facial deformity, fine corneal opacities, impaired hearing, dental hypoplasia, ligamentous laxity, and hepatomegaly. Patients develop severe myelopathy that may result in obstructive and restrictive airway disease, paralysis of the muscles of respiration, and involvement of the heart valves. In some cases the myelopathy has been attributed to spinal compression at the levels of C_1 and C_2 vertebrae secondary to hypoplasia of the dens of C_2 and dislocation of the dens dorsad (27).

It has been shown that the primary defect of Morquio's syndrome B is a structural mutation that is allelic with that seen in the infantile and adult type GM_1 gangliosidosis (sphingolipidosis). Although these two conditions involve the same enzyme deficiency, their clinical manifestations are distinct (41). The multiplicity of phenotypic expression of acid beta-galactosidase deficiency may be due to the heterocatalytic characteristic of this enzyme. This enzyme cleaves galactose not only from keratosulfate but also from glycosaminoglycans, galactose oligosaccharides, and glycoproteins (11). In Morquio's syndrome type B, beta-galactosidase deficiency results in defective degradation of keratan sulfate. Thus, a diagnosis is suspected when keratan sulfate is found in high quantities in the urine. In mild cases, however, keratan excretion decreases with age and may reach normal levels in the second decade of life, in which case demonstration of deficient enzymatic activity in leukocytes and fibroblasts will help in the diagnosis (11).

To differentiate between Morquio's syndrome B and GM_1 gangliosidosis, clinical characteristics have to be considered. In the infantile type of GM_1 gangliosidosis, there are severe neurological changes, whereas in Morquio B skeletal deformities are more predominant, with no motor or mental retardation (42). Studies on the kinetic properties of this enzyme revealed that in Morquio's syndrome there is a low affinity of beta-galactosidase for substrate. On the other hand, in GM_1 gangliosidosis affinity is normal, but the kinetic properties (V_{max}) are markedly diminished (43).

Microscopic changes in Morquio's syndrome are evident in the brain, cartilage, skin, and bone. Large vacuoles are seen in the cells of the basal and malpighian layers of the epidermis and chondrocytes, but rarely in the brain and liver (11,44).

G. MPS V

Scheie's syndrome was classified as MPS V until it was found to be caused by deficiency of the same enzyme as MPS I (11). This syndrome was described above.

H. MPS VI (Maroteaux-Lamy Syndrome)

The basic defect in Maroteaux-Lamy syndrome is a deficiency of arylsulfatase B (N-acetyl galactosamine-4-sulfatase), which is required to hydrolyze the sulfate group from N-acetylgalactosamine-4-sulfate residues of dermatan sulfate (11). It is characterized by short stature that becomes evident at 2 years of age, at which time the dysostosis multiplex becomes apparent (4,11,27). Intelligence is normal but occasionally patients develop hydrocephalus and neurological complications due to atlantoaxial subluxation resulting from hypoplasia of the odontoid process. Severe myelopathy has been reported that occurred as a result of cervical spinal cord compression by a thickened dura (45). The corneas become cloudy early, but there are no retinal pigmentary changes described in MPS I, II, and III (27). Aortic valvular stenosis has been rarely associated with the syndrome (46).

Differentiation of Maroteaux-Lamy syndrome from Scheie's syndrome may be clinically difficult because both are inherited as autosomal recessive traits and are characterized by normal intellect. In Maroteaux-Lamy syndrome, however, the skeletal changes are more conspicuous (47). Moreover, there are typical cytoplasmic metachromatic granulations in a large proportion of neutrophils of patients with Maroteaux-Lamy syndrome, which are absent in Scheie's syndrome. In Scheie's syndrome, both dermatan and heparan sulfate are excreted in excess amounts in the urine, whereas in Maroteaux-Lamy syndrome only dermatan sulfate is excreted in excess.

Metachromatic lysosomal inclusions have also been found in the lymphocytes, Kupffer's cells, cornea, platelets, conjunctivae, and skin (11,48). Definitive diagnosis is made by demonstrating excess dermatan sulfate in the urine and a deficiency of the enzyme arylsulfatase B in leukocytes and fibroblasts (11). There is genetic heterogeneity, as in other mucopolysaccharidoses. In some, the mutant arylsulfatase B enzyme had similar antigenic cross-reactivity with the normal enzyme with undetectable activity, while in others there may be residual activity (49).

I. MPS VII (Sly's Syndrome)

The first case of MPS VII was first reported by Sly in 1973 (50). This occurred in a 7-week-old patient who presented for correction of metatarsus adductus. Initial clinical features, which included umbilical hernia, hepatosplenomegaly, thoracolumbar gibbus, and chondroitin sulfaturia, suggested a mucopolysaccharide storage disorder. Short stature became apparent at age 18 months, the head rapidly enlarged, pectus carinatum developed, and the lower costal margins flared outward. He also developed a heart murmur and cardiac enlargement. Psychomotor development was normal for the first 30 months but later deteriorated. There was no corneal clouding, but he had recurrent infections. Radiological changes of "dysostosis multiplex" were typical of those found in several of the classical mucopolysaccharidoses. This patient was found to have a virtual absence of the lysosomal hydrolase beta-glucuronidase activity. Mucopolysaccharide accumulation involved not only the liver and spleen but also the blood and bone marrow granulocytes.

Later reports of patients with beta-glucuronidase deficiency suggested a variation in clinical presentation including the presence of corneal clouding, varying age of onset of mucopolysacchariduria, with increase in chondroitin sulfate with or without an increase in dermatan and heparan sulfate (51). Those patients with an early age of onset had a more severe clinical manifestation; those patients with a later age of onset had a milder clinical picture. Severe beta-glucuronidase deficiency is the common denominator. Occasionally, the only manifestations are progressive kyphosis and scoliosis. Mental retardation or short stature may or may not be present (52).

Almost all patients have shown metachromatic inclusions in leukocytes and cultured skin fibroblasts. Liver biopsy may show giant cell transformation without inclusions and clear vesicles (53). Diagnosis is made only by demonstrating the absence of significantly diminished beta-glucuronidase activity.

J. Treatment

There have been various attempts to correct the specific enzymatic deficiencies in the lysosomal storage disorders (54). The first approach has been direct administration of the missing enzyme in the form of plasma infusion and leukocyte transfusion. Although reported to be successful by some in decreasing urinary excretion of mucopolysaccharides, plasma transfusion has resulted in short-lived or insignificant effects because the plasma contains only small amounts of the lysosomal enzyme needed (55,56). Leukocyte transfer has resulted in more significant clinical and biochemical response, such as improved joint mobility, increased alpha-L-iduronase activity, and decreased urinary excretion of acid mucopolysaccharides (57).

The second approach, which is transplantation of fibroblast or bone marrow, has shown varying success. Dean et al. demonstrated a marked increase in breakdown of glycosaminoglycans subsequent to skin transplantation with increase in Hunter corrective enzyme activity (58). They also reported marked improvement in their patients' general behavior, with no detectable deterioration in intellectual function or increase in liver size. It is assumed that these transplanted fibroblasts can release enough corrective enzyme to induce the observed results. On the other hand, attempts to correct the enzyme deficiency of Hunter's or Hurler's disorders by fetal fibroblast transplantation has also been reported to fail to induce prolonged biochemical or chemical improvement (59).

Bone marrow transplantation has been successfully used in the treatment of Maroteaux-Lamy syndrome (60). This resulted in increased arylsulfatase beta activity in peripheral lymphocytes and granulocytes with decrease in urinary excretion of glycosaminoglycans. Long-term follow-up revealed substantial decrease in liver and spleen size and normalization of cardiac function. Despite the few reported successes with fibroblast and bone marrow transplant, the problems that face any other form of organ or tissue transplantation remain: immunological rejection and graft versus host reactions. The mortality rate associated with bone marrow transplantation of such patients has been reportedly high (over 40%). This high mortality rate and the lack of evidence that the enzyme present in the blood can reach the brain have been deterrents to the use of this form of treatment (54).

II. GLYCOPROTEIN STORAGE DISORDERS

Glycoproteins are a major component of mammalian tissues, both intracellularly and extracellularly. These consist of oligosaccharide chains that are covalently linked to the peptide bone. Because of its abundance, a large amount of this material is produced even in normal turnover. A defect in the degradation of glycoprotein could result in accumulation of oligosaccharides in the organic matrix of bone and result in skeletal changes. Most of the process of degradation occurs in the lysosome, mainly through a series of hydrolytic steps in which each unit is removed from the nonreducing ends of the oligosaccharide. These hydrolases include alpha-mannosidase, alpha-fucosidase, beta-galactosidase, alpha-neuraminidase (sialidase), beta-N-acetylhexosaminidase, and aspartylglycosaminidase (Fig. 2). A deficiency of any of these enzymes results in accumulation of the partially degraded glycoprotein and the clinical manifestations of the various deficiency disorders, which will be discussed below (Table 3). These conditions are inherited as autosomal recessive traits with specific ethnic predilections (61).

A. Mannosidosis

A deficiency of the acidic form of alpha mannosidase results in mannose-rich accumulation of oligosaccharides in tissues. This disorder was first described by Ockerman in 1967 in a patient who had characteristics similar to Hurler's syndrome but had accumulation of mannose-containing oligosaccharides instead of mucopolysaccharides (62,63). Two types of mannosidosis have been described, type I or infantile form and type II or juvenile-adult form. Type I is characterized by more severe neurological and skeletal manifestations with earlier onset of symptoms and death between 3 and 10 years of age. Type II is characterized by absence of symptoms until later childhood or adolescence.

The skeletal manifestations include short stature, platyspondyly, coxa valga, limitation of interphalangeal joint extension, lumbar gibbus, and congenital hip dislocation. The radiological skeletal changes show dysostosis multiplex. Most of the radiological changes remain static after 4 years of age, with normalization of some skeletal defects. Other clinical manifestations include coarse facies, hearing loss, hepatosplenomegaly, hypotonia, inguinal and umbilical hernias, lenticular opacities, recurrent infections, and hypogammaglobulinemia (64–67).

Microscopically, there is generalized ballooning of the cytoplasm of nerve cells throughout the cerebral cortex, brain stem, and spinal cord, but not in the basal ganglia (60). Large foam cells that stain with periodic acid–Schiff are seen in the bone marrow, neuronal storage cells, lymphocytes, Kupffer's cells, and reticuloendothelial cells. This periodic-acid–Schiff-staining material represents mannose-rich oligosaccharides (65).

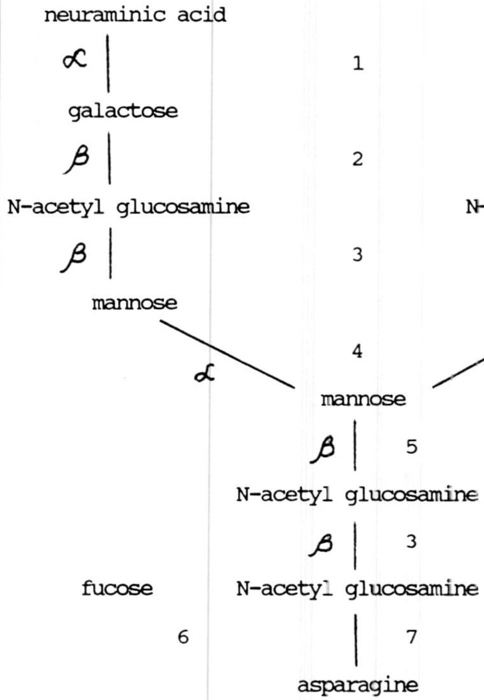

Cleavage Site	Enzyme	Deficiency State
1	α-neuraminidase (sialidase)	Sialidosis
2	β-galactosidase	GM_1 gangliosidosis
3	hexosaminidase A and B	GM_2 gangliosidosis
4	α-mannosidase	mannosidosis
5	β-mannosidase	
6	α-L-fucosidase	fucosidosis
7	N-aspartyl-β-glucosaminidase	aspartyl glycosaminuria

Figure 2 Steps in the degradation of a glycoprotein.

There are three distinct forms of human alpha-mannosidase in the liver, two of which are lysosomal with acidic optimal activity (pH 4.0–4.5), the third is nonlysosomal and optimally active at pH 6.0 (68). Aside from the clinical manifestations, the diagnosis of alpha-mannosidosis is made by demonstrating the periodic-acid–Schiff-staining material in lymphocytes or other tissues, mannose in the urine, and a complete deficiency or a reduced activity of the acidic iso-

Table 3 Glycoprotein Storage Disorders

Type	Enzyme Defect	Skeletal changes	Neurological Changes	Hepato-splenomegaly	Others
Mannosidosis I	Alpha-mannosidase	Platyspondyly, coxa valga, limitation of phalangeal extension	+++	+++	Hearing loss, corneal opacities, cataracts
Mannosidosis II	Alpha-mannosidase	Milder than I	++	++	Same as I
Fucosidosis I	Alpha-L-fucosidase	Lumbar kyphosis, short trunk, short neck, pectus carinatum	++	++	Increased sweat CI
Fucosidosis II	Alpha-L-fucosidase	Same as I	++	++	Normal sweat, CI, angiokeratoma
Aspartylglycosaminuria	N-aspartyl-beta-glycosaminidase	Widened ribs, widened tubular bone diaphysis, thickened skull, coarse trabeculation	++	+/-	Lens opacity, acne
Sialidosis I	Alpha-neuraminidase	None	+++	-	Blindness, cherry-red spot
Sialidosis II Infantile	Alpha-neuraminidase	Kyphoscoliosis, pectus carinatum, joint flexion, pes cavus, dolichocephaly, hypoplastic sinuses	++	+/-	Cherry-red spot renal disease
Juvenile	Alpha-neuraminidase	Milder than infantile type	++	-	Cherry-red spot, angiokeratoma, visual and hearing loss
Congenital	Alpha-neuraminidase	Same as in infantile type	++	++	Hydrops fetalis
Galactosialidosis	Combined alpha-neuraminidase and beta-galactosidase	Acetabular dysplasia, coxa valga, scoliosis, platylspondyly, eroded lumbar vertebrae	++	+/-	Cherry-red spot, angiokeratomas, Hurler's facies

enzymes, but a normal activity of the neutral isoenzyme. The latter may explain the residual enzyme activity in some patients and mild clinical manifestations (69). A striking chemical abnormality in this disorder is storage of the glycopeptide containing 3 mol of mannose and 1 mol of N-acetyl glucosamine (70).

B. Fucosidosis

Fucose, a deoxy sugar, is a constituent of oligosaccharides in the mucopolysaccharides and mucolipids of various human and animal tissues. Fucosidosis was first reported as an autosomal recessive neurovisceral disease by Durand et al. in 1966 in two siblings who had progressive cerebral degeneration and mental deterioration (71). Laboratory evaluation revealed increased sweat and salivary chloride and sodium content, gallbladder dysfunction, and glycolipid accumulation in lymphocytes, skin, liver, and other tissues. The excess glycolipid consisted of ceramide tetrahexosides, with fucose as the last hexose group (72). The basic defect of this disease is a complete absence of alpha-L-fucosidase (73).

There are two forms of fucosidosis. Sixty percent of cases have type I or the fatal infantile form, which is characterized by more severe manifestations than type II or the adult disease. Aside from the signs reported by Durand, the clinical features may also include psychomotor retardation, dysostosis multiplex, hepatosplenomegaly, and seizures. Aside from a milder disease, type II fucosidosis is distinguished mainly by the presence of angiokeratoma, a longer survival, often to the adult years, and a normal sweat chloride level (74).

Skeletal findings are characterized by dysotosis multiplex including lumbar kyposis contractures of the hips, knees, ankles, and elbows; marked shortening of the trunk, pectus carinatum, and short neck (74). Roentgenological changes are closely similar to those of the Sanfilippo syndrome (75). A case of fucosidosis has been reported in which the disease appeared to be limited to bone (76). This 9-year-old child had normal intelligence and no visceromegaly but had spondyloepiphyseal metaphyseal dysplasia and a deficiency of alpha-L-fucosidase activity.

Aside from the presence of the above clinical and radiological findings, and the demonstration of excess fucose in the urine, the diagnosis of fucosidosis is confirmed by demonstrating the absence of alpha-L-fucosidase activity in cultured cells (77) or even in plasma or serum (78). However, since some normal individuals can have low plasma alpha-L-fucosidase activity but normal leukocyte activity (79), it is necessary to demonstrate the enzyme deficiency in both plasma and leukocytes (80). The assay of alpha-L-fucosidase activity in the liver may be misleading since it may demonstrate up to 50% of normal alpha-L-fucosidase activity. This could be due to a small amount of normal enzyme present or to inhibition of regular amounts of the normal enzyme (81). The carrier state may also be detected by direct determination of alpha-L-fucosidase activity in mononuclear cells. However, in serum or plasma there is a wide overlap between normal subjects and heterozygotes (82).

C. Aspartyl Glycosaminuria

Aspartyl glycosaminuria is another autosomal recessive glycoprotein storage disease caused by a deficiency of the enzyme N-aspartyl-beta-glycosaminidase (83). This enzyme is involved in hydrolyzing the GlcNAc–Asn linkage in lysosomes and its deficiency results not only in excessive urinary excretion of aspartyl glycosamine but also in a clinical syndrome that results from accumulation of this material.

The skeletal manifestations include short stature, brachycephaly, and mild dysostosis multiplex, which includes widened ribs and tubular bone diaphyses, thickened skull, and coarse trabeculation (84). Other associated findings are uncontrolled behavior, psychomotor retardation, seizures, transient hepatosplenomegaly, cardiac valvular lesions, coarse facies, recurrent infections, diarrhea, lens opacities, joint laxity, macroglossia, and umbilical hernia (61,85). Life expectancy could extend to the fourth decade.

Microscopic evaluation revealed vacuolated cells in the bone marrow, small intestines, skin, lymph nodes, kidney, liver, and brain. There are lysosomal abnormalities, which include granular matrix, electronlucent droplets (lipid), and membrane bound electrondense structures (84).

Since GlcNAc-Asn may be excreted in minimal amounts in the urine of normal individuals (86), more definitive tests are necessary to make the diagnosis. Absent or decreased activity of N-aspartyl-beta-glycosaminidase in plasma, leukocytes, seminal fluid, liver, brain, spleen, or fibroblasts should be demonstrated before a diagnosis of aspartyl glycosaminuria is made. The carrier state may also be detected by demonstrating a deficiency of the enzyme in plasma or white blood cells (87).

D. Sialidosis Type II

Primary deficiency of the enzyme N-acetyl neuramine acid hydrolase (neuraminidase) results in accumulation and excretion of sialylated oligosaccharides called sialidosis. In 1979, Lowden and O'Brien classified sialidosis into two types. Type I includes the group of patients with an isolated primary neuraminidase deficiency who have no somatic manifestations, that is, normal physical appearance and body proportions and normal intelligence, but have cherry red spots in the retina and myoclonic seizures (88). On the other hand, sialidosis type II describes patients who have short stature and dysostosis multiplex. Some of the original patients with type II sialidosis also demonstrated a deficiency of beta-galactosidase, but later studies have shown that this may be a separate genetic disorder and will, therefore, be discussed later under a different category (89).

Patients with sialidosis type II appear normal at birth, with skeletal changes occurring at about 9 months of age (90). The skeletal changes include short stature, severe kyphoscoliosis, pectus carinatum, joint flexion, and pes cavus. The skull is thickened with a slight dolichocephaly. The sinuses are hypoplastic. The long bones are osteopenic and trabeculate, the iliac wings dysplastic, and the hips dislocated (90). Features resembling those of Hurler's syndrome develop much later, at about 10 years of age. Intelligence starts to lag behind at around the same time. There is also progressive visual and hearing loss, cherry-red spots, punctate lenticular opacities, esotropia, and occasional corneal opacities. Patients may also have hepatosplenomegaly and peripheral neuropathy (61,90). Seizures may not start until the second year of life (91).

Microscopically, lymphocytes and Kupffer's cells appear vacuolated and the bone marrow contains foam cells in sialidosis type II that are not present in type I (61). Analysis of neuraminidase activity in skin fibroblast cultures reveals absence or marked deficiency of the enzyme. Patients with type II disease have a lower enzyme activity than those with type I (92). This would explain their more severe clinical course, marked dysmorphism, and bone abnormalities. On the other hand, patients with type I sialidosis may have a normal enzyme activity or demonstrate up to 12.4% activity of neuraminidase (93).

E. Combined Neuraminidase-Beta-Galactosidase Deficiency

A deficiency of both neuraminidase and beta-galactosidase may occur. This is a genetic disorder that is clinically distinct from sialidosis, which is due to an isolated neuraminidase deficiency, or from GM_1 gangliosidosis and Morquio syndrome type B, both of which are due to an isolated deficiency of beta-galactosidase. It has been postulated that the combined neuraminidase-beta-galactosidase deficiency is the result of a defective 32 kD glycoprotein that is required to protect these enzymes from excessive intralysosomal degradation and to give them their full hydrolytic capacity (94). This combined deficiency disorder is characterized by a normal structural gene located in chromosome 10 but a defective gene in chromosome 20, which apparently codes for this important 32 kD glycoprotein, resulting in a defective posttranslational modification of these enzymes (95). In contrast, in sialidosis the defect is in the structural gene for neuraminidase (96).

Skeletal abnormalities include acetabular dysplasia, subluxation of the hip with coxa valga, scoliosis, platyspondyly, and erosion of the anterior margins of the lumbar vertebral bodies (97).

Other characteristics of the combined neuraminidase-beta-galactosidase deficiency disorder include facies resembling those in Hurler's syndrome with large tongue and lips, generalized angiokeratomas, mostly in the lips, jaws, limbs, elbows, knees, and genitalia. Cherry-red spots are seen in the macula.

There is visual impairment, tortuous vasodilatation of the bulbar conjunctivae with slight corneal and lenticular opacities. Neurological manifestations include ataxia, ballism movements of the fingers, resembling dysmetria, and adiadokinesia. Skeletal abnormalities include acetabular dysplasia, subluxation of the hip with coxa valga, scoliosis, platyspondyly, and erosion of the anterior margins of the lumbar vertebral bodies (97).

Microscopic examination reveals vacuoles in vascular endothelial cells dermal histiocytes, Schwann's cells, and perineural cells, but not in the axons. Lipid-like homogeneous materials are occasionally seen. The angiokeratomatous lesions display an intense dilatation of blood vessels with swollen endothelial cells similar to foam cells.

Diagnosis is based on the demonstration of a marked decrease in the activities of beta-galactosidase and neuraminidase in the cultured skin fibroblasts and leukocytes (96).

Prenatal diagnosis of the combined enzyme deficiency disorder has been reported with use of a rapid and reliable assay using the fluorogenic 4-methylumbelliferyl substrates to detect diminished levels of neuraminidase and beta-galactosidase (98). Prenatal diagnosis can also be done for mannosidosis, aspartyl-glycosaminuria, and sialidosis, and decisions regarding termination of pregnancy may be based on the degree of enzyme deficiency from cultured amniotic cells (61).

F. Treatment

There is no specific treatment for any of the above glycoprotein storage disorders. However, fibroblast and bone marrow transplantation have been tried in the treatment of mannosidosis. Studies have shown that mannose-containing oligosaccharides were degraded after transfer of the missing enzyme from normal lymphocytes to mannosidosis fibroblasts on direct contact in tissue culture. This effect can be prolonged if there was repeated contact with the donor lymphocytes, is a result of endocytosis by cell-to-cell contact, and is not mediated by mannose-6-phosphate receptors (99,100). The addition of human liver alpha-D-mannosidase to cultured fibroblasts from mannosidosis patients resulted in partial correction of the metabolic defect (101).

Much earlier, Desnick et al. demonstrated that the residual activity of alpha-D-mannosidase in the liver could be improved more than 2-1/2-times when assayed in the presence of cobalt and zinc. Although this finding suggests that there may be a therapeutic value of cobalt and/or zinc supplementation in these patients, there has been no further report on their usefulness in vivo (102).

Apart from these attempts to treat alpha-mannosidase deficiency, no definitive treatment is available for the other glycoprotein storage diseases. Studies have indicated that leupeptin and EP 475, which are inhibitors of lysosomal thiolproteases in restoring partial beta-galactosidase activity; have significantly increased the neuraminidase levels in conditions with combined neuraminidase–beta-galactosidase deficiency. Moreover, other studies have shown that addition of fibroblasts from patients with isolated deficiency of either of the two enzymes resulted in restoration of the enzymatic activities of the enzymes. These studies further support the proposal made by D'Azzo et al. that the combined neuraminidase-beta-galactosidase deficiency is due to a deficiency in a glycoprotein normally required to protect the two enzymes from being degraded (103).

III. GANGLIOSIDE STORAGE DISORDERS

Gangliosides are a major component of brain tissue but are also present in most other body cells including the skeletal system. These compounds are glycosphingolipids containing sialic acid in their oligosaccharide chains, which are catalyzed by exohydrolases by a stepwise removal of sugar molecules. If one of the hydrolases is deficient, further breakdown is blocked, resulting in accumulation of ganglioside (104).

Three types of ganglioside storage disease have been described, but only the infantile type of GM_1 gangliosidosis results in predominant skeletal changes. Tay-Sachs disease and Sandhoff's disease have predominantly neurological manifestations and will, therefore, not be discussed in this chapter.

GM_1 gangliosidosis is an autosomal recessive disease that results from a deficiency of the lysosomal acid beta-galactosidase. Accumulation of glycolipids and oligosaccharides with a terminal beta-galactosidic linkage results (Fig. 3). Recent studies have shown that the mechanism behind the enzymatic defect in GM_1 gangliosidosis is an interference with the phosphorylation of precursor beta-galactosidase (105). This results in secretion of the precursor rather than its compartmentalization into the lysosomes.

Type 1 GM_1 gangliosidosis is the infantile or generalized disease in which symptoms begin at birth or shortly afterwards. Patients are usually born with edematous extremities. There is generalized hypotonia, respiratory difficulty, and convulsions. Internal strabismus and lateral nystagmus may be present. Cherry-red spots may be seen in the macula. Macrocephaly may develop. Hepatosplenomegaly is present in over 80% of patients by 6 months of age (106).

The most important skeletal changes are seen in the spine and upper extremities and resemble the dystosis multiplex in Hurler's syndrome (106–108). There is thoracolumbar gibbus and/or kyphosis, coarse trabeculation of long bones, iliac flaring, and mild coxa valga. There is generalized rarefaction of the cortex of most bones, beaking of the vertebral bodies, widening of the midshaft of the humeri and long bones, and proximal and distal tapering of these long bones.

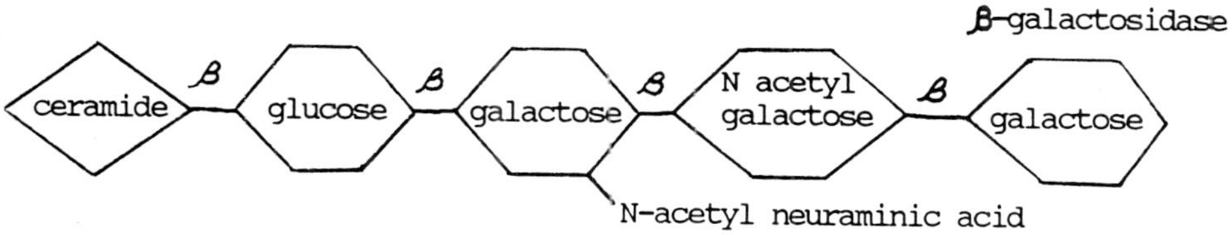

Figure 3 Structure of GM_1 ganglioside showing site of normal cleavage by beta-galactosidase. A deficiency of beta-galactosidase in GM_1 gangliosidosis results in accumulation of gangliosides with a terminal beta-galactosidic linkage.

The metacarpal bones are wedge-shaped with proximal constriction of the lateral metacarpals. There is cloaking of the humerus indicating subperiosteal new bone formation. In the skull, the sella appears shoe-shaped and elongated. The ribs are spatulate. Patients usually die at about 2 years of age.

An unusual variant of infantile GM_1 gangliosidosis has been described in which an infant presented with cardiomyopathy and progressive neurological deterioration starting at 4 months of age with no associated skeletal changes (109).

Type 2 (juvenile type) GM_1 gangliosidosis has a later onset of clinical manifestations (usually after 1 year of age), after which psychomotor retardation becomes rapidly progressive (104). The somatic manifestations present in infantile GM_1 gangliosidosis are either absent or very mild. The radiological changes include mild inferior beaking of the vertebral bodies and pelvic deformities. Patients may survive up to 3–10 years. Death is usually due to complications of respiratory failure.

Type 3 (adult type) GM_1 gangliosidosis is characterized by late-onset neurological impairment usually as dysarthria and gradual loss of intellectual function. Seizures are uncommon and normal vision is maintained. These patients usually have a normal life span (110).

Microscopic examination reveals vacuolation of lymphocytes in the peripheral blood and vacuolation of histiocytes in the bone marrow, parafollicular zones of the lymph nodes, red pulp of the spleen, and sinusoids of the liver and intestinal mucosa. The most striking pathological changes are visceral histiocytosis, neuronal lipidosis, and cytoplasmic vacuolation of renal glomerular epithelial cells (106). Ultrastructural studies demonstrate two types of membrane-bound vacuoles: one containing lamellar membranes and the other containing finely granular material (111).

Diagnosis is made clinically and confirmed by enzyme assay of beta-galactosidase in leukocytes and cultured skin fibroblasts in the absence of urine mucopolysaccharides. Prenatal diagnosis is performed by enzyme analysis of cultured amniotic fluid cells and by detection of galactosyl oligosaccharides in amniotic fluid by high-pressure liquid chromatography (112). Since pathological changes have been demonstrated even in a 24 week fetus, any attempts at intrauterine treatment must be started before the second trimester of pregnancy.

There is no specific treatment available for any of the ganglioside storage disorders. Intrathecal injection of hexosaminidase A has been tried in Tay-Sachs disease without clear success. Prenatal diagnosis by amniotic fluid enzyme assay has been the only effective preventive method (104).

IV. MUCOLIPID STORAGE DISORDERS

The mucolipidoses are a group of disorders that result from defects in carbohydrate and lipid metabolism and affect the organic matrix of bones. These conditions share some features of mucopolysaccharidosis as well as sphingolipidosis (113). These include mucolipidoses I, II, and III. The underlying defect in mucolipidosis I (also called sialidosis type II) is a deficiency of alpha-neuraminidase, which differs from the two other mucolipidoses and was, therefore, discussed separately in another section of this chapter.

Mucolipidoses II and III are due to defects in the synthesis of a marker necessary for the intracellular transport of acid hydrolases into lysosomes (114). Normally, hydrolases have mannose-6-phosphate residues that guide them to lysosomes by a receptor-mediated process. In mucolipidosis II, acid hydrolases are not phosphorylated and in mucolipidosis III these are either not phosphorylated or have a reduced phosphate content (113). As a consequence, the hydrolases are secreted rather than translocated to lysosomes. Moreover, these hyrolases do not undergo proteolysis, which is their usual fate within lysosomes.

Although mucolipidoses II and III are clinically similar, the electrophoretic mobility patterns of their lysosomal hydrolases are different, suggesting that these two disorders are genetically distinct (115). Moreover, it has also been shown that patients with mucolipidoses II and III have kinetic differences in their neutral N-acetylglucosaminyl phosphotransferase with respect to its catalytic activity and affinity for substrate (116).

A. I-Cell Disease (Mucolipidosis II, ML II)

I-cell disease (ML II) is an autosomal recessive disorder due to a defect in a recognition marker that enables acid hydrolases to reach lysosomes. This condition presents after birth with congenital hip dislocation, umbilical or inguinal hernia, facial and skeletal abnormalities, a tight thickened skin, low birthweight, and hypotonia (117). Patients are later noted to have delayed psychomotor development and recurrent respiratory infections. The facial features include a high forehead, prominent epicanthal folds, puffy eyelids, flat bridge of the nose, anteverted nostril, wide philtrum, and corneal clouding. There is restriction of joint motion in the shoulders, hips, and wrists. There is hepatomegaly and rarely, splenomegaly. As the child grows older, the coarse features and psychomotor retardation progress and patients more closely resemble those with Hurler's syndrome.

The skeletal features are similar to those found in GM_1 gangliosidosis type I and, in the later phases, like those in Hurler's syndrome. There is "cloaking" of the long tubular bones, particularly in the femur and humerus. The phalanges are bullet-shaped, the distal end of the radius and ulna tilted. There is iliac flaring, and anterior and inferior beaking of the vertebral bodies. The ribs have a broad and spatulate appearance. The cranial vault is thickened and there may be premature closure of the sagittal sutures (117). There is metaphyseal fragmentation and irregularity (118). Aside from moderate dysostosis multiplex evident in early infancy, clubfoot and immobile thumb may be present (119).

The term I-cell disease was derived from the cytoplasmic inclusion bodies found in skin fibroblasts ("I cells"). These inclusions are periodic and acid-Schiff positive, oil-red-O-positive, granular, and represent lysosomes containing heterogeneous materials. Other microscopic findings include lipid inclusions in hepatocytes but not in Kupffer cells. The glomerular epithelial cells and fibrocytes contain a few clear inclusions. In the neurons and astrocytes are seen mostly dense inclusions with occasional clear inclusions, but other cell organelles are normal (120). Ultrastructural studies of the inclusions showed that they are membrane-bound and weakly metachromatic, in contrast to the intense metachromasia of the Hurler–Hunter's inclusions. The lipid content of the inclusions in I-cell disease is high. They are also comprised of multivesicular and pleiomorphic membranes, with electron-dense and some electronlucent material (121). A high cystine content was also demonstrated in cultured fibroblasts of patients with I-cell disease, which appeared to be a result of an altered membrane structure, the presence of undigested inclusions, and increased degradation of protein in the lysosomal pathway (122).

The diagnosis of I-cell disease is made when the pathognomonic feature of Sudan-B-black-staining cytoplasmic inclusion in cultured fibroblasts is observed. Moreover, the level of activity of glucosaminyl-N-acetyl phosphotransferase activity in cultured fibroblasts is below the normal range but does not correlate with the severity of clinical manifestations (119).

B. Pseudo-Hurler's Polydystrophy (Mucolipidosis III, ML III)

The primary defect in ML III is a deficiency of glucosaminyl-N-acetyl phosphotransferase, which catalyzes the transfer of alpha-N-acetylglucosamine 1-phosphate residues to high-mannose oligosaccharide units of lysosomal enzymes. The enzymes affected include beta-hexosaminidase, iduronate sulfatase, and arylsulfatase B. These enzymes cannot enter the lysosomes and thus remain in high levels extracellularly (123).

The clinical characteristics of ML III include growth retardation, severe dysostosis multiplex, restricted joint motion, tight skin, swollen eyelids, late-onset hepatosplenomegaly, umbilical hernia, hyperopia, astigmatism, optic nerve abnormalities, corneal opacities, and normal or only slightly impaired mental and neurological development (123,124).

Radiological evaluation shows bullet-shaped metacarpals, deformity of the distal radius, widened shaft of the radius and ulna, anterior compression of L_1 with decreased anterioposterior (AP) dimension, slight kyphosis, inferior beaking of vertebral bodies, vagus deformity of the femoral neck, flared iliac wings, and flattened proximal femoral epiphysis (125).

Biochemical findings include deficient intracellular levels of multiple lysosomal hydrolases in cultured fibroblasts, increased levels of the same lysosomal hydrolases in serum or culture media, and normal levels of urine acid mucopolysaccharides (125). Just as in ML II, there is clinical and biochemical heterogeneity (123,126). In some instances, a variant of this disorder has been identified involving a catalytically active N-acetyl glucosaminyl phosphotransferase that is defective in its ability to recognize lysosomal enzymes as specific substrates for phosphorylation (121).

Clinically, ML II can be differentiated from ML III because of the earlier onset of symptoms and clinical changes in the former. Children with ML II are affected at birth with severe psychomotor retardation, dysostosis multiplex, hypotonia, and organomegaly and rarely survive the first decade of life. On the other hand, ML III patients have subclinical symptoms until about 3-5 years of age and have milder somatic manifestations and mental retardation. Affected individuals may reach adulthood (114).

Biochemically, ML II can be distinguished from ML III by differences in the extent of intracellular deficiency and extracellular elevation of lysosomal enzyme activities in fibroblast cultures. For example, the intracellular activity of alpha-fucosidase, beta-galactosidase, alpha-mannosidase, and neuraminidase is very low or almost completely absent in ML II and also low but slightly higher in ML III. Extracellularly, alpha-fucosidase and alpha-mannosidase activities are slightly higher than normal in both conditions, but beta-glucuronidase, hexosaminidase-A, and alpha-mannosidase levels are markedly elevated in both ML II and ML III (116) (Table 4).

C. Treatment

There is no definitive treatment for any of the phosphotransferase deficiency disorders. Sucrose loading has been reported to normalize multiple deficiencies of intracellular lysosomal hydrolases in I-cell disease fibroblasts (128). The degree of induction of hydrolases, however, varies, suggesting heterogeneity in this disorder (129). Some studies have produced correction of I-cell defect by hybridizing I cells with different types of fibroblasts with a single enzyme defici-

Table 4 Intracellular and Extracellular Enzyme Activities[a] in Normal and Fibroblast Cultures from Patients with I-Cell Disease and Pseudo-Hurler's Polydystrophy

Enzyme	Normal controls (n=12)	I-cell disease (n=5)	Pseudo-Hurler's polydystrophy (n=3)	Variant of Pseudo-Hurler's (n=5)[b]
Intracellular				
Alpha-fucosidase	72 ± 18	2.2 ± 0.5	16 ± 3.2	19 ± 3.0
Beta-galactosidase	584 ± 183	5.7 ± 3.2	63 ± 19	87 ± 27
Alpha-mannosidase	98 ± 31	9.3 ± 3.9	17 ± 5.0	14 ± 4.1
Neuraminidase	39 ± 16	0.5 ± 0.3	7.6 ± 2.8	13 ± 4.1
Acid phosphatase	2954 ± 480	2620 ± 467	2889 ± 355	3036 ± 612
Beta-glucosidase	162 ± 37	148 ± 50	207 ± 58	271 ± 107
Extracellular				
Alpha-fucosidase	0.8 ± 0.3	2.7 ± 0.6	1.9 ± 0.3	1.6 ± 0.2
Beta-glucuronidase	41 ± 13	345 ± 73	136 ± 23	121 ± 23
Hexosaminidase A	97 ± 24	878 ± 221	279 ± 38	314 ± 57
Alpha-mannosidase	2.3 ± 0.6	24 ± 4.6	13 ± 2.1	12 ± 3.0
Beta-glucosidase	0.2 ± 0.1	0.2 ± 0.1	0.2 ± 0.1	0.3 ± 0.1

[a]Extracellular activities represent the activities of enzymes secreted into serum-free medium, in 24 hr, by mg cell protein.
[b]Pseudo-Hurler's polydystrophy cell lines that express normal N-acetyl-glucosaminyl phosphotransferase activity toward alpha-methylmannoside acceptor.
Source: From Ref. 116.

ency, such as GM_1 gangliosidosis type I cells, Sandhoff's fibroblasts, and fibroblasts from mannosidosis patients. This complementation may be the result of the presence of normal polypeptide chains in I cells whereas the other cell types provide a factor that causes intracellular retention of the enzymes (130).

V. SPHINGOLIPID STORAGE DISORDERS

A few conditions with abnormalities in lipid metabolism result in prominent skeletal changes. These conditions generally affect the metabolism of sphingolipid, a polar lipid whose core structure is provided by the long-chain amino alcohol, sphingosine. Sphingolipids are present in almost all tissues of the human body. The highest concentrations are in the white matter of the central nervous system. Sphingolipids are normally degraded within lysosomes of phagocytic cells particularly the reticuloendothelial system. This pathway is illustrated in Figure 4. A series of hydrolases cleaves specific bonds in the compounds that form the pathway for removing sugars and sulfates in a stepwise manner.

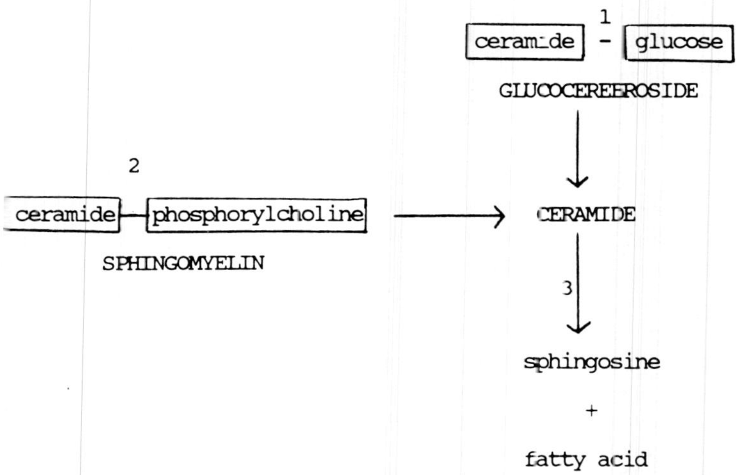

Site of Action	Enzyme	Deficiency State
1	β- glucuronidase	Gaucher's disease
2	sphingomyelinase	Niemann-Pick disease
3	ceramidase	Farber's granulomatosis

Figure 4 Steps in the degradation of sphingolipids that affect the skeletal system.

Inability to catabolize certain lipids due to a deficiency of a hydrolytic enzyme results in accumulation of lipids in the reticulodenothelial cells of the spleen, liver, and bone marrow (131). This resultant increasing mass of reticuloendothelial cells accounts not only for the hepatosplenomegaly and lymph node enlargement but also for the bone lesions due to expansion of the bone marrow (132). These skeletal changes are outlined in Table 4. In some conditions, the brain is severely affected; this is believed to be due to local accumulations of lipid from tissue turnover (131).

Of the known disorders of lipid metabolism, three conditions are characterized by major skeletal aberrations: Gaucher's disease, Niemann-Pick disease, and Farber's disease (Table 5). In contrast, the other lipid storage disorders such as metachromatic leukodystrophy, Tay Sach's, and Krabbe's disease affect the central nervous system primarily (133). All of these disorders are inherited in an autosomal recessive fashion.

Table 5 Skeletal Manifestations of Sphingolipid Storage Disorders

Gaucher's Disease	Niemann-Pick Disease	Farber's Disease
Aseptic necrosis of femoral head Vertebral collapse Erlenmeyer-flask deformity of distal femur Osteopenia Osteosclerosis Subarticular osteonecrosis Osteomyelitis	Osteoporosis Coxa valga Widening of diaphyses and metaphyses of metacarpals and distal phalanges	Periarticular bone erosions Joint contractures and subluxations Osteopenia

A. Gaucher's Disease

Gaucher's disease is the most common heritable disorder of glycolipid metabolism and is due to a deficiency of a lysosomal acid hydrolase, glucosyl ceramide-beta-glucosidase (glucocerebrosidase), which catalyzes the cleavage of glucose from the glucocerebroside (134). Glucocerebrosides arise mainly from the degradation of sphingoglycolipids in both leukocytes and erythrocytes. These compounds are not a normal structural component of membranes but are only observed during synthesis and degradation of more complex glycosphingolipids (135). Glucocerebrosides are composed of equimolar portions of sphingosine, a long-chain fatty acid, and glucose. When not hydrolyzed, this material accumulates in reticuloendothelial cells causing the latter to expand, called "Gaucher's cells."

The clinical disorder has been classified into three categories based on the differences in their phenotypic expressions: Type 1 (adult or chronic nonneuronopathic), type 2 (infantile, acute neuronopathic), and type 3 (juvenile, subacute neuronopathic).

The adult form, which is the most common type of the disorder, may be evident at any age and manifest with organomegaly, hypersplenism, pingueculae, and bone lesions (132). There is usually no involvement of the central nervous system (134).

The bone complications are prominent and occur in 50–75% of all patients with Gaucher's disease. The hip is the usual site of pain and orthopedic disability in these patients, which may be due to aseptic necrosis of the femoral head (136). Pathological fractures frequently involve the proximal femur and occasionally vertebral collapse may occur. Roentgenograms reveal expanded cortex of the distal femur (Erlenmeyer-flask deformity) with bone erosion, cyst-like cavities, and cortical thinning (137). Other skeletal manifestations include osteopenia, osteosclerosis, infarction of the marrow, subarticular osteonecrosis, modeling deformities, and even osteomyelitis (138).

Computed tomography and ^{99}Tc sulfur colloid bone marrow scans that reveal areas of decreased density have been shown to be effective in assessing the extent and severity of skeletal involvement (139). Later studies have shown that magnetic resonance imaging is more sensitive in demonstrating the extent of the abnormalities (140).

Retardation of growth and development has been observed in some patients, for which no hormonal basis is known. However, there has been a report of a patient with Gaucher's cells in the pituitary (134).

Children with the infantile form of the disease usually become symptomatic before 6 months of age and die by 2 years of age (134). There is severe involvement of the central nervous system.

The juvenile form of the disease is slowly progressive and becomes evident in childhood. The manifestations are intermediate between types 1 and 2 patients, both skeletal and neurologic manifestations occur.

The most striking microscopic finding in Gaucher's disease is the predominance of Gaucher's cells, which are lipid-laden cells found in most organ systems and all parts of the reticuloendothelial system particularly in the red pulp of the spleen, the sinusoids of the liver and lymph nodes, and the bone marrow (134). The cells stain with periodic acid–Schiff and are positive for acid phosphatase.

1. Diagnosis

The diagnosis of Gaucher's disease may be established by demonstration of Gaucher's cells in the bone marrow, liver, and lymph node biopsy in a patient with hepatosplenomegaly. More specifically, diminished glucocerebrosidase activity in cultured leukocytes or skin fibroblasts may help in establishing the diagnosis (137). Recently, lymphocytes have been used to demonstrate a deficiency of the enzyme using a fluorescent analog (141).

Prenatal diagnosis of Gaucher's disease has been done with reliability. A few fetuses with type 3 Gaucher's disease could be identified correctly, but the fetus with type 1 disease is more difficult to identify. The fetus at risk for type 2 disease can be identified on the basis of normal glucosidase activity measured with a fluorogenic material: 4-methylumbelliferyl-beta-D-glucopyranoside (142).

2. Treatment

The management of patients with Gaucher's disease is mainly supportive, directed at alleviating and preventing complications. Bone pain may be relieved with the use of strong analgesics. Infections should be treated with appropriate antibiotics. Because hypersplenism may lead to anemia, thrombocytopenia, and hemorrhage, splenectomy is sometimes necessary. Partial splenectomy has been shown to work, leaving a functioning remainder of the spleen (143–145). However, total splenectomy has been blamed for the acceleration of pulmonary, renal, and skeletal complications (146–148). Hence, partial splenectomy is recommended.

Bone marrow transplantation has been done in an attempt to provide a permanent source of enzymatic competent cells (149). It carries the same risk as any tissue transplantation, but has been shown to be effective in increasing the production of beta-glucocerebrosidase by hematopoietic cells. However, normalization of plasma cerebroside levels and disappearance of Gaucher's cells from the bone marrow occurred more slowly (150). Moreover, there is no evidence that bone marrow transplantation will increase the glucocerebrosidase activity in the central nervous system. This might limit the use of bone marrow transplantation to nonneuronopathic cases of Gaucher's disease.

B. Niemann-Pick Disease

Niemann-Pick disease is an autosomal recessive disorder that is characterized by excessive accumulation of sphingomyelin in various tissues and organs. It may be caused by a deficiency of sphingomyelinase, the enzyme that catalyzes the cleavage of phosphorylcholine from sphingomyelin. Aside from sphingomyelin, there may also be an increase in the amount of unesterified cholesterol, lyso-bisphosphatidic acid, and glycosphingolipids (151). The most consistent findings are hepatosplenomegaly and foam cells in the bone marrow.

There are five clinically distinct forms of this condition depending on the age of onset, neurologic manifestations, and demonstrable enzymatic deficiency. Types A (acute, neuronopathic) and B (chronic nonneuronopathic) have a generalized deficiency of sphingomyelinase, whereas the causes for types C (chronic neuronopathic), D (Nova Scotia variant), and E (adult, nonneuronopathic) are still poorly understood. Among these five types of Niemann-Pick disease, type B is characterized by prominent somatic manifestations without neurological deterioration. These patients have skeletal changes not present in the other types. They also have hepatosplenomegaly, growth retardation, skin lesions, and delayed puberty (152).

The skeletal changes include osteoporosis, coxa valga, and widening of the diaphysis and the metaphysis, particularly in the metacarpal bones and distal phalanges. Pulmonary involvement is not infrequent, with exertional dyspnea being the most common complaint, accompanied by susceptibility to infections and pneumonia. A 48-year-old woman was diagnosed as having type B Niemann-Pick disease histologically and by enzyme studies; she presented with coronary artery disease and hepatosplenomegaly (153).

Types A and B Niemann-Pick disease are characterized by an accumulation of sphingomyelin and moderate elevation of unesterified alcohol levels, while type C disease is characterized by an accumulation of unesterified cholesterol with less accumulation of sphingomyelin. A cellular cholesterol homeostasis malfunction might also be responsible for the deficient esterification and excessive accumulation of cholesterol in Niemann-Pick disease type C (154,155). Acid lipase activity was noted to be absent in both hepatocytes and macrophages in type C cells; this deficiency probably plays a role in its pathogenesis (156).

Patients with type D disease have clinical manifestations identical to those with type C. The difference, however, lies in the sphingomyelinase activity in type D, which is normal. These patients are exclusively descendants of an Acadian couple born in Yarmouth, Nova Scotia (157). The defect in this disorder has been shown to resemble that in type C: patients are unable to esterify cholesterol derived from low-density lipoproteins and nonlipoprotein sources. However, type D cells showed a significantly lower accumulation of cellular cholesterol than type C cells, suggesting that these two types of Niemann-Pick disease differ in the segment of cholesterol homeostasis pathway affected (158).

Patients with type E Niemann-Pick disease are adults who have some degree of hepatosplenomegaly and foam cells but no neurological manifestations. Although they have elevated levels of sphingomyelin in the liver and spleen, they may show either low or normal sphingomyelinase activity (151,159).

Microscopic examination reveals foam cells in the bone marrow, liver, lungs, spleen, and lymph nodes. These cells can be differentiated from Gaucher's cells in that the stain test for acid phosphatase is weakly positive, unlike the strong reaction in Gaucher's cells (151). The foam cells in patients with Niemann-Pick disease have eccentric nuclei and black, granular cytoplasmic inclusions. The ganglion cells in the central nervous system of patients with the neuronopathic types of Niemann-Pick disease are frequently swollen, with vacuoles in the cytoplasm. There are membrane-bound inclusions. There is loss of cells in the cerebral and cerebellar cortex, with gliosis and secondary demyelination in some portions of the white matter.

1. *Diagnosis*

Prenatal diagnosis of types A and B has been successfully achieved by assaying the sphingomyelinase activity in cultured amnictic fluid cells. Diagnosis of type C disease, however, might be difficult because of the normal or intermediate activity of this enzyme (160,161).

2. *Treatment*

There is still no specific treatment for Niemann-Pick disease. Supportive therapy, such as splenectomy, may alleviate the complications of hypersplenism. Bone marrow transplantation has been tried in mice, but the same problem exists that has been observed in this form of treatment of other inborn errors of metabolism. Although there appeared to be a decrease in the accumulation of sphingomyelin and cholesterol in the spleen and bone marrow, there was no improvement in the neurological manifestations. This drawback is probably caused by the inability of leukocytes to pass the blood–brain barrier and enter the necessary areas of the brain (162,163). Despite attempts to alter the blood–brain barrier temporarily with the use of mannitol and arabinose to allow passage of larger molecules such as enzymes, only 1% of the infused enzymes actually entered the brain (164).

C. Farber's Disease (Lipogranulomatosis)

Farber's disease is a rare, progressive, autosomal recessive disorder of lipid metabolism characterized by excessive accumulation of ceramide in various tissues of the body as a result of a deficiency of the lysosomal enzyme acid ceramidase. This catalyzes the degradation of ceramide to sphingosine and fatty acid by hydrolysis at the amide bond. There is minimal involvement of the bone itself although, occasionally, there is local infiltration of the bone adjacent to the involved joint (165).

The prominent clinical features of Farber's disease are progressive arthropathy with periarticular and subcutaneous nodules, hoarseness, nutritional and growth failure, pulmonary failure, and psychomotor retardation (166,167). Radiographs of hands and feet show periarticular bone erosions, joint contractures, subluxations, and generalized osteopenia (166,167). The liver may be enlarged and cardiac murmurs may be heard. The eyes may be involved and may show retinal opacifications with a cherry-red center or conjunctival granulomatous lesions and corneal or lenticular opacifications (165). The disease may have a variable course, with death occurring before 2 years of age in some and as late as the third decade in others (168).

Microscopic examination of the nodules shows granulomatous infiltration at varying stages. Early lesions are characterized by infiltration of histiocytes surrounded by lymphocytes and plasma cells (169). The histiocytes have finely granular cytoplasm with eccentric or centrally located nuclei. Older lesions show larger histiocytes with basophilic granular cytoplasm and some fibrosis, vacuolation, and necrosis.

The reticuloendothelial system is minimally involved. The central nervous system shows cytoplasmic ballooning of the large neurons and glial cells with formation of granuloma. Lysosomal inclusions are lamellar, rectilinear, or curvilinear (170).

Diagnosis is strongly suspected in a child who develops the clinical features described above and is confirmed by the typical histological appearance of the nodules, the demonstration of ceramide accumulation in these lesions, and the decreased or absent acid ceramidase activity in cultured fibroblasts (170,171). Prenatal diagnosis is possible and may help in making the decision to terminate a pregnancy as early as the 16th week of gestation (172).

No specific therapy is available. Joint swelling and pain may be relieved by corticosteroids. Since manifestations are mainly somatic and involvement of the central nervous system is minimal, the use of enzyme replacement appears encouraging (172).

VI. HOMOCYSTINURIA

Homocystinuria is an autosomal recessive disorder of methionine metabolism that results in alterations in the collagen structure of connective tissue. This condition is caused by an abnormality in either of two pathways: transsulfuration or methylation of homocysteine (Fig. 5). Homocysteine is converted to cystathionine by condensation of serine. This reaction is catalyzed by cystathionine-beta-synthase, which depends on pyridoxal phosphate for activity. Homocysteine may also be methylated to form methionine, either by the help of beta-homocysteine methyltransferase or 5, methyltetrahydrofolate homocysteine methyltransferase. This latter reaction needs the cosubstrate 5, methyltetrahydrofolate, which is formed with the help of another coenzyme 5,10-methylenetetrahydrofolate reductase. A deficiency of any of the above enzymes can result in excessive accumulation of homocysteine, the metabolically active form of homocystine that is responsible for the clinical syndrome of homocystinuria (173-176) (Table 6).

The best-described form of homocystinuria is that due to a deficiency of cystathionine beta-synthase. The most consistent finding is ectopia lentis or dislocation of the lens, which results from disruption of the zonular fibers that connect the lens to the ciliary body.

Skeletal manifestations in cystathionine beta-synthase-deficient patients are quite significant; osteoporosis is the most common. Osteoporosis frequently involve the spine and the long bones and may result in pathological fractures or vertebral collapse (177). Patients are generally very tall and their long bones are very long and thin. There is arachnodactyly with relative shortening of the 4th metacarpal (178). The metaphyses and epiphyses of long bones are often widened. There may be kyphoscoliosis, bowing of long bones, genu valgum, enlargement of the carpal bones, and elongation of the talus. There may be pectus carinatum or excavatum (179,180).

The most common neurological manifestation is mental retardation, although about 20% of patients have normal or almost normal intelligence (181,182). There may be convulsions with electroencephalographic (EEG) changes (183). Sometimes, neurological abnormalities develop after a cerebrovascular accident (184). Thromboembolism is the most life-threatening complication of homocystinuria. Studies have shown that homocysteine results in an increased platelet thromboxane product without a compensatory increase in antithrombotic vascular prostacyclin in vitro (185).

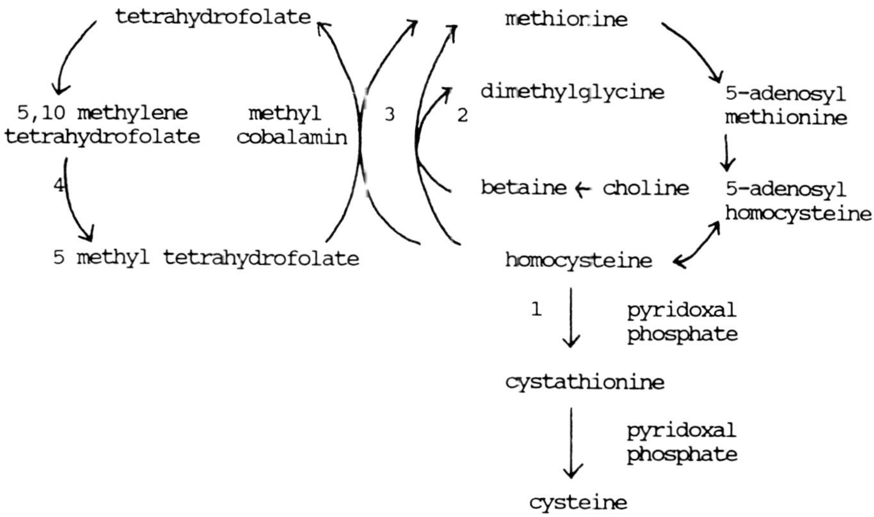

Reaction	Enzyme
1	cystathionine β-synthase
2	betaine:homocysteine methyltransferase
3	5-methyl tetrahydrofolate:homocysteine methyltransferase
4	5,10-methylene tetrahydrofolate reductase

Figure 5 The transulfuration pathway in the metabolism of methionine and homocysteine.

Homocystinuria secondary to a disorder in homocysteine methylation presents in a somewhat different manner that cystathionine beta-synthase deficiency. Neurological manifestations predominate and the physical features of patients with cystathionine beta-synthase deficiency are absent (186). Stature is normal, but mental retardation is severe and death occurs at an early age.

Diagnosis of homocystinuria is suspected in a child presenting with the clinical features noted above. However, this should be differentiated from Marfan's syndrome, which may similarly present with arachnodactyly, tall stature, and ectopia lentis. In cystathionine beta-synthase deficiency, large amounts of homocysteine are found in the urine. This is not normally detected in human urine. Plasma levels of homocystine and methionine are also elevated, with low or absent levels of cystine. These can be determined either by amino acid analyzer or by isotachophoretic analysis (187). In defects of homocysteine methylation, however, methionine levels are low or low-normal (188). Occasionally, a false-negative result may be obtained. This usually happens when a patient is ingesting even low doses of supplemental vitamin B_6 (177).

Table 6 Differentiation Between the Two Types of Homocystinuria

Enzyme Deficient	Elevated Amino Acid in Plasma	Eye Findings	CNS Changes	Skeletal Changes	Cerebrovascular Changes
Cystathionine-beta synthase	Homocysteine Methionine	Ectopia lentis Iridodonesis Myopia Astigmatism Cataracts Optic atrophy Retinal degeneration and detachment	Mental retardation in 20%	Tall stature Long tubular bones Genu valgum Pectus carinatum or excavatum	Intimal fibrosis Atherosclerosis Thrombi
5,10 Methylene tetrahydrofolate reductase	Normal plasma and CSF methionine but elevated urine methionine levels	None	Severe mental retardation	Normal stature Normal skeletal system	None

The characteristic histopathological picture of the eye in cystathionine beta-synthase deficiency includes retinal degeneration, atrophy of the non-pigmented ciliary epithelium, and disruption of zonular fibers (189). In the skeletal system there is a defect in endochondral epimetaphyseal ossification (180). Vascular changes include thickening and fibrosis of the intima and even atherosclerotic changes of large arteries and the aorta. Occasionally, thrombi are seen (174). The liver may show fatty changes. The most common findings in the central nervous system are infarcts secondary to thromboembolic events (184). Other reports include spongy degeneration and demyelination of the white matter (190).

Definitive diagnosis is made by demonstrating reduced activity of cystathionine beta-synthase or one of the methylation enzymes in liver biopsy specimens or cultured lymphocytes and fibroblasts.

The management of homocystinuria is aimed at correcting the biochemical abnormalities that probably lead to the disease's manifestations and the treatment of complications (177). Some patients have shown diminishing levels of homocysteine with administration of large amounts of pyridoxine, a precursor of the cofactor pyridoxal phosphate that works with cystathionine beta-synthase to exert its effect (191). Doses between 250 and 1200 mg/day have been used. Response in terms of decrease in homocysteine levels have not been dose-related (192). In patients who do not respond to pyridoxine supplementation, diet modification may be helpful. Diets low in methionine are expected to diminish levels of homocysteine, which is believed to be responsible for the clinical effects. The amount of methionine in the diet will be determined by the ability to maintain blood methionine levels below 0.04 μmol/ml and keep the blood and urine showing little or no homocysteine. Supplementation with L-cystine may be necessary. The efficacy of dietary therapy has not been proven, although there have been reports of improved psychomotor development, prevention of thromboembolic episodes, and normalization of growth (177).

The use of betaine has been shown to be successful in producing biochemical and clinical improvement in patients who do not respond to pyridoxine. Betaine or trimethylglycine is a cofactor in the remethylation of homocysteine to methionine. By preventing the elevation of homocysteine levels, it is hoped that vascular complications are reduced (193,194).

Complications such as pathological fractures, vitreous hemorrhage, retinal detachment, and acute glaucoma are treated by conventional measures such as surgery. Thromboembolic phenomena are usually avoided by the use of dipyridamole and acetylsalicylic acid, which are antithrombotic agents.

VII. CLINICAL ASSESSMENT

Making a definite diagnosis in a patient with a skeletal abnormality is an important but difficult task. Although there is usually no definite cure, particularly for an inherited metabolic abnormality, genetic counseling and prenatal diagnosis are the two most helpful means of preventing recurrences in affected families and can best be done with the proper diagnosis available. Moreover, in conditions in which a primary metabolic disorder could be identified, an experimental therapeutic method is usually tried, particularly when the anticipated benefits of treatment greatly outweigh the risks of nontreatment.

A patient who presents with skeletal defects and other organ involvement should make one suspect an inherited metabolic disorder that affects connective tissues. Stature should be accurately measured. In the presence of short stature, the urine should be screened for mucopolysaccharides. Those who show mucopolysacchariduria could either have dysostosis multiplex with stiff joints or loose joints. The former type of skeletal involvement is seen in all types of mucopolysaccharide storage disorders except Morquio's syndrome. These mucopolysaccharide storage disorders could be differentiated clinically on the basis of the presence or absence of mental retardation and corneal clouding. Mental retardation and corneal clouding are seen in Hurler's and Hurler-Scheie's syndromes, but micrognathia is seen only in the latter. Patients with Scheie's and Maroteaux-Lamy syndromes usually have corneal clouding but have normal intelligence. These two conditions could be differentiated on the basis of the type of mucopolysaccharide in the urine. On the other hand, patients with Hunter's syndrome usually have normal intelligence and no corneal clouding.

The presence of dysostosis multiplex in a patient with normal stature also calls for testing the urine for mucopolysaccharides. If the urine shows mucopolysaccharides, the patient has either Scheie's syndrome or Sly's syndrome, the presence of metatarsus adductus is more suggestive of Sly's syndrome. Since both conditions result in excretion of both dermatan and heparan sulfate, the diagnosis can only be made after enzyme analysis of cultured skin fibroblasts. If the urine does not show mucopolysaccharides, the presence of hepatosplenomegaly, dysostosis multiplex, and oligosaccharides in the urine narrow down the differential diagnosis to mannosidosis, fucosidosis I and II, and congenital sialidosis II. Clinically, patients with mannosidosis have a characteristic spoke-like lenticular opacity, patients with fucosidosis I have an abnormal sweat chloride test, patients with fucosidosis II have angiokeratoma, while patients with sialidosis II have cherry-red spots in the retina. If no hepatomegaly is noted in a patient with oligosaccharides in the urine, aspartylglycosaminuria and sialidosis should be considered. The former is characterized by lens opacities, while sialidosis I and II are characterized by cherry-red spots in the retina.

If no oligosaccharides are noted in the urine, ganglioside storage disorder or mucolipidosis should be considered. I-cell disease can be diagnosed if skin fibroblasts reveal sudanophilic periodic-acid-Schiff-positive inclusions, while GM_1 gangliosidosis can be diagnosed by the presence of cytoplasmic vacuolation of renal glomerular epithelial cells on renal biopsy.

When other skeletal abnormalities are identified in the child instead of dysostosis multiplex, lipid storage disorders should be considered. Gaucher's disease is likely if an Erlenmeyer-flask deformity is noted in the long bones. Bone marrow infiltration, coxa valga, and widening of long bone diaphyses and metaphyses are characteristics of Niemann-Pick disease. Joint contractures and periarticular nodules and erosions are seen in Farber's disease.

Finally, when faced with a patient with tall stature, arachnodactyly and disproportionate lengthening of long bones, homocystinuria should be differentiated from Marfan's syndrome.

Since many of the clinical, skeletal, and laboratory features of metabolic disorders overlap, making a definitive diagnosis by measuring enzyme activity in cultured skin fibroblasts is imperative. These clinical differences can help in narrowing down the possibilities so that the enzymes most likely to be deficient are assayed.

REFERENCES

1. Rimoin, D. L., and Lachman, R. S. The chondrodysplasias. In: *Principles and Practice of Medical Genetics*. A. E. Emery and D. L. Rimoin (eds.). Churchill Livingston, New York, 1983.
2. International nomenclature of constitutional diseases of bone, revision, May 1983. *Ann. Radiol.* 26:456 (1983).
3. Schwartz, N. B. Carbohydrate metabolism II. Special pathways. In: *Textbook of Biochemistry with Clinical Correlations*. T. M. Devlin (ed.). John Wiley and Sons, New York, 1982.
4. Resnick, D. Additional congenital or heritable anomalies and syndromes. In: *Diagnosis of Bone and Joint Disorders*. D. Resnick and G. Niwayama (eds.). W. B. Saunders, Philadelphia, 1981.
5. Coster, L., Carlstedt, I., Kendall, S., Malstrom, A., Schmidtchen, A., and Fransson, L. Structure of proteoheparan sulfates from fibroblasts. *J. Biol. Chem.* 261:12079 (1986).
6. White, A., Handler, P., Smith, E. L., Hill, R. L., and Lehman, I. R. *Principles of Biochemistry*, 6th ed. McGraw-Hill, New York, 1978.
7. Horton, W. A., Chou, J. W., and Machado, M. A. Cartilage collagen analysis in the chondrodystrophies. *Collagen Rel. Res.* 5:349 (1985).
8. Stanescu, V., Stanescu, R., and Maroteaux, P. Pathogenic mechanisms in osteochondrodysplasias. *J. Bone Joint Surg.* 66A:817 (1984).
9. Stob, H., and Pesch, H.-J. Structural changes of collagen fibrils in skeletal dysplasias. *Virchows Arch. (Pathol. Anat.)* 405:341 (1985).
10. Spranger, J. Pattern recognition in bone dysplasias. *Prog. Clin. Biol. Res.* 200:315 (1985).
11. McKusick, V. A., and Neufeld, E. F. The mucopolysaccharide storage diseases. In: *The Metabolic Basis of Inherited Disease*, 5th ed. J. B. Stanbury, J. B. Wyngaarden, D. S. Fredericksen, J. L. Goldstein, and M. S. Brown (eds.). McGraw-Hill, New York, 1983.

12. McKusick, V. A., and Pyeritz, R. E. Genetic heterogeneity and allelic variation in the mucopolysaccharidoses. *Johns Hopkins Med. J.* 146:71 (1980).
13. Huang, K.-C., Sukegawa, K., and Orii, T. Screening test for urinary glycosaminoglycans and differentiation of various mucopolysaccharidoses. *Clin. Chim. Acta* 151:147 (1985).
14. Savage, A., and Applegarth, D. A. Diagnosis of mucopolysaccharidoses using H-n.m.r. spectroscopy of glycosaminoglycans. *Carbohydrate Res.* 149:471 (1986).
15. Horton, W. A., and Schimke, R. N. A new mucopolysaccharidosis. *J. Pediatr.* 77:252 (1970).
16. Maroteaux, P., and Lamy, M. Hurler's disease, Morquio's disease, and related mucopolysaccharidoses. *J. Pediatr.* 67:312 (1965).
17. Renteria, V. G., Ferrans, V. J., and Roberts, W. C. The heart in Hurler's syndrome: Gross, histologic, and ultrastructural observations in 5 necropsy cases. *Am. J. Cardiol.* 38:487 (1976).
18. Parfrey, N. A., and Hutchins, G. M. Hepatic fibrosis in the mucopolysaccharidoses. *Am. J. Med.* 81:825 (1986).
19. Bach, G., Friedman, R., Weissman, B., and Neufeld, E. F. The defect in the Hurler and Scheie syndromes: Deficiency of alpha-L-iduronidase. *Proc. Natl. Acad. Sci. U.S.A.* 69:2048 (1972).
20. Lamon, J. M., Trojak, J. E., and Abbott, M. H Bone cysts in mucopolysaccharidosis I S (Scheie syndrome). *Johns Hopkins Med. J.* 146:73 (1980).
21. Mueller, O. T., Shows, T. B., and Opitz, J. M. Apparent allelism of the Hurler, Scheie, and Hurler/Scheie syndromes. *Am. J. Med. Genet.* 18:547 (1984).
22. Den Tandt, W. R., Sharpe, S., Giesberts, M., and Poorthuis, B. J. Microtest for determination of alpha-L-iduronidase in plasma and leucocytes and its potential for diagnosing alpha-L-iduronidase deficiency. *Lancet* 1:794 (1984).
23. Kajii, T., Matsuda, I., Oshaw, A. T., Katsunuma, H., Ichida, T., and Arashima, S. Hurler-Scheie genetic compound (MPS IH-IS) in Japanese brothers. *Clin. Genet.* 6:394 (1974).
24. Winters, P. R., Harrod, M. J., Molenick-Heetred, S. A., Kirkpatrick, J., and Rosenberg, R. N. Alpha-L-iduronidase deficiency and possible Hurler/Scheie genetic compound: Clinical, pathological, and biochemical findings. *Neurology* 26:1003 (1976).
25. McKusick, V. A., Kaplan, D., Wise, D., Hanley, W. B., Suddarth, S. B., Sevick, M. E., and Maumanee, A. E. The genetic mucopolysaccharidoses. *Medicine* 44:445 (1965).
26. Shapiro, J., Strome, M., and Crocker, A. C. Airway obstruction and sleep apnea in Hurler and Hunter syndromes. *Ann. Otol. Rhinol. Laryngol.* 94:458 (1985).
27. Caffey, J. P. *Pediatric X-Ray Diagnosis*, 7th ed. Year Book Medical Publishers, Chicago, 1978.
28. Ballenger, C. E., Swift, T. R., Leshner, R. T., El Gammal, T. A., and McDonald, T. F. Myelopathy in mucopolysaccharidosis type II (Hunter syndrome). *Ann. Neurol.* 7:382 (1980).

29. Young, I. D., and Harper, P. S. Long-term complications in Hunter's syndrome. *Clin. Genet.* 16:125 (1979).
30. Elsner, B. Ultrastructure of the rectal wall in Hunter's syndrome. *Gastroenterology* 58:856 (1970).
31. Liebaers, I., DiNatale, P., and Neufeld, E. F. Iduronate sulfatase in amniotic fluid: an aid in the prenatal diagnosis of the Hunter syndrome. *J. Pediatr.* 90:423 (1977).
32. Kleijer, W. J., Mooy, P. D., Liebaers, I., Van De Kamp, J. J. P., and Niermeijer, M. F. Prenatal monitoring for the Hunter syndrome: The heterozygous female fetus. *Clin. Genet.* 15:113 (1979).
33. Kresse, H., Mucopolysaccharidosis IIIA (Sanfilippo A disease): Deficiency of heparan sulfamidase in skin fibroblasts and leukocytes. *Biochem. Biophys. Res. Commun.* 54:1111 (1973).
34. Von Figura, K., and Kresse, H. The Sanfilippo B corrective factor: An N-acetyl alpha-D-glucosaminidase. *Biochem. Biophys. Res. Commun.* 48:262 (1972).
35. Pallini, R., Leder, I. G., and DiNatale, P. Sanfilippo type C diagnosis: assay of acetyl CoA: Alpha-glucosaminide N-acetyltransferase using [^{14}C] glucosamine as substrate and leukocytes as enzyme source. *Pediatr. Res.* 18:543 (1984).
36. Kresse, H., Paschke, E., Von Figura, K., Gilberg, W., and Fuchs, W. Sanfilippo disease type D, deficiency of N-acetylglucosamine-6-sulfate sulfatase required for heparan sulfate degradation. *Proc. Natl. Acad. Sci. U.S.A.* 77:6622 (1980).
37. Uvebrant, P. Sanfilippo type C syndrome in two sisters. *Acta Pediatr. Scand.* 74:137 (1985).
38. Haust, M. D., and Gordon, B. A. Ultrastructural and biochemical aspects of the Sanfilippo syndrome, type III genetic mucopolysaccharidosis. *Connect. Tissue Res.* 15:57 (1986).
39. Van De Kamp, J. J. P., Niermeijer, M. F., Von Figura, K., and Giesberts, M. A. H. Genetic heterogeneity and clinical variability in the San Filippo syndrome (types A, B, and C). *Clin. Genet.* 20:152–160 (1981).
40. Kleijer, W. J., Janse, H. C., Vosters, R. P. L., Niermeijer, M. F., and Van De Kamp, J. J. P. First trimester diagnosis of mucopolysaccharidosis IIIA (Sanfilippo A disease). *N. Engl. J. Med.* 314:185 (1986).
41. Van der Horst, G. T. J., Kleijer, W. J., Hoogeveen, A. T., Huijmans, J. G. M., Blom, W., and Van Diggelen, O. P. Morquio B syndrome: A primary defect in B-galactosidase. *Am. J. Med. Genet.* 16:261 (1983).
42. Trojak, J. E., Ho, C.-K., Roesel, R. A., Levin, L. S., Kopits, S. E., Thomas, G. H., and Toma, S. Morquio-like syndrome (MPS IVB) associated with deficiency of a B-galactosidase. *Johns Hopkins Med. J.* 146:75 (1980).
43. Czartoryska, B., Gorska, D., and Abramowicz, T. Kinetic properties of B-galactosidase in Morquio B disease. *Acta Anthropogenet.* 7:301 (1983).
44. Koto, A., Horwitz, A. L., Suzuki, K., and Tiffany, C. W. The Morquio syndrome: Neuropathology and biochemistry. *Ann. Neurol.* 4:26 (1978).
45. Peterson, D. I., Bacchus, H., Seaich, L., and Kelly, T. E. Myelopathy associated with Maroteaux-Lamy syndrome. *Arch. Neurol.* 32:127 (1975).

46. Wilson, C. S., Mankin, H., and Pluth, J. R. Aortic stenosis and mucopolysacchridosis. *Ann. Intern. Med.* 92:496 (1980).
47. Di Ferrante, N., Hyman, B. H., Klish, W., Donnelly, P. V., Nichols, B. L., and Dutton, R. V. Mucopolysaccharidosis VI (Maroteaux-Lamy disease) clinical and biochemical study of a mild variant case. *Johns Hopkins Med. J.* 135:42 (1974).
48. Levy, L. A., Lewis, J. C., and Sumner, T. E. Ultrastructures of Reilly bodies (metachromatic granules) in the Maroteaux-Lamy syndrome (mucopolysaccharidosis VI). *Am. J. Clin. Pathol.* 73:416 (1980).
49. Black, S. H., Pelias, M. Z., Miller, J. B., Blitzer, M. G., and Shapira, E. Maroteaux-Lamy syndrome in a large consanguineous kindred: Biochemical and immunologic studies. *Am. J. Med. Genet.* 25:273 (1986).
50. Sly, W. S., Quinton, B. A., McAlister, W. H., and Rimoin, D. L. Beta glucuronidase deficiency: Report of clinical, radiologic, and biochemical features of a new mucopolysaccharidosis. *J. Pediatr.* 82:249 (1973).
51. Lee, J. L. S., Falk, R. E., Ng, W. G., and Donnell, G. N. Beta-glucuronidase deficiency. A heterogeneous mucopolysaccharidosis. *Am. J. Dis. Child.* 139:57 (1985).
52. Sewell, A. C., Gehler, J., Mittermaier, G., and Meyer, E. Mucopolysaccharidosis type VII (Beta-glucuronidase deficiency): A report of a new case and a survey of those in the literature. *Clin. Genet.* 21:366 (1982).
53. Beaudet, A. L., Di Ferrante, N., Ferry, G. D., Nichols, B. L., Jr., and Mullins, C. E. Variation in the phenotypic expression of beta-glucuronidase deficiency. *J. Pediatr.* 86:388 (1975).
54. Adinolfi, M., and Brown, S. Strategies for the correction of enzymatic deficiencies in patients with mucopolysaccharidoses. *Dev. Med. Child. Neurol.* 26:401 (1984).
55. Di Ferrante, N., Nichols, B. L., Donnelly, P. V., Neri, G., Hrgovcic, R., and Berglund, R. K. Induced degradation of glycosaminoglycans in Hurler's and Hunter's syndromes by plasma infusion. *Proc. Natl. Acad. Sci.* 68:303 (1971).
56. Erickson, R. P., Sandman, R., Robertson, W. B., and Epstein, C. J. Inefficacy of fresh frozen plasma treatment of mucopolysaccharidosis II. *Pediatrics* 50:693 (1972).
57. Nishioka, J., Mizushima, T., and Ono, K. Treatment of mucopolysaccharidosis. Clinical and biochemical aspects of leucocyte transfusion as compared with plasma infusion in patients with Hurler's and Scheie's syndromes. *Clin. Orthop. Rel. Res.* 140:194 (1975).
58. Dean, M. F., Muir, H., Benson, P. F., Button, L. R., Roylston, A., and Mowbray, J. Enzyme replacement therapy by fibroblast transplantation in a case of Hunter syndrome. *Nature* 261:323 (1976).
59. Adinolfi, M., McColl, I., Chase, D., Fensom, A. H., Welsh, K., Brown, S., Marsh, J., Thick, M., and Dean, M. Transplantation of fetal fibroblasts and correction of enzymatic deficiencies in patients with Hunter's or Hurler's disorders. *Transplantation* 42:271 (1986).

60. Krivit, W., Pierpont, M. E., Ayaz, K., Tsai, M., Ramsay, N. K. C., Kersey, J. H., Weisdorf, S., Sibley, R., Snover, D., McGovern, M. M., Schwartz, M. F., and Desnick, R. J. Bone-marrow transplantation in the Maroteaux-Lamy syndrome (mucopolysaccharidosis type VI). *N. Engl. J. Med.* 311:1606 (1984).
61. Beaudet, A. L. Disorders of glycoprotein degradation: Mannosidosis, fucosidosis, sialidosis, and aspartylglycosaminuria. In: *The Metabolic Basis of Inherited Disease*. J. B. Stanbury, J. B. Wyngaarden, D. S. Fredricksen, J. L. Goldstein, and M. S. Brown (eds.). McGraw-Hill, New York, 1983.
62. Ockerman, P. A. A generalized storage disorder resembling Hurler's syndrome. *Lancet* 1:239 (1967).
63. Abraham, D., Blakemore, W. F., Jolly, R. D., Sidebotham, R., and Winchester, B. The catabolism of mammalian glycoproteins. Comparison of the storage products in bovine, feline, and human mannosidosis. *Biochem. J.* 215:573 (1983).
64. Booth, C. W., Chen, K. K., and Nadler, H. L. Mannosidosis: Clinical and biochemical studies in a family of affected adolescents and adults. *J. Pediatr.* 88:821 (1976).
65. Yunis, J. J., Lewandowski, R. C., Sanfilippo, S. J., and Tsai, M. Y. Clinical manifestations of mannosidosis–a longitudinal study. *Am. J. Med.* 61: 841 (1976).
66. Spranger, J., Gehler, J., and Cantz, M. The radiographic features of mannosidosis. *Radiology* 119:401 (1976).
67. Kjellman, B., Gamstorp, I., Brun, A., Ockerman, P. A., and Palmgren, B. Mannosidosis: A clinical and histopathologic study. *J. Pediatr.* 75:366 (1969).
68. Carrol, N., Dance, N., Masson, P. K., Robinson, D., and Winchester, B. G. Human mannosidosis–the enzyme effect. *Biochem. Biophys. Res. Commun.* 49:579 (1972).
69. Bach, G., Kohn, G., Lasch, E. E., El Massri, M., Ornoy, A., Sekeles, E., Legum, C., and Cohen, M. M. A new variant of mannosidosis with increased residual enzymatic activity and mild clinical manifestations. *Pediatr. Res.* 12:1010 (1978).
70. Tsay, G. C., Dawson, G., and Matalon, R. Glycopeptide storage in skin fibroblasts cultured from a patient with alpha-mannosidase deficiency. *J. Clin. Invest.* 56:711 (1975).
71. Durand, P., Borrone, C., Della Cella, G., and Philippart, M. Fucosidosis. *J. Pediatr.* 75:665 (1969).
72. Borrone, C., Gatti, R., Trias, X., and Durand, P., Gucosidosis. Clinical, biochemical, immunologic, and genetic studies in two new cases. *J. Pediatr.* 84:727 (1974).
73. Van Hoof, F., and Hers, H. G. Mucopolysaccharidosis by absence of alpha fucosidase. *Lancet* 1:1198 (1968).
74. Borrone, C., Gatti, R., Trias, X., and Durand, P. Fucosidosis: Clinical biochemical, immunologic, and genetic studies in two new cases. *J. Pediatr.* 84:727 (1974).

75. Brill, P. W., Beratis, N. G., Kousseff, B. G., and Hirschhorn, K. Roentgenographic findings in flucosidosis type 2. *Am. J. Roentgenol.* 102:747 (1968).
76. Schafer, I. A., Powell, D. W., and Sullivan, J. C Lysosomal bone disease. *Pediatr. Res.* 5:391 (1971).
77. Kousseff, B. G., Beratis, N. G., Strauss, L., Brill, P. W., Rosenfeld, R. E., Kaplan, B., and Hirschhorn, K. Fucosidosis type 2. *Pediatrics* 57:205 (1976).
78. Zielke, K., Okada, S., and O'Brien, J. S. Fucosidosis: Diagnosis by serum assay of alpha-L-fucosidase. *J. Lab. Clin. Med.* 79:164 (1972).
79. Ng, W. G., Donnell, G. N., and Koch, R. Serum alpha-L-fucosidase activity in the diagnosis of fucosidosis. *Pediatr. Res.* 7:391 (1973).
80. Ng, W. G., Donnell, G. N., Koch, R., and Bergren, W. R. Biochemical and genetic studies of plasma and leukocyte alpha-L-fucosidase. *Am. J. Hum. Genet.* 28:42 (1976).
81. Alhadeff, J. A., Andrews-Smith, G. L., and O'Brien, J. S. Biochemical studies on an unusual case of fucosidosis. *Clin. Genet.* 14:235 (1978).
82. Beratis, N. G., Turner, B. M., and Hirschhorn, K. Fucosidosis: Detection of the carrier state in peripheral blood leukocytes. *J. Pediatr.* 87:1193 (1975).
83. Maury, P. Accumulation of two glycoasparagines in the liver in aspartylglycosaminuria. *J. Biol. Chem.* 254:1513 (1979).
84. Isenberg, J. N., and Sharp, H. L. Aspartylglycosaminuria: Psychomotor retardation masquerading as a mucopolysaccharidosis. *J. Pediatr.* 86:713 (1975).
85. Pollitt, R. J., Jenner, F. A., and Merskey, H. Aspartylglycosaminuria. An inborn error of metabolism associated with mental defect. *Lancet* 1:253 (1968).
86. Maury, P. Quantitative determination of 4-N-2-acetamido-2-deoxy-B-D-glycopyranosyl-L-asparagine in the urine of patients with aspartylglycosaminuria by gas liquid chromatography. *J. Lab. Clin. Med.* 93:718 (1979).
87. Aula, P., Raivio, K., and Autio, S. Enzymatic diagnosis and carrier detection of aspartylglycosaminuria using blood samples. *Pediatr. Res.* 10:625 (1976).
88. Lowden, J. A., and O'Brien, J. S. Sialidosis: A review of human neuraminidase deficiency. *Am. J. Hum. Genet.* 31:1 (1979).
89. Rapin, I., Goldfischer, S., Katzman, R., Engel, J., Jr., and O'Brien, J. S. The cherry-red-spot–myoclonus syndrome. *Ann. Neurol.* 3:234 (1978).
90. Winter, R. M., Swallow, D. M., Baraitser, M., and Purkiss, P. Sialidosis type 2 (acid neuraminidase deficiency): Clinical and biochemical features of a further case. *Clin. Genet.* 18:203 (1980).
91. Kelly, T. E., and Graetz, G. Isolated acid neuraminidase deficiency: A distinct lysosomal storage disease. *Am. J. Med. Genet.* 1:31 (1977).
92. O'Brien, J. S., and Warner, T. G. Sialidosis: Delineation of subtypes by neuraminidase assay. *Clin. Genet.* 17:35 (1980).
93. Thomas, G. H., Tipton, R. E., Ch'jen, L. T., Reynolds, L. W., and Miller, C. S. Sialidase (alpha-N-acetyl neuraminidase) deficiency: The enzyme defect in an adult with macular cherry-red spots and myoclonus without dementia. *Clin. Genet.* 13:369 (1978).

94. D'Azzo, A., Hoogeven, A., Reuser, A. J. J., Robinson, D., and Galjaard, H. Molecular defect in combined beta-galactosidase and neuraminidase deficiency in man. *Proc. Natl. Acad. Sci. USA* 79:4535 (1982).
95. Hoogeven, A. T., Verheijen, F. W., D'azzo, A., and Galjaard, H. Genetic heterogeneity in human neuraminidase deficiency. *Nature* 285:500 (1980).
96. Mueller, O. T., Henry, W. M., Haley, L. L., Byers, M. G., Eddy, R. L., and Shows, T. B. Identification and chromosome location of genes involved in glycoprotein neuraminidase deficiency disorders. *Am. J. Hum. Genet.* 36: 2055 (1984).
97. Ishibashi, A., Tsuboi, R., and Shinmei, M. Beta-galactosidase and neuraminidase deficiency associated with angiokeratoma corporis diffusum. *Arch. Dermatol.* 120:1344 (1984).
98. Kleijer, W. M., Hoogeven, A., Verheijen, F. W., Niermeijer, M. F., Galjaard, H., O'Brien, J. S., and Warner, T. G. Prenatal diagnosis of sialidosis with combined neuraminidase and beta-galactosidase deficiency. *Clin. Genet.* 16:60 (1979).
99. Abraham, D., Muir, H., Olsen, I., and Winchester, B. Direct enzyme transfer from lymphocytes corrects a lysosomal storage disease. *Biochem. Biophys. Res. Commun.* 129:417 (1985).
100. Olsen, I., Dean, M. F., Harris, G., and Muir, H. Direct transfer of a lysosomal enzyme from lymphoid cells to deficient fibroblasts. *Nature* 291: 244 (1981).
101. Chester, M. A., Hultberg, B., Norden, N. E., and Szabo, L. The nature of mannose-containing material which accumulates in cultured fibroblasts from patients with mannosidosis. *Biochem. Biophys. Acta* 627:244 (1980).
102. Desnick, R. J., Sharp, H. L., Grabowski, G. A., Brunning, R. D., Quie, P. G., Sung, J.H., Gorlin, R. J., and Ikonne, J. U. Mannosidosis: Clinical, morphologic, immunologic, and biochemical studies. *Pediatr. Res.* 10: 985 (1976).
103. Strisciuglio, P., Creek, K. M., and Sly, W. S. Complementation, cross correction, and drug correction studies of combined beta-galactosidase neuraminidase deficiency in human fibroblasts. *Pediatr. Res.* 18:167 (1984).
104. O'Brien, J. S. The gangliosidoses. In: *The Metabolic Basis of Inherited Disease*, 5th ed. J. B. Stanbury, J. B. Wyngaarden, D. S. Fredrickson, J. L. Goldstein, and M. S. Brown (eds.). McGraw-Hill, New York, 1983.
105. Hoogeven, A. T., Reuser, A. J. J., Kroos, M., and Galjaard, H. GM_1 gangliosidosis. Defective recognition site on beta-galactosidase precursor. *J. Biol. Chem.* 261:5702 (1986).
106. O'Brien, J. Generalized gangliosidosis. *J. Pediatr.* 75:167 (1969).
107. Grossman, H. and Danes, S. Neurovisceral storage disease. Roentgenographic features and mode of inheritance. *Am. J. Roentgenol.* 103:149 (1968).
108. Rabinowitz, J. G., and Sacher, M. Gangliosidosis (GM_1). A re-evaluation of the vertebral deformity. *Am. J. Roentgenol.* 121:155 (1974).

109. Charrow, J., and Hvizd, M. G. Cardiomyopathy and skeletal myopathy in an unusual variant of GM_1 gangliosidosis. *J. Pediatr.* 108:729 (1986).
110. Wenger, D. A., Sattler, M., Mueller, O. T., Myers, G. G., Schneider, R. S., and Nixon, G. W. Adult GM_1 gangliosidosis. Clinical and biochemical studies on two patients and comparison to other patients called variant or adult GM_1 gangliosidosis. *Clin. Genet.* 17:323 (1980).
111. Alroy, J., Orgad, U., Ucci, A. A., Schelling, S. H., Schunk, K. L., Warren, C. D., Raghavan, S. S., and Kolodny, E. H. Neurovisceral and skeletal GM_1-gangliosidosis in dogs with beta-galactosidase deficiency. *Science* 229:470 (1985).
112. Bieber, F. R., Mortimer, G., Kolodny, E. H., and Driscill, S. G. Pathologic findings in fetal GM_1 gangliosidosis. *Arch. Neurol.* 43:736 (1986).
113. Neufeld, E. F., and McKusick, V. A. Disorders of lysosomal enzyme synthesis and localization: I-cell disease and pseudo-Hurler polydystrophy. In: *The Metabolic Basis of Inherited Disease*, 5th ed. J. B. Stanbury, J. B. Wyngaarden, D. S. Fredricksen, J. R. Goldstein, and M. S. Brown (eds.). McGraw-Hill, New York, 1983.
114. Mueller, O. T., Honey, N. K., Little, L. E., Miller, A. L., and Shows, T. B. Mucolipidosis II and III. The genetic relationships between two disorders of lysosomal enzyme biosynthesis. *J. Clin. Invest.* 72:1016 (1983).
115. Honey, N. K., Miller, A. L., and Shows, T. B. The mucolipidoses: Identification by abnormal electrophoretic patterns of lysosomal hydrolases. *Am. J. Med. Genet.* 9:239 (1981).
116. Ben-Yoseph, Y., Pack, B. A., Mitchell, D. A., Elwell, D. G., Potier, M., Melancon, S. B., and Nadler, H. L. Characterization of the mutant N-acetylglucosaminylphosphotransferase in I-cell disease and pseudo-Hurler polydystrophy: Complementation analysis and kinetic studies. *Enzyme* 35:106 (1986).
117. Leroy, J. G., Spranger, J. W., Feingold, M., Opitz, J. M., and Crocker, A. C. I-cell disease: A clinical picture. *J. Pediatr* 79:360 (1971).
118. Patriquin, H. B., Kaplan, P., Kind, H. P., and Giedion, A. Neonatal mucolipidosis II (I-cell disease): Clinical and radiologic features in three cases. *AJR* 129:37 (1977).
119. Okada, S., Owada, M., Sakiyama, T., Yutaka, T., and Ogawa, M. I-cell disease: clinical studies of 21 Japanese cases. *Clin. Genet.* 28:207 (1985).
120. Tondeur, M., Vamos-Hurwitz, E., Mockel-Pohl, S., Dereume, J. P., Cremer, N., and Loeb, H. Clinical, biochemical, and ultrastructural studies in a case of chondrodystrophy presenting the I-cell phenotype in tissue culture. *J. Pediatr.* 79:366 (1971).
121. Hanai, J., Leroy, J., and O'Brien, J. S. Ultrastructure of cultured fibroblasts in I-cell disease. *Am. J. Dis. Child.* 122:34 (1971).
122. Greene, A. A., Jonas, A. J., Harms, E., Smith, M. L., Pellett, O. L., Bump, E. A., Miller, A. L., and Schneider, J. A. Lysosomal cystine storage in cystinosis and mucolipidosis type II. *Pediatr. Res.* 19:1170 (1985).
123. Little, L. E., Mueller, O. T., Honey, N. K., Shows, T. B., and Miller, A. L. Heterogeneity of N-acetylglucosamine 1-phosphotransferase within mucolipidosis III. *J. Biol. Chem.* 261:733 (1986).

124. Traboulsi, E. I. and Maumenee, I. H. Ophthalmologic findings in mucolipidosis III (pseudo-Hurler polydystrophy). *Am. J. Ophthalmol.* 102:592 (1986).
125. Herd, J. K., Dvorak, A. D., Wiltse, H. E., Eisen, J. D., Kress, B. C., and Miller, A. L. Mucolipidosis type III. Multiple elevated serum and urine enzyme activities. *Am. J. Dis. Child.* 132:1181 (1978).
126. Gehler, J., Sewell, A. C., and Spranger, J. Clinical variability in mucolipidosis type III. *Clin. Genet.* 19:504 (1981).
127. Varki, A. P., Reitman, M. L., and Kornfeld, S. Identification of a variant of mucolipidosis III (pseudo-Hurler polydystrophy): A catalytically active N-acetylglucosaminylphosphotransferase that fails to phosphorylate lysosomal enzymes. *Proc. Natl. Acad. Sci. USA* 78:7773 (1981).
128. Kato, T., Okada, S., Oshima, T., Inui, K., Yutaka, T., and Yabuuchi, H. Normalization of intracellular lysosomal hydrolases in I-cell disease filbroblasts with sucrose loading. *J. Biol. Chem.* 257:7814 (1982).
129. Okada, S., Kato, Tomochika, K., Oshima, T., Yutaka, T., and Yabuuchi, H. Heterogeneity in mucolipidosis II (I-cell disease). *Clin. Genet.* 23:155 (1983).
130. D'Azzo, A., Halley, D. J. J., Hoogeveen, A., and Galjaard, H. Correction of I-cell defect by hybridization with lysosomal enzyme deficient human fibroblasts. *Am. J. Hum. Genet.* 32:519 (1980).
131. Brady, R. O. Lipid storage disorders enzyme replacement therapy: Current status and future strategies. In: *Congenital Metabolic Diseases.* (R. Wapnir, ed.). Marcel Dekker, New York, 1985.
132. Lachiewicz, P. F. Gaucher's disease. *Orthop. Clin. North Am.* 15:765 (1984).
133. Stern, J. Hereditary and acquired mental deficiency. In *Biochemistry in Clinical Practice.* D. L. Williams and V. Marks (eds.). Elsevier Science, New York, 1985.
134. Brady, R. O., and Barranger, J. A. Glycosylceramide lipidosis: Gaucher's disease. In: *The Metabolic Basis of Inherited Disease*, 5th ed. J. B. Stanbury, J. V. B. Wyngaarden, D. S. Fredricksen, J. L. Goldstein, and M. S. Brown (eds.). McGraw-Hill, New York, 1983.
135. Glew, R. H. Lipid metabolism II. Pathways of metabolism of special lipids. In: *Textbook of Biochemistry with Clinical Correlations.* T. M. Devlin (ed.). John Wiley, New York, 1982.
136. Goldblatt, J., Sacks, S., and Beighton, P. The orthopedic aspects of Gaucher's disease. *Clin. Orthop.* 137:208 (1978).
137. Pastakia, B., Brower, A. C., Chang, V. H., and Barranger, J. A. Skeletal manifestations of Gaucher's disease. *Semin. Roentgenol.* 21:254 (1986).
138. Bell, R. S., Mankin, H. J., and Doppelt, S. H. Osteomyelitis in Gaucher disease. *J. Bone Joint Surg.* 68A:1380 (1986).
139. Hermann, G., Goldblatt, J., Levy, R. N., Goldsmith, S. J., Desnick, R. J., and Grabowski, G. A. Gaucher's disease type 1: Assessment of bone involvement by CT and scintigraphy. *AJR* 147:943 (1985).

140. Rosenthal, D. I., Scott, J. A., Barranger, J., Mankin, H. J., Saini, S., Brady, T. J., Osier, L. K., and Doppelt, S. Evaluation of Gaucher disease using magnetic resonance imaging. *J. Bone Joint Surg.* 68A:802 (1986).
141. Midorikawa, M., Okada, S., Yutaka, T., Yabuuchi, H., Naoi, M., Kiuchi, K., and Yagi, K. Assay of glucocerebrosidase using a fluorescent analogue of glucocerebroside for the diagnosis of Gaucher disease. *Biochem. Int.* 11: 327 (1985).
142. Kitagawa, T., Owada, M., Sakiyama, T., Aski, K., Kamoshita, S., Amenomori, Y., and Kobayashi, T. In utero diagnosis of Gaucher's disease. *Am. J. Hum. Genet.* 30:322 (1978).
143. Bar-Maor, J. A., and Govrin-Yehudain, J. Partial splenectomy in children with Gaucher's disease. *Pediatrics* 76:398 (1985).
144. Rubin, M., Yampolski, I., Lambrozo, R., Zaizov, R., and Dintsman, M. Partial splenectomy in Gaucher's disease. *J. Pediatr. Surg.* 21:125 (1986).
145. Shiloni, B. D., Rachmilewitz, E., and Durst, A. L. The role of splenectomy in Gaucher's disease. *Arch. Surg.* 118:929 (1983).
146. Schneider, E. L., Epstein, C. J., Kaback, M. M., Brandes, D. Severe pulmonary involvement in adult Gaucher's disease: Report of 3 cases and review of literature. *Am. J. Med.* 63:475 (1977).
147. Chander, P. N., Nurse, H. M., and Pirani, C. L. Renal involvement in adult Gaucher's disease after splenectomy. *Arch. Pathol.* 103:440 (1979).
148. Rose, J. S., Grabowski, G. A., Barnett, S. H., and Desnick, R. J. Accelerated skeletal deterioration after splenectomy in Gaucher type 1 disease. *AJR* 139:1202 (1982).
149. Rappeport, J. M., and Ginns, E. I. Bone-marrow transplantation in severe Gaucher's disease. *N. Engl. J. Med.* 311:84 (1984).
150. Rappeport, J. M., Barranger, J. A., and Ginns, E. I. Bone marrow transplantation in Gaucher disease. *Birth Defects* 22:101 (1986).
151. Brady, R. O. Sphingomyelin lipidoses: Niemann-Pick disease. In: *The Metabolic Basis of Inherited Disease*, 5th ed. J. B. Stanbury, J. B. Wyngaarden, D. S. Fredrickson, J. L. Goldstein, and M. S. Brown (eds.). McGraw Hill, New York, 1983.
152. Pavone, L., Fiumara, A., and LaRosa, M. Niemann-Pick disease type B: Clinical signs and follow-up of a new case. *J. Inherited Metab. Dis.* 9:73 (1986).
153. Landas, S., Foucar, K., Sando, G. N., Ellefson, R., and Hamilton, H. E. Adult Niemann-Pick disease masquerading as sea blue histiocyte syndrome: Report of a case confirmed by lipid analysis and enzyme analysis. *Am. J. Hematol.* 20:391 (1985).
154. Kruth, H. S., Comly, M. E., Butler, J. D., Vanier, M. T., Fink, J. K., Wenger, D. A., Patel, S., and Pentchev, P. G. Type C Niemann-Pick disease. Abnormal metabolism of low density lipoprotein in homozygous and heterozygous fibroblasts. *J. Biol. Chem.* 261:16769 (1986).
155. Pentchev, P. G., Kruth, H. S., Comly, M. E., Butler, J. D., Vanier, M. T., Wenger, D. A., and Patel, S. Type C Niemann-Pick disease. A parallel loss of regulatory responses in both the uptake and esterification of low density lipoprotein-derived cholesterol in cultured fibroblasts. *J. Biol. Chem.* 261:16775 (1986).

156. Lageron, A. A comparison between the hepatocytes and macrophages of sphingomyelin, cholesterol, and acid lipase in various types of Niemann-Pick disease. *J. Inherited Metab. Dis.* 9 Suppl. 2:311 (1986).
157. Matthews, J. D., Weiter, J. J., and Kolodny, E. H. Macular halos associated with Niemann-Pick type B disease. *Ophthalmology* 93:933 (1986).
158. Butler, J. D. B., Comly, M. E., Kruth, H. S., Vanier, M., Filling-Katz, M., Fink, J., Barton, N., Weintroub, H., Quirk, J. M., Tokoro, T., Marshall, D. C., Brady, R. O., and Pentchev, P. G. Niemann-Pick variant disorders: comparison of errors of cellular cholesterol homeostasis in group D and group C fibroblasts. *Proc. Natl. Acad. Sci. USA* 84:556 (1987).
159. Yatziv, S., Liebovitz-Ben Gershon, Z., Ornoy, A., Bach, G. Clinical heterogeneity in a sibship with Niemann-Pick disease type C. *Clin. Genet.* 23: 125 (1983).
160. Schneider, E. L., Ellis, W. G., Brady, R. O., McCullock, J. R., and Epstein, C. J. Prenatal Niemann-Pick disease: Biochemical and histological examination of a 19-gestational week fetus. *Pediatr. Res.* 6:720 (1972).
161. Vanier, M. T., Boue, J., and Dumez, Y. Niemann-Pick disease type B: First trimester prenatal diagnosis on chorionic villi and biochemical study of a foetus at 12 weeks of development. *Clin. Genet.* 28:348 (1985).
162. Sakiyama, T., Tsuda, M., Owada, M., and Joh, K. Bone marrow transplantation for Niemann-Pick mice. *Biochem. Biophys. Res. Commun.* 113: 605 (1983).
163. Sakiyama, T., Tsuda, M., Kitagawa, T., Miyawaki, S., Shinagawa, T., and Tadakoro, M. Bone marrow transplantation in Niemann-Pick mice. *J. Inherited Metab. Dis.* 9:305 (1986).
164. Barranger, J. A., Rapoport, S. I., Fredericks, W. R., Pentchev, P. G., MacDermott, K. D., Steusing, J. K., and Brady, R. O. Modification of the blood brain barrier: Increased concentration and fate of enzymes entering the brain. *Proc. Natl. Acad. Sci. USA* 76:481 (1979).
165. Moser, H. W. and Chen, W. W. Ceramidase deficiency: Farber's granulomatosis. In: *The Metabolic Basis of Inherited Disease*, 5th ed. J. B. Stanbury, J. B. Wyngaarden, D. S. Fredrickson, J. L. Goldstein, and M. S. Brown (eds.). McGraw-Hill, New York, 1983.
166. Sagita, M., Dulaney, J. T., and Moser, H. W. Ceramidase deficiency in Farber's disease (Lipogranulomatosis). *Science* 178:1100 (1972).
167. Pavone, L., Moser, H. W., Mollica, F., Reitano, C., and Durand, P. Farber's lipogranulomatosis: Ceramidase deficiency and prolonged survival in three relatives. *Johns Hopkins Med. J.* 147:193 (1980).
168. Pachman, L. M., Frank, J., Liu, M., and Moser, H. W. Lipogranulomatosis (Farber disease). *J. Pediatr.* 93:320 (1978).
169. Abul-Haj, S. K., Martz, D. G., Douglas, W. F., and Geppert, L. J. Farber's disease. Report of a case with observations on its histogenesis and notes on the nature of the stored material. *J. Pediatr.* 61:221 (1962).
170. Rutsaert, J., Tondeur, M., Vamos-Hurwitz, E., and Dustin, P. The cellular lesions of Farber's disease and their experimental reproduction in tissue culture. *Lab. Invest.* 36:474 (1977).

171. Dulaney, J. T., Milunsky, A., Sidbury, J. B., Hobolth, N., and Moser, H. W. Diagnosis of lipogranulomatosis (Farber disease) by use of cultured fibroblasts. *J. Pediatr.* 89:59 (1976).
172. Fensom, A. H., Neville, B. R. G., Moser, A. E., Bensom, P. F., Moser, H. W., and Dulaney, J. T. Prenatal diagnosis of Farber's disease. *Lancet* 2: 990 (1979).
173. Skovby, F. Homocystinuria. *Acta Paediatr. Scand.* Suppl. 321:1 (1985).
174. Mudd, S. H., and Levy, H. L. Disorders of transsulfuration. In: *The Metabolic Basis of Inherited Disease*, 5th ed. J. B. Stanbury, J. B. Wyngaarden, D. S. Fredrickson, J. L. Goldstein, and M. S. Brown (eds.). McGraw-Hill, New York, 1983.
175. Kang, A. H., and Trelstad, R. L. A collagen defect in homocystinuria. *J. Clin. Invest.* 52:2571 (1973).
176. Pinnell, S. R., and Murad, S. Disorders of collagen. In: *The Metabolic Basis of Inherited Disease*, 5th ed. J. B. Stanbury, J. B. Wyngaarden, D. S. Frederickson, J. L. Goldstein, and M. S. Brown (eds.). McGraw-Hill, New York, 1983.
177. Schimke, R. N., McKusick, V. A., Huang, T., and Pollack, A. D. Homocystinuria. *J.A.M.A.* 193:71 (1965).
178. Tamburrini, O., Bartolomeo-De Iuri, Andria, G., Strisciuglio, P., and Del Giudice, E. Short fourth metacarpal in homocystinuria. *Pediatr. Radiol.* 15:209 (1985).
179. Schedewie, H., Willich, E., Grobe, H., Schmidt, H., and Muller, K. M. Skeletal findings in homocystinuria: A collaborative study. *Pediatr. Radiol.* 1:12 (1973).
180. Brenton, D. P., Dow, C. J., James, J. I. P., Hay, R. L., and Wynne-Davis, R. Homocystinuria and Marfan's syndrome: A comparison. *J. Bone Joint Surg.* 54B:277 (1972).
181. Valle, D., Pai, G. S., Thomas, G. H., and Pyeritz, R. E. Homocystinuria due to cystathionine B synthase deficiency. Clinical manifestations and therapy. *Johns Hopkins Med. J.* 146:110 (1980).
182. Wilcken, B., and Turner, G. Homocystinuria in New South Wales. *Arch. Dis. Child.* 53:242 (1978).
183. Dunn, H. G., Perry, T. L., and Dolman, C. L. Homocystinuria. *Neurology* 16:407 (1966).
184. White, H. H., Rowland, L. P., Araki, S., Thompson, H. L., and Cowen, D. Homocystinura. *Arch. Neurol.* 13:455 (1965).
185. Graeber, J. E., Scott, J. H., Ulane, R. E., Schulman, J. D., and Stuart, M. J. Effect of homocysteine and homocystine on platelets and vascular arachidonic acid metabolism. *Pediatr. Res.* 16:490 (1982).
186. Haan, E. A., Rogers, J. G., Lewis, G. P., and Rowe, P. B. 5,10-Methylenetetrahydrofolate reductase deficiency. Clinical and biochemical features of a further case. *J. Inherited Metab. Dis.* 8:53 (1985).
187. Mizobuchi, N., Ageta, T., Sasaki, K., and Kodama, H. Isotachophoretic analyses of cystine, homocystine and cystathionine in urine from patients with inborn errors of metabolism. *J. Chromatogr.* 382:321 (1986).

188. Brattstrom, L., Israelson, B., and Jeppson, J. O. Heterozygosity for homocystinuria in premature arterial disease. *N. Engl. J. Med.* 314:849 (1986).
189. Ramsey, M. S., Yanoff, M., and Fine, B. S. The ocular histopathology of homocystinuria: A light and electron microscopic study. *Am. J. Ophthalmol.* 74:377 (1972).
190. Chou, S. M., and Waisman, H. A. Spongy degeneration of the nervous system: Case of homocystinuria. *Arch. Pathol.* 79:357 (1965).
191. Barber, G. W., and Spaeth, G. L. Pyridoxine therapy in homocystinuria. *Lancet* 1:337 (1967).
192. Carson, N. A. J., and Carre, I. J. Treatment of homocystinuria with pyridoxine. A preliminary study. *Arch. Dis. Child.* 44:387 (1969).
193. Wilcken, D. E. L., Dudman, N. P. B., and Tyrrell, P. A. Homocystinuria due to cystathionine beta-synthase deficiency–the effects of betaine treatment in pyridoxine-responsive patients. *Metabolism* 34:1115 (1985).
194. Wilcken, D. E. L., Wilcken, B., Dudman, N. P. B., and Tyrrell, P. A. Homocystinuria–the effects of betaine in the treatment of patients not responsive to pyridoxine. *N. Engl. J. Med.* 309:448 (1983).

Index